Neuroethics

Neuroethics

Agency in the Age of Brain Science

JOSHUA MAY

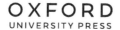

Oxford University Press is a department of the University of Oxford. It furthers
the University's objective of excellence in research, scholarship, and education
by publishing worldwide. Oxford is a registered trade mark of Oxford University
Press in the UK and certain other countries.

Published in the United States of America by Oxford University Press
198 Madison Avenue, New York, NY 10016, United States of America.

© Oxford University Press 2023

All rights reserved. No part of this publication may be reproduced, stored in
a retrieval system, or transmitted, in any form or by any means, without the
prior permission in writing of Oxford University Press, or as expressly permitted
by law, by license, or under terms agreed with the appropriate reproduction
rights organization. Inquiries concerning reproduction outside the scope of the
above should be sent to the Rights Department, Oxford University Press, at the
address above.

You must not circulate this work in any other form
and you must impose this same condition on any acquirer.

Library of Congress Cataloging-in-Publication Data
Names: May, Joshua, author.
Title: Neuroethics : agency in the age of brain science / Joshua May.
Description: New York, NY : Oxford University Press, [2023] |
Includes bibliographical references and index.
Identifiers: LCCN 2023006178 (print) | LCCN 2023006179 (ebook) |
ISBN 9780197648094 (paperback) | ISBN 9780197648087 (hardback) |
ISBN 9780197648124 (ebook) | ISBN 9780197648117 (epub)
Subjects: LCSH: Neurosciences—Moral and ethical aspects. |
Agent (Philosophy)
Classification: LCC RC343 .M395 2023 (print) | LCC RC343 (ebook) |
DDC 612.8—dc23/eng/20230315
LC record available at https://lccn.loc.gov/2023006178
LC ebook record available at https://lccn.loc.gov/2023006179

DOI: 10.1093/oso/9780197648087.001.0001

*To my parents and my students,
who have shaped my brain for the better.*

I note the obvious differences
between each sort and type,
but we are more alike, my friends,
than we are unalike.

– Maya Angelou
from the poem "The Human Family"

Contents

List of Figures — xi
List of Tables — xiii
Preface — xv
Acknowledgments — xix

PART I. INTRODUCTION

1. Ethics Meets Neuroscience — 3
    1.1 Kevin's Klüver–Bucy Syndrome — 3
    1.2 What Is Neuroethics? — 4
    1.3 What's to Come — 9
    1.4 Conclusion — 14
    Appendix: Philosophy and Brain Primers — 15
        A.1 Philosophy Primer — 15
        A.2 Brain Basics — 23

PART II. AUTONOMY

2. Free Will — 35
    2.1 Weinstein's Window — 35
    2.2 What in the World Is Free Will? — 38
    2.3 Determinism: No Choice? — 40
    2.4 Physicalism: No Control? — 43
    2.5 Epiphenomenalism: No Coherence? — 46
    2.6 Conclusion — 61

3. Manipulating Brains — 63
    3.1 A Parkinson's Patient — 64
    3.2 What's the Problem? — 65
    3.3 Patient Autonomy — 68
    3.4 Personal Identity — 70
    3.5 Unreliable Risk-Benefit Ratios — 80
    3.6 Conclusion — 88

PART III. CARE

4. Mental Disorder		93
4.1 Two Homicides in Texas		93
4.2 Two Theories		95
4.3 The Need for Nuance		99
4.4 Ethical Implications		109
4.5 Conclusion		116
5. Addiction		119
5.1 Reprimand for Relapse		119
5.2 What Is Addiction?		120
5.3 Loss of Control in Addiction?		128
5.4 Is Addiction a Brain Disease?		132
5.5 Addiction as a Disorder		138
5.6 Conclusion		144

PART IV. CHARACTER

6. Moral Judgment		149
6.1 Dugan's Defense		149
6.2 Are Gut Feelings Necessary?		151
6.3 Are Gut Feelings Always Reliable?		161
6.4 Conclusion		173
7. Moral Enhancement		175
7.1 Microdosing Morality		176
7.2 A Presumptive Case for Enhancement		178
7.3 Ethical Concerns		186
7.4 Conclusion		199

PART V. JUSTICE

8. Motivated Reasoning		205
8.1 Split-Brain Self-Deception		205
8.2 Reasoning Motivated by Values		208
8.3 Bias in (Neuro)Science		214
8.4 What Motivates Scientists?		219
8.5 Conclusion		227

9. Brain Reading 229
    9.1 Exoneration by EEG 229
    9.2 Unjust Verdicts 231
    9.3 Too Unreliable? 233
    9.4 Too Dangerous? 242
    9.5 Balancing and Parity 247
    9.6 Neuromarketing 251
    9.7 Conclusion 256

PART VI. CONCLUSION

10. Nuanced Neuroethics 261
    10.1 Back to Kevin's Brain Surgery 261
    10.2 Avoid Alarmism and Neurohype 263
    10.3 Approach Evidence With Vigilance 265
    10.4 Recognize the Complexity of Human Agency 266
    10.5 Emphasize Continuity Over Categories 268
    10.6 Blend Philosophy and Neuroscience 272

Bibliography 275
Index 307

Figures

A.1	The Hollow Mask Illusion	18
A.2	The Cerebral Cortex	27
A.3	Navigating the Brain	28
2.1	The Cyst in Weinstein's Brain	36
2.2	Libet's Experimental Setup	50
2.3	Summary of Libet's Brain Wave Data	51
3.1	Deep Brain Stimulation	65
3.2	Null Results After Preregistration	84
5.1	Three Dopamine Pathways	125
6.1	Key Brain Areas in Moral Cognition	152
6.2	The Switch Dilemma	164
6.3	The Push Dilemma	165
8.1	A Split-Brain Patient's Matching Task	207
9.1	High vs. Low Standard Deviation in a Population	234
9.2	High vs. Low Base Rates in a Population	236
9.3	Forward vs. Reverse Inference	240
10.1	The Great Cognitive Continuum	269

Tables

4.1	Pathological Effects on Agency	106
4.2	Nonpathological Effects on Agency	115
5.1	Some Key Elements of Addiction	121
5.2	Claims and Criticisms of the Brain Disease Model	139
6.1	Functional Contributions of Brain Areas to Moral Cognition	156
7.1	Potential Methods of Moral Bioenhancement	184
8.1	A Taxonomy of Motivated Reasoning	212
8.2	Some Sources of Motivated Reasoning in Science	221
10.1	Lessons for Human Agency	267

Preface

Immanuel Kant famously proclaimed: "Two things fill the mind with ever-increasing wonder and awe . . . the starry heavens above me and the moral law within me." I would add the three-pound organ between my ears. It's no understatement to say we're in the age of brain science. We've come so far since the days of lobotomies and phrenology, and yet we remain largely ignorant of how these billions of neurons generate the mind. Since the brain is the seat of the self, this new frontier brings forth new ethical conundrums and forces us to reconsider the conception of ourselves as rational, virtuous creatures with free will.

As with all frontiers, there is the risk of excessive zeal and overreach. Unlocking the mysteries of the brain and deploying novel neurotechnologies is both alluring and scary. Many scientists and ethicists are led to speculate about and oversell the prospects or perils of the science. We're sometimes told that advances in neurobiology reveal that free will is a farce but that these same advances also have the power to make us superhuman. Ethical alarm bells ring with urgency.

My aim in this book is to take the brain science seriously while carefully and soberly scrutinizing its ethical concerns and implications. The "nuanced neuroethics" that emerges is modest, not alarmist, yet we'll see that our present understanding of the human brain does force us to see our minds as less conscious and reliable—though more diverse and flexible—than we might otherwise think. This balanced conception of human agency has direct implications for how we address the ethical concerns raised by this new frontier. Ultimately, I hope a more nuanced approach to the entire field helps us appreciate the abundant forms of agency made possible by the human brain.

Ambitions

The text aims to be a contribution, as well as an introduction, to the literature. We will not merely raise tantalizing ethical questions, which is all too common in neuroethics, but also attempt to answer them. So the tour of this burgeoning field will be a rather opinionated one. Similar to the book's goal of dismantling dubious divisions between the neurologically typical and atypical, the book itself openly challenges the distinction between a research monograph and a textbook.

For years, I have taught an undergraduate neuroethics course at the University of Alabama at Birmigham (a sample syllabus is available on my website, joshdmay.com). It's the sort of class that cries out for a textbook that's accessible to both neuroscience and philosophy majors. Neuroscience is an increasingly popular major on college campuses, and these students deserve a philosophically rich discussion of the ethical issues, informed by the latest scientific evidence and its limitations.

For the philosophy majors, in my experience, neuroethics serves as an excellent special topics course, even a capstone for the major. It tackles a range of cutting-edge philosophical problems that span not just ethical issues (such as autonomy, justice, and virtue) but also other subfields, such as the metaphysics of mind (free will, personal identity, the mind-body problem) and epistemology, especially the philosophy of science (drawing sound scientific inferences, understanding the role of values in science). The present text in particular draws on recent insights from metaphysics (transformative experience, the moral self), philosophy of science (medical nihilism, reverse inference), and disability advocacy (neurodiversity). Thus, neuroethics requires philosophy students to apply their broad philosophical knowledge to contemporary problems.

Students will find that, although this book introduces neuroethics, it is not introductory. The field is relatively new, situated at the cutting edge of philosophical and scientific debates. The many controversial issues require readers to dig into both data and the bread and butter of philosophy: arguments. Alongside this comparatively dry main course, however, will be rich stories and savory science (with an occasional sip of word play as a digestif). The book also employs some handy expository tactics from the sciences, such as figures and tables. I hope readers will see the value in clearly representing, breaking down, and analyzing both scientific evidence and arguments with premises.

The style of the book assumes readers are comfortable with philosophical writing and argumentation. Moreover, since I aim to point readers to the relevant literatures, and situate my own views well within them, citations are not kept to a minimum. I've tried to write the book so that it's suitable for adoption in classes that, like my own neuroethics course, are comprised of students who already have some philosophy under their belts. Nevertheless, the topics may be enticing and palatable enough for a wide range of students and scholars to digest.

Readers should take home the message that philosophy and neuroscience help one another. I hope neuroscientists will see that philosophical analysis helps us to clarify murky debates, draw important distinctions, and clearly construct and evaluate arguments. However, as the neuroscientists might be quick to point out, philosophical analysis must be properly informed by the science.

Philosophers are often dubious of the relevance of neuroscience to philosophical questions. Sure, philosophers from antiquity have cared about how the human mind works, but shouldn't we just look directly to the brain's software (the field of psychology) rather than its hardware (neuroscience)? Throughout this book we'll see that neurobiology reveals psychological functions and limits, especially in cases of brain damage. Direct interventions on the brain's hardware also yield novel treatments that raise important ethical questions. And studying the brain directly can sometimes provide a more direct line to the mind that bypasses the mouth, which is prone to rationalizations or outright lies. Another balm to the philosopher's skepticism about brain science is the recognition that it's not all about brain imaging. Neuroscience includes psychopathology, brain damage, neurochemistry, and brain stimulation technologies. When the evidence about the brain's hardware converges with psychological science, philosophical analysis, and other fields of inquiry, we start to gain a handle on the mysteries of the mind and the ethical issues they raise.

Format

The main chapters share some recurring features. Each kicks off with a case study to help ground abstract issues in the lives of real people. Neuroethics often inspires speculations about moral problems of a distant future when humans can skillfully manipulate their brains with great precision, like cyborgs in a sci-fi thriller. Against this trend, I stick to case studies from the present or recent past in order to avoid alarmism and undue attention to problems the human species may never live to face.

I have also compiled a companion website (visit joshdmay.com). There readers will find discussion questions for each chapter, which can help spark dialogue in a class or reading group.

The grouping of chapters is a bit unorthodox. Discussions of neuroethics often divide its topics into the more theoretical and the more practical issues (the "neuroscience of ethics" and the "ethics of neuroscience"). I have opted instead to switch back and forth between the two sorts of questions in neuroethics, for several reasons. First, the divide between the theoretical and practical is often blurry and boundaries are arbitrary. Second, the answers to some questions in one domain rely on answers from another. The practical question of whether it's ethical to alter our brains to become better people, for instance, depends on a more theoretical understanding of how moral cognition works in the brain. Finally, interweaving the topics helps shake things up and minimize the fatigue that comes from repetition.

Throughout the book, I discuss other theorists' answers to these questions, but I also develop my own take. I will serve as both a tour guide and interlocutor, for this is no ordinary trip through the annals of history but an active debate rife with arguments and ethical implications. If you're more of a student than a scholar and find yourself adamantly disagreeing with my view, congratulate yourself on having a philosophically active mind! Indeed, if you find yourself readily agreeing with me on the controversial issues of neuroethics, perhaps you should take pause and reevaluate your tendencies toward credulity. (For those active in these scholarly debates, on the other hand, capitulations are most welcome.)

Acknowledgments

Although I've worked across disciplinary boundaries in the past, neuroethics is different. Neuroscience is significantly larger than psychological science and involves studying the mind at radically different levels and angles, from the chemistry of the brain to its gross anatomy, from computational mechanisms to therapeutic interventions. Neuroscience also deploys complicated cutting-edge technologies (such as magnetic resonance imaging and optogenetics) and trades in highly technical terminology (What is a G protein-coupled receptor? What does the ventromedial prefrontal cortex do exactly?). This book would not have been possible without some formal training and the time to complete it.

Fortunately, for two weeks in the summer of 2017, I was able to participate in the fantastic Summer Seminars in Neuroscience and Philosophy (SSNAP) at Duke University. There, I and about a dozen other fellows learned a great deal about neuroscience from leading researchers while getting hands-on experience with brain anatomy and technologies like transcranial magnetic stimulation. (There also may have been some karaoke.) Special thanks to Felipe de Brigard and Walter Sinnott-Armstrong who run those transformative seminars, and to the John Templeton Foundation for funding them. Well beyond these seminars, Walter has been formative throughout my philosophical and neuroscientific endeavors. Always encouraging and supportive, he has been an inspiring model of how to do interdisciplinary work with philosophical rigor and humor. A true utilitarian, he makes sure work is a joy.

My (joyful) work on this book was also made possible through the support of a paid sabbatical at UAB and then an Academic Cross-Training Fellowship from the John Templeton Foundation (grant #61581). I am ever grateful for this sabbatical-fellowship combo, which freed me from teaching for five semesters (from 2020 to

2022) so that I could learn much more about brain science and write this book. (The opinions expressed in this work are mine, of course, and do not necessarily reflect the views of the Templeton Foundation.) During this research leave, I attended lab meetings to see how the neuroscience sausage is made, presented at interdisciplinary conferences, talked with neuroscientists and others outside my discipline, and audited the courses required for UAB's Behavioral Neuroscience PhD. Special thanks go to my academic cross-training mentor Rajesh Kana (Professor of Psychology at the University of Alabama), who is an expert in neuroimaging and social cognition, and all-around a wonderful human being. Rajesh allowed this philosophical gadfly to participate in his weekly lab meetings, and he met regularly with me to discuss philosophy, neuroscience, and the vagaries of a global pandemic.

While working on this manuscript, I received valuable feedback from many philosophers, scientists, lawyers, and clinicians. Though memory in the human brain is certainly imperfect, my slightly more reliable notes suggest I profited from discussions or correspondence with Kenton Bartlett, Robyn Bluhm, Mary M. Boggiano (Dr. B!), Jonathan Buchwalter (and his 2021 Debate Class at Tuscaloosa County High School), Emily Cornelius, Veljko Dubljevic, Jeremy Fischer, Rachel Fredericks, Frederic Gilbert, Andrea Glenn, Hyemin Han, Julia Haas, Rajesh Kana, Matt King, Victor Kumar, Robin Lester, Neil Levy, Andrew Morgan, Mariko Nakano, Patrick Norton, Greg Pence, Jonathan Pugh, Kristen Sandefer, Katrina Sifferd, Walter Sinnott-Armstrong, Michael Sloane (who provided wonderfully detailed comments on every chapter), Macarena Suarez Pellicioni, and Clifford I. Workman. Thank you all. Wholehearted thanks also go to three philosophy majors at UAB—and former Ethics Bowl debate team members—who served as research assistants: Kimberly Chieh, Carly Snidow, and Mohammad Waqas. They helped proofread drafts of chapters, come up with discussion questions, and research case studies. I am grateful for their assistance and so very proud of their many achievements at UAB and beyond. Thanks also to my editor, Peter Ohlin, at Oxford University Press who early on was enthusiastic and supportive of this project.

Three chapters of this book draw from previously published articles of mine. Chapter 4 draws from and expands on "Moral Responsibility and Mental Illness: A Call for Nuance" published in *Neuroethics* and co-authored with my friend and colleague Matt King. Our work on that article first started me down the path to developing a more nuanced approach to neuroethics. Chapter 6 borrows a little from my article "Moral Rationalism on the Brain" published in *Mind & Language*. Chapter 8 draws from and expands on my paper "Bias in Science: Natural and Social" published in *Synthese*. My thanks to the publishers (and, in one case, my co-author) for the permission to republish portions of the material here.

Finally, a heartfelt thanks to my wonderful daughter, Juliana. Although too young to provide feedback on more than the cover art for this book, she regularly helped me recharge by being my hiking partner, climbing buddy, sous-chef, and primary source of comic relief.

PART I
INTRODUCTION

1
Ethics Meets Neuroscience

1.1 Kevin's Klüver–Bucy Syndrome

On a Friday in 2006, at his home in New Jersey with his wife standing by, a man in his 50s was arrested by federal authorities for downloading child pornography. Kevin, as we'll call him, later remembers first being asked, "You know why we're here?" to which he replied, "Yeah, I do, I was expecting you" (Abumrad & Krulwich 2013). He immediately took the agents to his computer and handed it over.

Ever since he was a teenager, Kevin suffered from epilepsy, which caused debilitating seizures. Neurological scans indicated that the focal point was in the right temporal lobe, a portion of the brain that stretches approximately from the temples to behind the ears. Kevin decided in his early 30s to have neurosurgery to remove a portion of this area (Devinsky et al. 2010). While the operation seemed to help by removing a small tumor, within a year the seizures returned. One incident occurred while driving on the freeway, which led to a crash and the loss of his driver's license. That prompted Kevin to undergo brain surgery again to remove even more of his temporal lobe.

Although the second surgery kept the seizures at bay for much longer, almost immediately Kevin noticed significant changes in his desires and behavior. He became more easily irritated, distracted, and angry—what he described as "mood swings"—and his cravings for food and sex became frequent, intense, and insatiable. He wanted intercourse with his wife daily, and, after frequently viewing legal pornography, his intense desires eventually led him to download increasingly perverse forms. These symptoms were consistent with *Klüver–Bucy syndrome*, so named after the eponymous psychologist and neurosurgeon duo who in the 1930s observed changes such as hypersexuality and hyperorality in rhesus monkeys after portions of their temporal lobes were removed.

Clearly, Kevin's illicit behavior was at least partially due to his brain surgery. Does he then deserve punishment or even blame? Orrin Devinsky, Kevin's neurologist at New York University's Langone School of Medicine, argued before the court that his patient was not in control and thus not to blame. The prosecution ultimately persuaded the judge that Kevin was at least partially in control, since he only downloaded the illegal material at home, not at work. Kevin's Klüver–Bucy syndrome, however, was taken to be a mitigating factor, and he received the shortest allowable sentence: "26 months in prison, 25 months of home confinement, and then a 5-year period of supervision" (Devinsky et al. 2010: 143).

This case illustrates how improved treatment and understanding of the human brain raises important ethical questions. Some are more *theoretical*—e.g., Does a patient like Kevin have free will and can we hold him morally responsible for his awful actions? Even if Kevin does lack self-control, are any of us much different, given that all our actions are determined by our brains? Other questions are more *practical*—e.g., Is it ethical to remove parts of a patient's brain to treat seizures or other symptoms even if it changes their personality?

In this chapter, we see how these two types of questions are related and form the backbone of neuroethics and subsequent chapters. This book's main aim is to provide a picture of this burgeoning field, with serious attention paid to both the philosophical issues and scientific evidence. To soberly scrutinize the empirical literature and avoid basing philosophical conclusions on alarmist reactions, we need tools from multiple disciplines. So the chapter ends with an appendix describing some basic philosophical and neurobiological concepts necessary for navigating neuroethics.

1.2 What Is Neuroethics?

1.2.1 Origins

Put simply, *neuroethics* is the study of moral issues that are either raised or answered by neuroscience. The field is similar to bioethics, which concerns ethical issues of life, death, and health that are largely spurred by advancements in medicine, especially life-sustaining treatment and assisted reproduction. For much of human history, life and death were largely dictated by nature. Children were born via sexual reproduction, and people with diseases or disorders simply lived with the symptoms or died. Advancements in medicine—from ventilators to in vitro fertilization—gave us the power to partially control life and death.

With great power, though, comes great responsibility. More specifically, new moral problems come along with great technology, and thus in the mid-20th century a new field was born. In addition to addressing present issues, bioethics aims to consider future moral problems so that our ethics is ahead of the science. Lest we find ourselves in a scenario like *Jurassic Park* in which, as one character from that 1993 film laments, "Your scientists were so preoccupied with whether or not they could, they didn't stop to think if they should."

The story is similar for neuroethics. By manipulating and illuminating the brain, neuroscience immediately raises philosophical, especially ethical, issues. The reason is simple: the brain is seat of the self—of one's personality, memories, even moral character. Studying and manipulating the brain directly involves human autonomy, identity, rationality, and mental health. Like any powerful technology or piece of knowledge, neuroscience can be a force for good or evil.

Another reason neuroscience raises moral problems is that it is rapidly advancing and poised to powerfully shape society. Neuroscience may rightly be regarded as the science of the century. The great interest in neurobiology is no doubt driven in part by the rise in neurodegenerative disorders in rapidly aging populations around the developed world. For much of the 20th century, medicine was aimed at curing the body's ailments, but now many of us will live long enough to experience brain diseases. Around 6 million Americans and 30 million people worldwide have Alzheimer's disease (Alzheimer's Association 2019), and the Centers for Disease Control and Prevention reported in 2017 that the disease is America's sixth-leading cause of death, responsible for ending more lives than diabetes and about as many as strokes (Heron 2019).

Research funding in neuroscience has swelled as well. In 2013, the Obama administration launched an unprecedented financial investment in neuroscience research called the BRAIN Initiative (short for Brain Research Through Advancing Innovative Neurotechnologies). Its mission is to fund research that will "deepen understanding of the inner workings of the human mind" and "improve how we treat, prevent, and cure disorders of the brain." By 2018, after just four years of funding, almost $1 billion had been awarded under the BRAIN Initiative (with a small portion going to projects in neuroethics specifically). Support for this level of investment by the U.S. government does not seem to be waning (Sanders 2020). Also in 2013, the European Union launched a similar funding initiative—the Human Brain Project—which has also awarded over $1 billion. The project's ambitious goal is to ultimately reverse engineer the human brain so that it can be simulated on supercomputers.

1.2.2 Two Branches, Intertwined

Neuroethics could just be conceived as an extension of bioethics. However, the field is importantly different in that neuroscience also clearly advances our understanding of how the mind works, which directly illuminates ancient moral problems. Neuroethics is "more than just bioethics for the brain" but a "brain-based philosophy of life," as Michael Gazzaniga puts it (2005: xv). Accordingly, from its inception around the turn of the 21st century, the field of neuroethics has been conceived as having two importantly distinct but connected branches (Roskies 2002).

The more practical branch, the *ethics of neuroscience*, concerns moral issues that arise from the use of emerging technologies and findings in neuroscience, such as brain manipulation, cognitive enhancement, mind reading, and the use of brain images as legal evidence. Questions along this branch, which we will cover in this book, include the following:

- When do brain stimulation treatments impair a patient's autonomy or sense of self?
- Are pills and brain stimulation appropriate methods of moral improvement?

- Should we trust brain science to read the minds of criminals and consumers?

Some of these questions raise issues about the treatment of patients, but neuroscience and its technologies are also opening up new moral problems for consumers and defendants.

The second branch is *the neuroscience of ethics*, which uses research on the brain to illuminate classic theoretical issues in moral philosophy, such as free will, responsibility, and moral knowledge. Examples of questions along this branch include the following:

- Does neuroscience show that free will is an illusion?
- Does having a neurological disorder exempt one from blame?
- Does neuroscience show we shouldn't trust our gut feelings in ethics?

As we saw, the case of Klüver–Bucy syndrome raises issues that intertwine both branches. We saw practical questions arise about how to ethically use neurosurgery to treat a patient, as well as theoretical questions about free will and moral responsibility. Although the two branches are often segregated in neuroethics, a main theme of this book is that they inform one another and are thus best addressed in tandem.

1.2.3 Why Neuroethics?

One might argue that neuroscience, particularly research on the human brain, raises few novel moral problems and sheds little light on theoretical questions in ethics. There are several sources of this worry. One comes from those who believe that philosophical questions are somehow isolated from empirical ones. Another rationale is that while scientific evidence is relevant to ethics, psychology is more useful than neuroscience, since our primary concern is with people's beliefs, desires, values, self-control, and autonomy, not their neuronal activity. In other words, neuroscience directly examines only the brain's "hardware," yet its "software," which is the province of psychology, is what's relevant to ethics.

Rather than respond to these skeptics now, the book as a whole is meant to diffuse such worries. We will see that examining the brain's hardware does shed light on psychological phenomena like beliefs, motivation, and self-control, which informs philosophical questions about free will, the self, and right action.

Other critics might press further and argue that the mind arises from more than just neuronal activity in the brain (Levy 2007). Because the peripheral nervous system spreads throughout the body, you can reduce anxiety by breathing deeply or gain confidence by standing tall. The environment is equally important. It is well-established that many addictive drugs act directly on the functioning of neurotransmitters, such as dopamine (more on this in Chapter 5). Yet it is equally well-established that addiction is exacerbated by changes in one's conditions and circumstances, such as poverty and isolation. In general, since our minds are shaped by what happens in our bodies and environments, we should avoid neurocentrism. Some philosophers maintain that one's thoughts and memories can be literally stored outside of one's body—say, in a smartphone or notebook—such that the mind extends beyond one's skull and skin (Clark & Chalmers 1998). Compare taking a second to retrieve a birthdate stored in your brain to taking a second to retrieve a birthdate stored in your smartphone. One counts as a memory, and so should the other, according to proponents of the *extended mind hypothesis*. If our minds are so embodied and embedded, why do we need a distinctive field of *neuro*ethics?

A satisfactory answer might seem to require addressing the extended mind hypothesis. Yet we can side-step the issue. Our focus will be primarily, though not exclusively, on the brain as the key organ of the mind, for it happens to be at the center of most relevant research and interventions in neuroscience. If important and distinctive issues arise from this approach, then we have some defense of neuroethics as a distinctive field. Although the book as a whole is meant to be the defense, let me begin by saying a little bit now by way of preview. There are two main sources of support, tied to the two branches of neuroethics.

First, although neuroscience is still a relatively new discipline, already there is a history of pressing moral problems. Patients have been subjected to dubious and disabling lobotomies, sometimes without informed consent (more on this in Chapter 3). Despite such recklessness, neuroscience and allied disciplines are now poised to considerably improve neurological symptoms that have long been resistant to treatment. The potential for success and failure in the treatment of mental ailments makes it imperative to consider the ethical possibilities as well as the limits of neurotechnologies, including whether to go beyond treatment to enhance our capacities. Even if the mind extends beyond the brain, direct brain interventions are here to stay and deserve ethical analysis.

The second reason why neuroethics matters is that neuroscience is advancing our understanding of the mind and ourselves, including what makes us moral or immoral. Many classical questions in moral philosophy turn on human nature, the mind, and the self. Do we have enough free will to warrant punishment? Do disorders, such as addiction and depression, compromise one's agency and thus make blame inappropriate? How can we learn right from wrong and become more virtuous? These questions span time and cultural traditions in the East and West. Our best answers will be informed by our latest sciences of the mind.

1.3 What's to Come

This book provides an opinionated introduction to neuroethics. The chapters each begin with one or two case studies that, like Kevin's brain surgery, are stories of real people—typically patients or defendants—whose brains and experiences exhibit the ethical issues at hand. In each chapter, we dig into a core issue and canvas the main positions, scientific evidence, and arguments. I ultimately defend my own views on these issues, but I aim to provide a comprehensive and balanced discussion.

Nevertheless, neuroethics encompasses a wide range of topics, and this book can't cover them all (or always in sufficient detail). Some important topics in neuroethics overlap closely with those familiar from bioethics, such as unethical experiments on humans and other animals (e.g., the Bucharest Early Intervention Study); consciousness in fetal development and nonhuman animals (including brain organoids); and incidental findings in neuroimaging research. Such topics receive little or no treatment here, only because our focus is on the more novel questions that neuroethics raises.

Below I provide a brief summary of the chapters to follow and highlight connections among them. My general approach is to rely on theoretical insights from the neuroscience of ethics to help adjudicate practical questions in the ethics of neuroscience. Accordingly, each part of the book pairs discussion of a more theoretical issue in one chapter with another chapter in which relevant practical questions arise. For example, what we should say about cognitive and moral enhancement (Chapter 7) depends greatly on how moral judgment and decision-making work in the brain (Chapter 6).

1.3.1 Autonomy

We begin in Chapter 2 with the story of an ad executive who pushed his wife off a balcony while a large brain tumor wreaked havoc on his frontal lobe. The case leads to an assessment of various threats to free will grounded in neuroscientific findings, particularly famous studies of unconscious influences on choice. Partly based on philosophical analysis of the studies as well as results in experimental philosophy, neuroscientific challenges to free will do not fully succeed. Nevertheless, agency comes in degrees, and some findings do suggest that we are less free than we tend to think.

Chapter 3 then turns to a key issue in the ethics of neuroscience: the manipulation of people's brains, from electrical stimulation to drugs that alter neurotransmitters. We encounter a patient with Parkinson's disease whose brain stimulation treatment led to marked changes in his personality. In this chapter, we only address treatment of brain disorders, not enhancement. Manipulating the brain, however, is ethically hazardous given how it can change one's personality, and even identity, to the point of compromising a patient's autonomy. We'll see that, like free will, personal identity comes in degrees and is pliable.

Nevertheless, our impoverished understanding of the brain suggests that we proceed with caution and don't oversell the benefits of medical interventions on patients' brains.

1.3.2 Care

The next pair of chapters move from autonomy and identity to closely related issues of agency among individuals suffering from mental maladies. Chapter 4 examines whether having a mental disorder—such as autism, depression, and obsessive-compulsive disorder—compromises one's agency enough to make blame (and praise) inappropriate. We start with two patients in Texas who were charged with homicide, but only one of whom was deemed not guilty by reason of insanity. Many people, including most philosophers, often assume that the most compassionate approach to mental disorders is to treat patients as categorically exempt from responsibility for their actions. However, our best understanding of human brains and of mental disorders suggests that they are so varied that we cannot infer from the mere fact that one has a mental disorder to anything about their agency or moral responsibility. In some contexts, symptoms flare up and mitigated blame can be appropriate, but this is also true for neurotypical individuals struggling with life's lemons, such as grief or divorce.

Chapter 5 features the case of a woman who repeatedly funds her addiction to opioids through theft. Even if individuals with, say, autism are praiseworthy and blameworthy for many of their actions, doesn't neuroscience warrant categorically excusing individuals with substance use disorder? Chapter 5 argues otherwise. Here too we should take a more nuanced approach to agency amid mental disorder. Our understanding of the neurobiology of addiction is fairly well developed, and many neuroscientists believe it categorically excuses immoral behavior since addictive drugs "hijack" the brain's reward system. Although this hijacking metaphor can be useful, it's easily misleading, for it overshadows how ordinary learning and motivation work similarly in the brain. Moreover, this conclusion is easier to swallow given the conclusions of previous chapters. Mitigated blame is warranted in many circumstances for both neurotypical individuals and those with mental disorders, so there are many circumstances in which blame will be inappropriate.

1.3.3 Character

The next part of the book asks what neuroscience reveals about how we form our moral attitudes and what that suggests about the enhancement of moral character. Chapter 6 includes the case of a vicious serial killer who exhibits the marked brain abnormalities of psychopathy. The case kicks off discussion of the neurobiological basis of moral judgment and decision-making. Early research suggested that many of our commonsense moral beliefs are formed automatically using emotional heuristics. The standard story is that our gut feelings in ethics are generally inflexible and often unreliable, which might even support certain moral theories over others. There is some truth in this standard picture, but we can resist its pessimistic conclusion. Many of our moral judgments may be based on automatic intuitions, but neuroscience increasingly suggests that these processes are sophisticated learning mechanisms that are inferential and flexible over time.

This picture of moral reasoning equips us to tackle debates about cognitive and moral enhancement in Chapter 7. Various smart drugs and do-it-yourself neurostimulation devices are becoming widely available and used by some not to treat disorders but to enhance their capacities beyond the norm. We focus on the case of a writer who temporarily self-medicated with psychedelics in an attempt to become a better person. Some ethicists worry that moral bioenhancement would be unsafe, curtail freedom, exacerbate inequality in society, or inculcate objectionable desires to perfect ourselves. Each of these worries is formidable but ultimately surmountable if we avoid alarmism and focus on how realistic moral bioenhancement can occur when individuals freely pursue their conception of the good life, uncoerced by others.

1.3.4 Justice

In the last major part of the book, we examine how neuroscience can promote or inhibit justice, although prior issues of harm, care, and character are not left behind.

We begin in Chapter 8 with a concession to the pessimists. While the brain is a reasoning machine, unfortunately this reasoning is often biased. Through self-deception, people often reason their way to conclusions they already want to accept. This is highlighted by the treatment of some patients with epilepsy who display a divided mind after the connection between their brain hemispheres is severed. But we'll see that self-deception and motivated reasoning are ubiquitous in ordinary life, even in science itself. Indeed, it can serve as a framework to explain the kind of fraud and questionable research practices that have led us into the current replication crisis in science, which afflicts not only psychology but also all other areas of science, including biology and neuroscience. Ironically, neuroscience suggests that humans are fallible even when doing neuroscience. This book, and the field of neuroethics itself, draws heavily on scientific evidence. Should we be skeptical that science can produce knowledge that informs such a controversial topic as ethics? I will argue that we shouldn't be skeptical, but that we must be exceedingly cautious, especially with neuroscience. It is still a relatively new and multifaceted discipline that is prone to misunderstanding and currently proceeds with little knowledge of how the brain gives rise to the mind.

Given that neuroscience is so abstruse and prone to misunderstanding, Chapter 9 asks whether it should be used to read the minds of individuals in the courtroom or consumers in the marketplace. Various forms of brain reading could be used to support a defendant's innocence (or guilt) or to understand consumer preferences. We dig into the case of an inmate wrongly convicted of murder whose exoneration was supported by "brain fingerprinting" evidence. The issues are decidedly ethical because poor evidence here can lead to injustice, either from false convictions, unwarranted acquittals, or violating consumer's rights to cognitive liberty. Juries might be unduly swayed by neuroscientific evidence, particularly brain images. I argue that neurobiological evidence is no weaker or liable to mislead than other forms of admissible evidence, and consistency reasoning requires us to treat like cases alike. Even if fairly weak on its own, neuroscience can serve a valuable role when combined with other evidence in a court of law. Neuromarketing, in contrast, is unlikely to profit from expensive investments in brain reading, given that corporations are already able to cheaply and effectively read our minds based on analyses of our search histories, purchases, and other elements of our digital footprints. So concerns about unprecedented invasions of privacy are generally overblown.

1.3.5 Nuanced Neuroethics

Chapter 10 brings the book to a close by drawing out some of the overarching lessons for neuroethics that emerge from the previous chapters. In the end, the book's subtitle might seem misleading, since agency is an explicit subject of only some chapters. However, all of them cover core aspects of human agency: free will, responsibility, self-control, moral judgment, reasoning, and character. Moreover, the central message of the book concerns human agency. On a "nuanced" approach, neuroscience forces us to rethink human agency as *less conscious and reliable* but *more diverse and flexible* than it is often supposed, which supports a measured approach to ethical issues in neuroscience that is *neither alarmist nor incredulous*. A central lesson for medicine, law, cognitive science, and public policy is that neurotypical and atypical brains are *more alike than unalike*.

1.4 Conclusion

You may be wondering about the case of Kevin that kicked off this chapter. Was he in control of downloading all of that heinous, illegal pornography? Should his neurological condition play a role in the court case at all? Should neurosurgeons have removed chunks of his brain in the first place, just to treat seizures? We'll have to wait for the answers—well, my answers—until the final chapter, where we are able to come full circle and apply the tools developed throughout our exploration of such distinct, but related, issues in neuroethics. To draw appropriate conclusions about Kevin's case, we need to further explore issues of agency, autonomy, justice, and mental health.

Appendix: Philosophy and Brain Primers

Before we embark on our neuroethics voyage, let's lay some groundwork for the rest of the book. Neuroethics is an interdisciplinary field that draws heavily from the sciences, but our primary approach will be philosophical. The controversial ethical issues require critical thinking about arguments on both sides, which is a specialty of philosophers. So let's begin with some key philosophical concepts and issues that are particularly useful for navigating neuroethics. Afterward we add some basic information about the brain to our neuroethics toolkit.

A.1 Philosophy Primer

A1.1 Metaphysics & Epistemology

It is fitting to begin by touching on a classic philosophical issue: *the mind-body problem*. Neuroscientists often treat the mind or mental phenomena as merely events, states, or processes of the brain or perhaps the whole nervous system. But there is a deep puzzle here.

Think for a second about your mind. Right now, you may be having certain experiences, such as a painful headache, sleepiness, or even happiness as you were recently interrupted by your pet's hilarious antics. Perhaps instead you're having trouble staying focused; your mind continues to wander off daydreaming about your upcoming weekend getaway or deliberating about how to confront your coworker about pulling his weight. On the one hand, from the inside these thoughts and experiences don't seem to be physical at all, let alone a storm of electrochemical processes in your brain. As René Descartes and other philosophers have long recognized, our intuitive conception of our minds is that they are related to, but distinct from, our bodies, including our brains. Indeed, such a *dualist* view is presumed by the popular belief in life after death (of the body). Or consider the very real phenomenon of out-of-body experiences in which people perceive themselves, or at least their consciousness, as floating above their lifeless bodies. Such experiences suggest that the mind is distinct from the corporeal self.

On the other hand, neuroscientists have shown that out-of-body experiences can be induced by stimulating a particular part of the brain, such as the temporoparietal junction (De Ridder et al. 2007). Indeed, new brain-machine interfaces have allowed paralyzed patients to control machines just by thinking. Cathy Hutchinson, for instance, suffered a stroke in her 40s that destroyed her ability to speak or move her own hands. Her tetraplegia was caused by damage to nerves in her brainstem, which prevented commands in her motor cortex from reaching her spinal cord and initiating movement in her limbs. Fifteen years later, researchers at Brown University developed a robotic arm with electrodes that connect directly to her motor cortex, allowing her to grab a bottle and bring it to her lips to drink, all without explicit training (Hochberg et al. 2012; videos are readily searchable on the internet).

Doesn't this all show that our thoughts and experiences are just states of the brain? Couldn't we discover that, while the mind doesn't seem physical from the inside, it actually is? Imagine Lois Lane insisting that it's impossible for Clark Kent to be Superman, because they don't seem identical from her perspective. New information can reveal that what seem like two distinct things—e.g., water and H_2O—are actually one. The mind's secret identity could be physical states of the brain. This alternative take on the mind-body problem is appropriately called *physicalism* (or *materialism*).

Fortunately for us, we needn't take a stand on this perennial dispute to delve fully into neuroethics. Even staunch dualists like Descartes, who was a serious anatomist himself, are *interactionists* who hold that the mind and body causally interact with one another and can be intimately connected. What physicalists and dualists would disagree vehemently about is a more basic metaphysical question about what kind of thing the mind is, not whether, say, stimulating the brain will have profound effects on the mind (or vice versa). No dualist, not even Descartes, would be surprised by the successes of brain-machine interfaces. Indeed, a common exclamation in neuroscience reporting is that a new study demonstrates that an activity—e.g., meditation, exercise, or drug use—"actually changes the brain!" Such surprise is warranted only if one assumes that the mind and brain do not causally interact, yet that assumption is rejected by physicalists and dualists alike.

Both theorists might be surprised, however, by how much the brain is involved in *constructing* not only our thoughts but also our experiences. Many people naïvely assume that our sense organs—eyes, ears, nose, etc.—provide all the information necessary to form our experiences, as if they are merely windows to the world. That is, we assume a form of *naïve realism* about perception, according to which the way things look, sound, or feel is a direct perception of reality (at least when our sense organs are working properly in normal conditions). The consensus among neuroscientists, however, is that our experiences are largely a construction of the brain—a model or prediction about what reality is like, based on extremely limited sensory information.

Vision illustrates this well. Many philosophers have long assumed that certain properties of objects, such as color, are something the mind paints onto reality, but the story is similar for all of our experiences, including that of shapes. If the brain simply used what the eyes provide as visual experience, then one would constantly see a blind spot in the center of one's visual field. After all, there are no photoreceptors on the retina where the optic nerve attaches to the back of the eye (Kandel et al. 2013: 580). Not only because of this inherent blind spot, but also because the photoreceptors in the eyes only provide a two-dimensional array of sensory information, the brain does a great deal of work to fill in the gaps and generate a three-dimensional visual experience. The eyes are not a window to the world at all. They are more like blackout curtains that let only some rays of light in, and the brain is like a scientist in that darkened room who does her best to predict what the outside world looks like with the help of a supercomputer. Although in any one instant she has precious little outside information, the computer has lots of prior experiences and expectations that help her build a model or prediction that can be updated in light of new (albeit limited) information over time.

Optical illusions help illustrate how the brain constructs these experiences. Consider the well-known "hollow mask illusion" (Figure A.1). The mask looks convex, like it is protruding toward the viewer, but this appearance doesn't match reality. The mask is in fact facing the opposite way and is thus "hollow" or concave. Yet your brain has seen many faces before, and its best model of them is that they are convex. So when presented with the hollow mask, your brain takes the facial features as powerful evidence that the mask is convex, like it has seen a million times before with similar objects. The result is an illusory experience. Interestingly, neurologists have found that patients with schizophrenia are not as subject to this illusion, apparently because their brains weigh the lower level sensory information more heavily than the "top-down" expectation that faces are generally convex (Dima et al. 2009). The illusion thus arises for

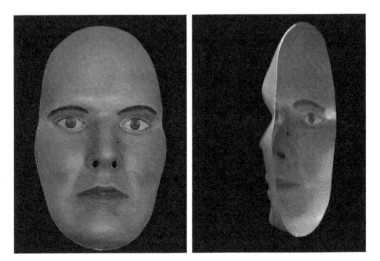

Figure A.1 The Hollow Mask Illusion
Mask of a face that appears convex (left panel) but is really concave (right panel).
Source: Papathomas & Bono 2004. Reprinted with permission of the publisher.

neurotypical individuals because the mask exploits an assumption the brain normally makes about faces.

We can illustrate the point with other sensory modalities too. One of the simplest audio illusions is the "McGurk effect," which demonstrates that the sounds we hear coming out of a person's mouth are partly dependent on what visual information we receive and our background beliefs about which mouth movements typically produce certain sounds. If you watch a video of a person vocalizing the sound "bah"—with the characteristic pressing of lips together to make a "b" sound—then you will hear "bah." However, if the very same sound is played while the person moves their mouth *as if* they are making an "f" sound—with the top teeth pressing down on the bottom lip—then you will hear "fah" (video demonstrations are readily searchable on the internet). This illustrates again how the brain constructs our experiences ("top down") given that only sparse sensory information is available, which is insufficient on its own to determine a particular experience (the "underdetermination problem" in perceptual psychology). The Buddha said, "Our life is the creation of our mind." Indeed.

Why should this matter for neuroethics? Isn't it well-known and uncontroversial that our brains help construct our experiences? Perhaps, but what is not well-known is the extent to which one's brain does this, and not only for experiences but also thoughts, emotions, and decision-making. Indeed, some philosophers and neuroscientist believe that all brain mechanisms boil down to the building of a model, and in particular a model of its own sensory input that predicts what input will come next, with the aim of minimizing errors in its predictions (Hohwy 2013; Clark 2016). We needn't take a stance on whether this grand unified "predictive processing" view of the brain is correct, let alone whether you're living in a computer simulation. Nevertheless, as we proceed to analyze ethical issues in neuroscience, we must keep in mind that even basic mental states and processes like vision arise from complex interactions among psychological states—such as beliefs, desires, and memories—which means we should expect most mental phenomena to arise from various networks of brain areas working together.

A1.2 Ethics

Unlike some controversies in metaphysics, we will delve into many controversies in moral philosophy. Questions in ethics are often divided up into three more or less discrete kinds, all of which can inform, or be informed by, the sciences of the mind. Start with the more concrete questions in ethics. In practical or *applied ethics*, we ask whether specific kinds of actions are right or wrong, typically controversial moral issues, such as abortion, euthanasia, war, and capital punishment. The ethics of neuroscience, and so roughly half of this book, falls squarely into this category, while the rest involves more theoretical issues in ethics.

Suppose we satisfied ourselves with answers to the applied or practical questions. We could then ascend to a more theoretical level of abstraction and ask: What in general makes a person or action good or bad, right or wrong, virtuous or vicious? Now we're in the realm of *normative ethics*, which attempts to discover a general explanation of right and wrong. Much like the physicist, who seeks a general explanation for why objects have the physical properties they do, the ethical theorist seeks a general explanation for why actions and individuals have certain moral properties.

There are three major theories in the running (which is about how many grand unifying theories we have in physics!). The simplest and perhaps most famous theory is *utilitarianism*, which John Stuart Mill expressed as: "actions are right in proportion as they tend to promote happiness, wrong as they tend to produce the reverse of happiness" (1863/1998: 55). In other words, the right thing to do is to maximize happiness. Should you sacrifice one innocent person to save five people, or instead let the five die in order to avoid killing the one? Mill would say—all else being equal—that you ought to kill the one for the greater good. As Spock famously put it on *Star Trek*: "Logic clearly dictates that the needs of the many outweigh the needs of the few." This view is one of a family of *consequentialist* theories because it says all that matters, morally speaking, are the consequences of one's action (Sinnott-Armstrong 2019). Imagine two individuals who both cause a fire that kills a dozen innocent people, but one of them does it intentionally while the other was merely negligent. Consequentialists say that the actors' intentions, in and of themselves, don't matter to the wrongness of their actions (although they may inform our evaluation of the actor's character). Both fire-starters did something wrong, but only one of them is a malicious person who is likely to do other terrible things.

Non-consequentialists balk at this bifurcation of morality into acts versus a person's motives or character. *Deontology* ("duty-based" ethics), for example, maintains that the morality of an act depends not only on its consequences but also on how one brought them about—e.g., on purpose or in a way that was unfair or failed to respect another's autonomy. One of Immanuel Kant's famous formulations of his fundamental principle of morality was "use humanity, whether in your own person or in the person of any other, always at the same time as an end, never merely as a means" (1785/1997: 38). Deontologists like Kant typically view morality as arising out of creatures with free will trying to get along rationally. Our endowment of rational autonomy requires us to treat one another fairly and respect each other's autonomy.

While deontology and utilitarianism were products of the Enlightenment, the final theory, *virtue ethics*, is ancient. Virtue ethicists, from Aristotle to Confucius, tend to be non-consequentialists but focus most on one's overall character. This tradition sees ethics as a matter of being an excellent person, and so character traits, not acts, should be the primary locus of moral evaluation. Virtues are like skills that allow a person to flourish, not merely happiness/harm and justice/unfairness, which are the exclusive focus of consequentialism and deontology. Virtue ethics embraces a wider range of basic moral values, such as bravery, prudence, loyalty, and (for some) even punctuality.

The foregoing is merely a sketch of theories in normative ethics, and we'll return to them later. However, we will not be relying much on them to resolve practical issues in the ethics of neuroscience. For example, we will not determine whether it's acceptable to manipulate a patient's brain simply by calculating the amount of happiness it would produce compared to alternative courses of action, disregarding whether the patient consented. That would assume that consequentialism, specifically utilitarianism, is true, which is just as controversial as any issue in neuroethics. It won't help to trade one controversy for another.

Nevertheless, it will be useful to keep these theories in mind for two reasons. First, some of the methods neuroscientists use for studying moral judgment rely on distinctions among these theories, and some philosophers have developed arguments for particular moral theories in light of research on how we form our moral beliefs in the first place (Chapter 6). Second, moral theories highlight core moral values—such as well-being, fairness, and loyalty—that we should consider when examining practical moral problems in neuroethics. We can recognize the importance of these moral values without taking a stance on which, if any, is fundamental or supersedes the others.

Bioethicists typically adopt this approach. The guiding *principles of bioethics*—autonomy, beneficence, non-maleficence, and justice—identify fundamental moral values without specifying how conflicts among them are to be resolved (Beauchamp & Childress 2019). This set of principles, however, is incomplete. Various aspects of virtue ethics are conspicuously absent, and more generally the list runs afoul of a core principle of moral psychology: "There's more to morality than harm and fairness" (Haidt 2012: 110). Other fundamental values that people hold dear also arise throughout ethics, including loyalty to one's group, respect for authority, and purity of mind and body. Perhaps these other moral foundations should be rejected or reduced to harm and fairness, but for our purposes it's useful to employ a broad ethical vocabulary. Indeed, although the book's chapters are grouped together under the heading of a single moral value, the discussions reveal that many other values are on the scene competing with it.

Finally, the last of the three main branches of moral philosophy ascends to an even higher level of theoretical abstraction. *Meta-ethics*, as the name suggests, examines ethics itself. We can ask whether the practice of praising and blaming each other is a matter of discovering objective truths or merely expressing our own emotions or our culture's set of social rules. We will not address that issue in this book. The arguments in the coming chapters are compatible with assuming that ethics is objective (a key element of "moral realism"), but also that it isn't completely. Consider the issue of moral enhancement (Chapter 7). The notion of enhancement assumes a moral metric on which people can improve or degrade. That's true, but the specifics of the metric are left wide open. The metric could be objective, entirely independent of human attitudes. But it could be subjective. For example, we might only be able to speak of improvement relative to a particular society's norms. Becoming more compassionate might amount to moral improvement in Western cultures but not others. We needn't settle that issue to talk about moral improvement generally.

A question in meta-ethics that we will address is whether we really know right from wrong—whether our moral beliefs aren't just the product of unreliable brain mechanisms that were instilled in humans long ago in their evolutionary history. Since such questions make empirical assumptions about human nature and how we form our moral beliefs, neuroscience becomes a relevant source of evidence to advance some meta-ethical debates. Again, it doesn't really matter whether moral knowledge is construed as knowledge of objective or subjective truths. All we need is a conception of moral truth. Compare truths that are relative to one's location. If I say "It's raining *here*" that can be true while I'm walking the streets of London but false if I'm standing in the dry Kalahari Desert. If I am in London, then it's true that I *know* that it's raining here, even if that truth is relative. Unless of course I believe it's raining in London for bad reasons, like a mere guess. So knowledge needn't be objective, and one can lack it even when the truths to be known aren't completely objective.

Now consider ethics. Suppose morality is relative to cultures and a man says, "It's wrong for a married woman to leave the house without her husband's permission." Even if morality is culturally relative, that statement can be true or false, and thus a potential object of knowledge, depending on which culture is at issue. If the man who utters that sentence is Australian, then cultural relativists will say that what this man says is false (relative to his culture) and thus not a piece of moral knowledge. So talk of knowing right from wrong needn't presume completely objective moral truths. The point isn't that morality is subjective (or not), but rather that we can remain *neutral* on that thorny issue in meta-ethics while addressing others.

A.2 Brain Basics

The philosophical substance of neuroethics often turns on the details of the science. Indeed, a mantra of this book will be: *Take seriously the details of the science (and philosophy).* If we are to learn from and critically evaluate a science, we must understand it in some depth. We'll focus on neuroscience specifically and ask whether it can raise or illuminate interesting moral problems. Often I will introduce technical neurobiological (and philosophical) concepts as they come up in the context for which they are used. However, some basics about the human brain will be useful to have on hand straight away (for useful resources, which I draw on here, see Kandel et al. 2013; Morrison 2018; Garrett & Hough 2018; de Brigard & Sinnott-Armstrong 2022).

A2.1 Electrochemical Cells

The crown jewel of the nervous system, the brain, is a truly wondrous organ. As we saw, your eyes can't even see by themselves; your brain does most of the work to build a rich three-dimensional image from a patchy smattering of light that hits the retina. None of your bodily organs can survive without the brain. It's responsible for constantly keeping your heart pumping, your lungs breathing, your hormones flowing, your body moving, and your mind wandering. It's no wonder the brain is a metabolic gas guzzler that consumes about 20% of the body's energy despite taking up only 2% of its weight.

This remarkable organ, which looks and feels like a gelatinous hunk of meat, is primarily made up of about 86 billion *neurons* (nerve cells), first posited in the late 19th century by the pioneering Spanish neuroscientist Santiago Ramón y Cajal. Although researchers are finding now that other cells in the nervous system are relevant for mental function, particularly neuroglia or glial cells, neurons are the star of the show. They communicate with one another by transferring electrical and chemical signals to different areas of the nervous system. Each neuron has many branches coming out from the cell body that stretch out to communicate with other neurons, sometimes stretching rather far given their minute size. So, although neurons are often depicted with short branches (to fit them on a single page or slide), they are often much, much longer. Signals coming into a given neuron hit its *dendrites*, while outgoing signals are transmitted through the *axon* to another neuron or target cell (e.g., a muscle or gland cell). A neuron that fires will send an electrochemical signal to another neuron's dendrites but does not touch it. A tiny gap, the *synapse*, exists between them through which the signal is passed on by chemicals called *neurotransmitters* (such as acetylcholine, dopamine, epinephrine, glutamate, and serotonin).

The past 100 years have seen an explosion of knowledge about neurons and the anatomy of the brain. Yet it remains largely a mystery how exactly these many tiny cells give rise to psychological phenomena, such as thoughts, emotions, decisions, and conscious experiences. It is clear that the brain takes in information from the senses to construct experiences and ideas, and these ultimately lead to judgments and decisions, when combined with motivations or goals. The brain may acquire some goals from experience, but others may be innate, instilled in us by evolution. For example, desires for food, water, affection, and eventually sexual activity may come "pre-wired" into our nervous systems.

Certain areas of the brain appear to be more involved in some basic psychological processes and events. In the early days, *phrenologists* erroneously thought that very specific parts of the brain were dedicated to very specific psychological phenomena—such as love, individuality, and even conscientiousness—in a kind of one-to-one mapping. The truth is somewhere in between. We now know, particularly from studies of patients with brain damage, that there is some *localization of function*: certain areas of the brain are involved in general functions, such as language, bodily movement, and vision. For instance, patients with brain lesions or damage to certain areas (e.g., Broca's or Wernicke's area) famously develop difficulties with the production or comprehension of speech, and patients who suffer certain temporal lobe damage acquire deficits in identifying animals but retain the ability to identify tools and other artifacts (Caramazza & Shelton 1998).

Then again, the brain is clearly a flexible organ that uses networks of areas holistically to perform psychological functions. Research on *neuroplasticity* suggests that some areas of the brain not normally used for a certain psychological function can learn to perform that function after long, repeated bouts of retraining. Humans born without arms can become archers, and dogs can learn to travel the ocean's waves on a surfboard (Eagleman 2020: 114). Even old brains can learn new tricks. Patients who lose the ability to move a limb after a stroke, for example, can regain that ability through intense physical therapy, and neuroimaging demonstrates that other parts of the brain pick up the slack from the stroke-damaged areas (Gauthier et al. 2008). So, while there is some localization of function, it only goes so far. It's tempting to think of the brain as fixed and specialized for specific tasks, but we're now realizing that it's fundamentally designed to learn, to adapt to different circumstances.

A2.2 Functional Systems

Since different areas of the human brain do seem to be preferentially involved in certain functions, some knowledge of neuroanatomy is necessary. We can identify regions using numbered areas of an atlas, such as the 52 Brodmann areas. But most brain research and case studies in neurology navigate the brain in terms of its anatomical regions. Start with our brain's outer layer, the *cerebral cortex*, which consists of four main lobes (which are, *very roughly speaking*, more involved in certain functions, indicated in parentheses):

- *Occipital lobe* (vision)
- *Parietal lobe* (touch, spatial and numerical processing, etc.)
- *Temporal lobe* (auditory processing, social and linguistic understanding, etc.)
- *Frontal lobe* (judgment, decision-making, aspects of personality, etc.)

These four lobes (see Figure A.2) contain many folds, which help increase the surface area of the brain within the limits of the skull. The cortex is thus like a mountainous terrain, where a ridge is referred to as a *gyrus* and a valley as a *sulcus*, which like Everest and Kilimanjaro have their own names (e.g., the Central Sulcus or Central Fissure). The frontal cortex is particularly important for neuroethics given its involvement in judgment, decision-making, and self-control. However, many other animals possess a frontal cortex as well. What's particularly developed in humans is the very front of the frontal cortex, and so it has a specific name as well—the *prefrontal cortex*.

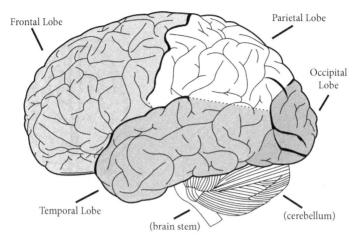

Figure A.2 The Cerebral Cortex
The four lobes of the outer layer of the human brain, which is the portion most advanced in humans. Our cerebral cortex contains many folds to increase its surface area.

The cerebral lobes are large areas that perform many functions. We can identify more specific areas within these lobes using anatomical terms:

- *Anterior* (front) vs. *posterior* (back)
- *Superior/dorsal* (above) vs. *inferior/ventral* (below)
- *Medial* (inner) vs. *lateral* (outward)

The structure of the brain in bipedal animals involves one marked departure from what is familiar in general anatomy. In other parts of the body, "dorsal" and "ventral" pair better with "anterior" and "posterior" since the dorsal/ventral distinction refers to above or below the spinal cord specifically. But in the human brain it's as if the spinal cord is making a roughly 90-degree turn once it hits the base of the brain, which forms a main line that is roughly parallel, rather than perpendicular, to the ground (see Figure A.3).

As an exercise, let's break down some areas that we'll encounter multiple times in this book. First consider the *ventromedial prefrontal*

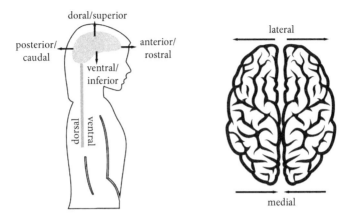

Figure A.3 Navigating the Brain

Anatomical terms used to locate and identify brain regions. E.g., the dorsolateral prefrontal cortex (dlPFC) is so named because it's the top outer portion of the front of the frontal lobe.

cortex. The term may sound like a nonsensical mouthful, but it's easy to get a sense of this area's location in the brain. Since it is part of the prefrontal cortex, we're somewhere in the front of the frontal lobe, behind the forehead. More specifically, it is the underside portion facing the ground (ventral) and not the outer portion but the inner portion (medial). And thus the ventromedial prefrontal cortex is roughly behind your eyes. Now consider the *posterior Superior Temporal Sulcus* (pSTS). We can infer that this is the rear (posterior) portion of an upper valley (superior sulcus) in the temporal lobe. That's a relatively large swath of cortex that can be identified by other subsections or overlapping regions as well (e.g., the temporoparietal junction, angular gyrus). Of course, we can't read the anatomical locations from the names of all brain areas. For example, all we can glean from "amygdala" is that it derives from the Latin term *almond*, as this pair of structures deep in the brain have an almond shape. (For a visualization of these brain areas, jump to Figure 6.1.)

The cerebral cortex is an important part of the human brain—a part that is exceptionally large and developed in humans—but it is only a fraction. Like many other animals, humans also have various *subcortical regions*, such as the basal ganglia and the thalamus. Another notable brain structure, the *cerebellum*, sits just under the occipital lobe at the back of the head and as its name suggests looks like a mini-brain (and appears to be necessary for balance and coordination, among other things). Farther down at the base is the *brain stem*, which plays a vital role in basic biological functions, such as breathing and heart rate. Very roughly speaking, the deeper within the brain a structure is, the more similarities it shares with analogous structures in many other vertebrates, particularly mammals. The portions of the brain that are more highly developed in humans tend to be near the brain's surfaces, especially in the prefrontal cortex. But it is easy to oversimplify, especially when discussing brain areas that are primarily identified anatomically. What is now clear is that the brain involves networks of areas that form circuits. The *limbic system*, for example, is at the crossroads of several cortical and subcortical areas, such as the amygdala, cingulate, hypothalamus, and hippocampus. This system appears to support emotion, motivation, long-term memory, and related functions found in many mammals. Yet these structures are not a group of islands isolated from the rest of the brain. The structures in the limbic system interact with other lobes and produce much more complex emotions in humans than most other animals experience.

Much of our understanding of brain function used to come from rare cases of brain damage in humans or the intentional lesioning of animal brains. But we now have functional neuroimaging that noninvasively detects neuronal activity in humans while they carry out mental tasks in the scanner. This technique has exploded onto the scene and dominated as a method in neuroscience since the 1990s. Some forms of brain imaging, such as positron emission tomography (PET scans), use chemical tracers to track neuronal activity. But a truly game-changing tool grew out of technologies that generate an image of the structure of bodily tissues using magnetic resonance imaging (MRI). *Functional* MRI (fMRI) allows researchers to detect changes in neuronal activity by tracking blood flow throughout the brain (Poldrack 2018). Neurons require more oxygenated blood after being activated, and fortunately for neuroscientists there appears to be a robust correlation between increased activity in neurons and an increase in blood flow to that area (two to six seconds afterward, at least). Another stroke of good luck is that the magnetic properties of oxygenated and deoxygenated blood are sufficiently different that they can be detected in MRI scanners. Researchers can then compare this blood oxygen level-dependent (BOLD) signal in different areas of the brain to infer which is likely more active.

The entire process of generating the colorful pictures we see in neuroimaging articles, and the reporting on them, are not really pictures at all. Unlike photographs, functional brain images are the result of many, many complex steps of experimental design and statistical inference (Roskies 2007).

Consider how complicated matters are with just a single statistical inference using relatively simple measures. Suppose researchers conclude that a dietary supplement is *probably* reducing anemia given that the blood samples from an experimental group exhibit higher iron levels than in the control group who ingested a placebo pill. The variable measured (iron level) is higher in one group compared to the other (say, 35 mcg/dL vs. 20 mcg/dL). But could this difference be due to chance? Statistical analyses can tell us whether it's reasonable to reject the *null hypothesis*: that a difference of that magnitude (or higher) would be observed in this sample even when there is no real difference in the population. Importantly, this rejection of the null is a probabilistic inference. There is always some probability that a similar (or greater) difference between these groups could be observed even when there is no real difference in the population (that is, even when the null hypothesis is true). However, if that probability is low enough—conventionally below 5% ($p < .05$)—then the difference is "statistically significant." But that term can be rather misleading, since it doesn't imply that the difference between groups is large, important, or significant (in the ordinary sense)—only that the difference, even if miniscule, is not likely due to chance. Matters are even worse with most experiments in neurobiology because there are many inferences, assumptions, and choices buried within the technology used, from the software packages that acquire the data to the decisions researchers make about which parameters to set. Moreover, neuroimaging data is extremely noisy with a low signal-to-noise ratio. In the end, the data that result, and the conclusions drawn on the basis of them, rely on many links in a long chain of statistical reasoning. That means there are many opportunities for errors to slip in (more on this in Chapters 8–9).

Nevertheless, neuroimaging has provided more evidence about the functions of brain areas and networks than we ever had before. Throughout the book, we will encounter more brain areas and neurobiological tools in context, as they become important for discussion of an ethical issue. But we have enough now to get us started. These brain basics are like a map that, along with our philosophical toolkit, equip us for the voyage.

PART II
AUTONOMY

2
Free Will

Fundamental to the many ways we hold one another accountable is the assumption that we have free will. We execute Ted Bundy for brutally killing young women and girls. We praise Oprah Winfrey for donating millions of dollars to fund scholarships at Morehouse College. Punishment and praise would seem unjustified if these individuals didn't make their choices freely, of their own free will.

Yet some theorists argue that neuroscience provides special reasons to believe that no one is truly free. In an opinion piece for *USA Today*, the biologist Jerry Coyne writes: "The debate about free will, long the purview of philosophers alone, has been given new life by scientists, especially neuroscientists studying how the brain works. And what they're finding supports the idea that free will is a complete illusion" (2012). Sam Harris has also joined the chorus and insists: "Free will *is* an illusion. . . . Thoughts and intentions emerge from background causes of which we are unaware and over which we exert no conscious control . . . your brain has already determined what you will do" (2012: 5, 9).

We'll see in this chapter that such skeptical conclusions are not necessarily foisted on us by the science. Free will can exist even if it turns out to be a bit different from what you might expect. Our decisions are driven largely by unconscious forces, but they facilitate human agency. To kick off the discussion, we begin with another legal case, one of the first in which brain-imaging evidence successfully reduced the sentence of a defendant in a homicide trial.

2.1 Weinstein's Window

The defendant, Herbert Weinstein (sounds like "wine stye-n"), was a 65-year-old retired advertising executive. On January 7, 1991,

Weinstein was charged with the murder of his second wife, Barbara. Her body lay 12 stories down from the window of their Manhattan apartment. When police arrived expecting to investigate a suicide, Weinstein acted as if he didn't know where his wife was. Eventually, the police informed Weinstein that witnesses saw a woman being thrown from the window. Weinstein then admitted that he and his wife had been arguing when she scratched his face and he impulsively strangled her to death, at which point he lifted the body up and out of the window to make it appear as if she had taken her own life (Davis 2017).

Weinstein had no prior history of violence. Those who knew him were shocked and considered the act wildly out of character. Indeed, after the incident, Weinstein was bizarrely calm and seemed unconcerned about the situation—his wife's death and the murder charge. Although psychiatric evaluations revealed no clear mental disorder and only slightly reduced dexterity in his right (dominant) hand, an MRI scan displayed an orange-sized obstruction on the left side of Weinstein's brain (see Figure 2.1). The obstruction turned out to be a large "arachnoid cyst," a rare growth in the spiderweb-like layer of the meninges, a membrane that protects the brain and spinal cord. The

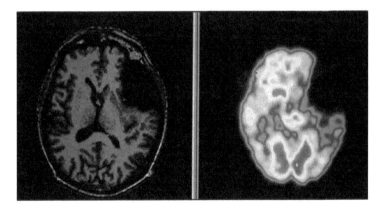

Figure 2.1 The Cyst in Weinstein's Brain

MRI and PET scans showing Herbert Weinstein's arachnoid cyst, which helped his legal team secure a lesser charge for the murder of his wife.

Source: Scans by Abass Alavi, in Rojas-Burke (1993). Reprinted with permission of the Society of Nuclear Medicine and Molecular Imaging.

cyst crowded out portions of his frontal and temporal lobes, which showed reduced function on two different measures of brain activity—electroencephalography (EEG) and a PET scan (Relkin et al. 1996).

Weinstein's defense team argued that he shouldn't be held responsible because, at least temporarily in the heat of the moment, "the cyst pressing on his brain had caused him to act out of character, irrationally, without control" (Davis 2017: 34). This isn't the first time an attorney successfully used neurological evidence to reduce or eliminate a defendant's culpability (more on this in Chapter 9). In 1981, the infamous John Hinckley Jr. attempted to assassinate Ronald Reagan in front of a hotel in Washington, DC. To the great consternation of many Americans, Hinkley was ultimately found not guilty by reason of insanity. While the defense introduced brain-imaging evidence from a CT scan, it's unclear whether it influenced the verdict. In Weinstein's case, however, it is clear that the prosecution became worried about a jury being swayed to acquit because of the large black spot on the brain scan. Since Weinstein's team was willing to settle for manslaughter instead of second-degree murder, the prosecutor agreed to pursue the lesser charge.

Our interest in this chapter is in the free will of ordinary individuals, not those with brain abnormalities or neurological conditions (discussed in Chapter 3). Nevertheless, Weinstein's case and others like it raise the question of whether any of us is truly free. After all, people without neurological damage still engage in misdeeds largely because of activity in their brains. What does it matter whether the brain activity is normal or abnormal, due to a cyst or a particular arrangement of neurons?

A number of neuroscientists believe that their field is the death of free will for us all. Joshua Greene and Jonathan Cohen, for example, assert that neuroscience is "beginning to characterize the mechanisms that underlie our sense of free will" and ultimately "a scientific understanding of these mechanisms can serve to dismantle our commitment to the idea of free will" (2004: 1781; see also Focquaert et al. 2012). We'll consider, in particular, the claim that neuroscience reveals that we lack free will because most of our decisions are driven by unconscious activity in the brain. The evidence is much less powerful than many assume, but it does suggest that we are often *less* free than we tend to think.

2.2 What in the World Is Free Will?

It might seem that the term *free will* simply means different things to different people, and so disputes over whether we have it devolve into semantics or merely verbal disputes. But studies of ordinary use of the term suggest a surprising amount of consensus.

One study found that, in participants' explanations of free will, most described either "making a choice, following one's desires, or being free of constraints" (Monroe & Malle 2009: 215). A wealth of other experiments have asked participants to rate how free an action was in various hypothetical scenarios. The results, while mixed, suggest that most people are willing to ascribe free will to individuals who are able to choose actions among genuine alternatives and control those actions in light of reasons (e.g., Sarkissian et al. 2010; May 2014a). The details are controversial, but such characterizations of free action fit well with much philosophical theorizing, particularly three central threads that we can alliteratively label *choice, control,* and *coherence* (King & May 2018).

Choice, conceived as a decision among genuine options, is central in many philosophical analyses. We do, after all, commonly excuse people from blame or praise when they couldn't have done otherwise. We don't praise ourselves for picking the bag of fair trade coffee when it's the only one available, and we don't blame the bank teller for handing over the money at gunpoint. The inappropriateness of blame or praise seems due to a lack of free choice. So free will seems to require selecting from alternative courses of action, electing and enacting one of them, unconstrained from external forces (Kane 1999). Accounts vary as to the strength and stringency of these requirements. Nevertheless, theorists often stress one's ability to consider a range of actions one might perform and to choose without constraint which one to execute.

Other theorists focus more on exercising effective *control* over one's actions. When a person does something entirely by accident, it looks as though they didn't choose it freely. A popular account of control involves appropriately recognizing and responding to the reasons one has for a course of action (Fischer & Ravizza 1998). Other views characterize control as a power to cause one's actions in a special way (Clarke 1993). Uniting these views is the thought that free will requires an ability to identify and assess reasons upon which one can then act.

In contrast to the way a decision is brought about, some theorists focus on whether one's choice expresses the right kind of *coherence* among one's psychological states (Frankfurt 1971; Wolf 1987). Deeply committed racists, for example, make bigoted remarks more freely than a person who blurts out an insensitive comment that's out of character. Similarly, we tend to treat the routine philanderer as choosing infidelity more freely than the spouse who is riddled with guilt over a one-off affair that quickly developed in the heat of the moment. In these ways, actions can reflect or express aspects of a person to varying degrees, and mental states can be more or less well integrated into an individual's overall beliefs, commitments, and values. The guiding thought here is that an action is free to the extent that it reflects one's real self, one's true values and intentions.

Although there is much disagreement as to whether choice, control, and coherence are exactly what's required for free will, these elements have much overlap, and a kind of "family resemblance." When a well-meaning man accidentally steps on your toes, for instance, his action seems less free (and less blameworthy) because it was not a choice he controlled and thus doesn't express any ill will. We can treat choice, control, and coherence as a cluster of elements relevant to the ordinary concept of free will, even without a precise and complete definition.

A useful model from the psychology of concepts is either a prototype or exemplar theory. Think about whether a television, lamp, or coatrack is a piece of furniture. You might try to precisely define the word "furniture" and see whether these items meet the criteria, but such definitions are notoriously difficult, if not impossible, to develop without controversy, imprecision, or incompleteness. Instead, we can treat a concept like *furniture* as characterized in terms of some prototypical instances of it, such as chairs and sofas, while marginal cases, such as a piano or a basket, are compared to a prototype or exemplar (Rosch 1975). A similar approach to the concept of free will would treat as prototypical, say, unconstrained choice that reflects one's values (May 2014a). The further from the prototype an action is, the less free it will be. Such an approach provides a clear model for how free will can come in degrees.

Now that we have some sense of what it is to act freely, we can ask whether neuroscience threatens it. Cases like Weinstein's, for instance, suggest that everyone's actions are determined by activity in their brains, which might be thought to undermine choice, control, or coherence. How can we formulate such challenges into a clear argument? We'll use the following schematic form (adapted from Nahmias 2014: 5), which begins with a *theoretical* or philosophical premise that is then combined with an *empirical* premise to yield skepticism about free will:

1. Having free will requires that X is *not* the case. [theoretical premise]
2. Neuroscience shows that X is the case (for human choice). [empirical premise] Therefore:
3. Neuroscience shows that humans lack free will.

Proponents of such skeptical arguments are often unclear what the X factor is exactly. Indeed, some discussions slide between different versions of the threat. Let's pry the threats apart and consider them on their own terms.

2.3 Determinism: No Choice?

Long before neuroscience was a distinct field, the classical threat to free will has been the theory that all events are determined by prior events. More precisely, *determinism* is the claim that, given the state of the universe and the laws of nature, there is only one possible future. It may seem, for example, that right before placing a food order you could choose either aloo gobi or biryani. Suppose you choose aloo gobi. If determinism is true, this is the only choice you could have made, at least given the laws of nature and the relevant facts leading up to your choice—e.g., that you had biryani yesterday and believe variety is the spice of life.

Determinism thus seems to make choice among genuine options impossible. This view that free will and determinism are incompatible (*incompatibilism*), appears to be a natural assumption among many cultures (Sarkissian et al. 2010). Although determinism is an ancient threat, many commentators seem to think that advances in our understanding of the brain make it more plausible. Determinism may thus be the key in an argument against free will:

1D. Having free will requires that **determinism** is *not* true.
2D. Neuroscience shows that **determinism** is true (for human choice). So:
3D. Neuroscience shows that humans lack free will.

Many philosophers would reject the first premise (1D) because most are *compatibilists* (Bourget & Chalmers 2013). That is, they believe that determinism, if true, poses no threat whatsoever to free will. On this picture, our actions are determined, sure, but by our own preferences, personalities, experiences, and so on. Compatibilists emphasize that deterministic processes do not *bypass* one's desires and deliberations but rather ensure that such mental states are the cause of one's action, rather than mere chance. Determinism does not entail *fatalism*—the idea that you will perform certain actions no matter what you think, feel, or desire. Although it may be that you will only choose aloo gobi on June 14 in the year 2050 at 6:45 p.m., it will be because you know you had biryani yesterday and prefer variety. Your choice is importantly dependent on your knowledge and preferences and thus controlled by them.

Compatibilism and incompatibilism are themselves logically incompatible. Yet each sits well with our ordinary conception of freedom. On the one hand, we tend to think that free will requires that determinism is false because only then do we have genuine alternatives from which to truly choose (that is, the ability to do otherwise). On the other hand, if determinism is false, then which alternative a person chooses seems to depend on an element of chance or luck. Suppose you live in an indeterministic world, and so the state of your brain and the laws of the universe allow for the possibility that you choose biryani again despite your desire for variety. If you do choose biryani again—despite preferring variety and having this dish recently—then the explanation for your choice will be largely a matter of randomness or mere probability (the neural processes will be "stochastic"). Making a choice by mere luck doesn't seem like free will either. So we are partly inclined to think that having free will depends on determinism being true (May 2014a). We are, in other words, intuitive incompatibilists *and* compatibilists. We could perhaps jettison one of these intuitive commitments while still retaining the core of our conception of freedom (Vargas 2013; Nichols 2015), but let us simply grant premise 1D for the sake of argument.

We'll focus instead on premise 2D. Does neuroscience show that the brain is a deterministic system? Determinism can seem particularly compelling given the development of systematic theories in physics, such as Newtonian mechanics in the 17th century. But a more recent and highly successful theory in physics, quantum mechanics, can be interpreted as involving indeterminacy at the subatomic level, which could bubble up to the neurological level.

Perhaps when we make significant choices that shape our lives there is some quantum indeterminacy in the brain that allows us to make different choices even holding fixed the laws of nature and prior facts about our preferences, memories, and beliefs (Kane 1999). For example, imagine you are deciding whether to speak up and defend your moral principles or keep quiet to avoid causing disruption. Even holding fixed the laws of nature, your timidity, and your desire to avoid confrontation, it could be that there is some probability that you will, against the odds, exhibit courage and fortitude.

Some neuroscientists have shown that activity in the brain can *predict* better than chance which of two simple options a person will select (e.g., Soon et al. 2008). However, even if we could predict people's choices with great accuracy, including important choices, that doesn't prove that determinism is true. Even with some indeterminacy, many choices may be very likely. Imagine that you have been working all year on an important personal project of building or constructing something—say, a sculpture, painting, or wooden desk. Once you've finally finished this masterpiece, you find yourself with a peculiar urge to burn it to the ground; yet you choose to keep it around. If determinism is false, you could have destroyed your prized possession, even given the laws of nature and your strong preference for it to remain intact. Sure, we can confidently predict that you won't destroy the fruit of your labor on a whim, even without recording your brain activity. But that doesn't prove that you couldn't have done otherwise. Determinism is the strict claim that, given the past and the laws of nature, it's *impossible* to do other than what you do, not merely that it's certain or predictable.

So, even if determinism undermines free will, neuroscience does not seem to have established it, and so premise 2D is not vindicated. Indeed, determinism remains primarily a dispute at the level of physics, not neuroscience (Roskies 2006). At the very least, our present understanding of the brain does not help settle this ancient question (Nahmias 2014).

2.4 Physicalism: No Control?

Perhaps the X factor is instead that our brains are merely physical and mechanistic. The renowned neuroscientist, Michael Gazzaniga (2012), seems to focus on this formulation of the argument: "Just as we have learned that the world is not flat, neuroscience, with its ever-increasing mechanistic understanding of how the brain enables mind, suggests that there is no one thing in us pulling the levers and in charge." On these grounds, Gazzaniga concludes, "It's time to get over the idea of free will and move on." Another eminent neuroscientist, P. Read Montague, writes: "Free will is the idea that we make choices and have thoughts independent of anything remotely resembling a physical process. . . . Consequently, the idea of free will is not even in principle within reach of scientific description" (2008: R584).

Here the assumption seems to be that free will requires a nonphysical self, a soul, that is able to control one's behavior unconstrained by physical laws. The threat becomes *physicalism*, which maintains that nothing, including the self or mind, is anything but a physical phenomenon (see the appendix to Chapter 1). (Some free will skeptics might insist that the threat to free will is something distinct from physicalism or determinism, such as "mechanism." But it is difficult to see what this would be if not the idea that the mind is non-physical or that our decisions are determined.)

Physicalism is distinct from determinism and can thus by plugged into a new version of the skeptical argument:

1P. Having free will requires that **physicalism** is *not* true.
2P. Neuroscience shows that **physicalism** is true (for human choice). So:
3P. Neuroscience shows that humans lack free will.

Like determinism, physicalism seems beyond the scope of neuroscience—an issue settled instead by physics or metaphysics. Nevertheless, let us grant the second empirical premise for the sake of argument and evaluate premise 1P instead. Must we conclude that free will is an illusion if the mind is simply the brain (or some combination of brain, body, and environment)?

It's possible to adjust and refine our concepts in light of scientific discoveries. Consider the concept of a *solidity*. In the 17th century, we may have assumed that an object, such as a table, isn't solid if it is mostly empty space. Yet, now that we know tables are mostly empty space at the molecular level, we don't treat this as discovering that tables aren't solid. Rather, the concept of solidity is refined (or perhaps discovered) to not require that solid objects be composed mostly of matter.

Of course, sometimes our ordinary concepts are so off the mark that we conclude there is nothing that satisfies them. This is presumably what happened with witches and phlogiston (see Vargas 2013; Nichols 2015). We discovered there is no magic and so concluded there are no witches, not that witches exist and turned out to be different from what we expected. Similarly, after discovering no need to posit a substance of phlogiston to explain combustion, we conclude that it doesn't exist, not that phlogiston just is a redox chemical reaction.

With respect to physicalism, is the concept of free will more like solidity or witches? We could try to settle this question from the armchair, but that has led to fundamental disagreements about how to conceive of free will. A more promising way forward is to probe ordinary usage of the concept to determine whether dualism is central to how we conceive of free will in the first place. Experimental philosophers have tackled precisely this question, and it turns out that most people think free will remains even if our minds are entirely physical processes. Participants read about hypothetical scenarios in which scientists discover that all mental processes are physical processes in the brain, and then answer whether a particular person had free will when making a decision. The vast majority of participants (75–90% across multiple studies) attribute free will in these circumstances (Mele 2014a), even if the brain processes perfectly predict what the person will do (Nahmias et al. 2014).

How could we conceptualize acting freely as a merely physical process? When researchers ask participants to define free will, there is little to no mention of a soul or immaterial mind (Monroe & Malle 2009). Instead, they describe core aspects of *agency*. Agents don't just move about in the world; they act for reasons, make and revise plans, and judge goals to be more or less worth pursuing. Agents also regulate themselves by reflecting on their motivations, distracting themselves from temptations, directing thoughts toward long-term goals, and so on. These are just psychological capacities that facilitate choice, control, and coherence, and we can easily understand them as generated by brains embedded in particular environments.

Indeed, exercising agency is not a merely internal, ephemeral process, exerted in a single moment of willpower. Few people beyond skilled Buddhists can directly tamp down their anger or anxiety through sheer force of will. Most of us primarily control our actions across time by taking a walk to calm down, committing to routines that inculcate good habits, and otherwise structuring our environments to help achieve goals. (Exercises of agency can thus be *diachronic* and *ecological*.) Consider the famous old story of Odysseus who tied himself to his ship's mast, thereby making it impossible to succumb to the song of the alluring sirens. Odysseus used pre-commitment to prevent an undesirable action. He still presumably felt the powerful desire to heed the sirens' call, but a properly structured environment can also control thoughts and desires. A simple but familiar example is deliberately choosing to banish junk food from the house in order to facilitate healthier eating. This has the advantage of preventing cravings in the first place, but we can also exercise control over mental states the moment they arise. For example, many people get irritable when they become tired or hungry. To become less "hangry," you can deploy breathing techniques that calm your nerves or tools from cognitive behavioral therapy that replace negative thoughts with positive ones. Other strategies are less direct and more external to the mind, such as keeping protein bars in the car or asking a loving partner for a reminder to snack (Jefferson 2022: 81). It's exceedingly difficult to mentally force the irritability away; much easier to just eat something or take a walk. In these ways, our environments provide "scaffolding" for agency, in the form of technology, supportive individuals, social institutions, and cultural norms (Clark 2016: 277; Vargas 2013: 243; Doris 2015: 129; Washington & Kelly 2016; Brownstein 2018). Whether direct and indirect, these are all exercises of agency in a physical world.

Many people do assume that the mind is disconnected from the ordinary physical world. Psychologists have found that from an early age humans across cultures are "intuitive dualists" (Chudek et al. 2018). Perhaps this informs the prototype many people have in mind when conceptualizing free will. Some will insist, with almost religious fervor, on reserving the term "free will" for something nonphysical, magical, spiritual. However, it looks as though conceptions of freedom can survive a thoroughly neurobiological view of the mind. At least the burden is on those who insist that physicalism precludes acting freely, rather than making freedom a bit different than we initially thought.

2.5 Epiphenomenalism: No Coherence?

So far free will doesn't seemed undermined by neuroscience, but a formidable threat remains. Numerous studies suggest that our decisions are largely driven by brain processes that are *unconscious* (simply not conscious), while our conscious intentions are merely along for the ride. Many of our conscious deliberations, intentions, and choices might be mere effects or byproducts ("epiphenomena"). As psychologist Daniel Wegner puts it: "It usually seems that we consciously will our voluntary actions, but this is an illusion" (2003: 1; see also Caruso 2012).

As with the other threats to free will, this one has a corresponding "ism." *Epiphenomenalism* is the thesis that our conscious mental states are merely *effects* of unconscious mental processes, not causes of our actions. On this picture, our conscious experiences of choice are like the steam rising from a boiling pot of water: a byproduct of the system, not a causal component.

Epiphenomenalism of this sort seems incompatible with free will. Wegner writes that our moral judgments of blame and punishment are based "not just on what people do but on what they consciously will" (2003: 335). Consider *somnambulism*, which is commonly known as "sleepwalking," but can involve much more than walking, including talking, writing, sexual intercourse, and even homicide (Schopp 1991; Siddiqui et al. 2009). One well-known case is that of Kenneth Parks who at the age of 23 killed his mother-in-law while sleepwalking (Broughton et al. 1994). On May 24 in 1987, at about 4:00 a.m., Ken stood up from the couch where he had fallen asleep watching *Saturday Night Live* and, in a state of somnambulism, drove about 14 miles to his in-laws' home in a Toronto suburb and attacked them. After strangling his father-in-law, Ken struck his mother-in-law over the head with a tire iron and stabbed her multiple times, leaving fatal wounds. By all accounts, Ken had an excellent relationship with his wife's parents, who were fond of him. Ken was apparently unconscious throughout the violence, becoming conscious around the time he began to leave the house. It was only when he sat down in his car that he realized he was holding a knife. Ken drove to the police station for help, saying he thought he "may have killed some people." Because there was no motive and Ken was apparently unconscious during the attack, a jury ultimately acquitted him of the murder charge, a verdict that was upheld in the Canadian Supreme Court.

If we're all really like Ken, then it seems no one has free will. Epiphenomenalism seems to imply that one's actions or their outcomes fail to reflect one's true self, even if they are controlled and chosen at some level by some part of one's brain. The skeptical argument now takes the following form:

1E. Having free will requires that **epiphenomenalism** is *not* true.

2E. Neuroscience shows that **epiphenomenalism** is true (for human choice). So:
3E. Neuroscience shows that humans lack free will.

Philosophical analysis and findings in neuroscience compel us to take seriously both premises. We'll consider each in turn, starting with 2E.

2.5.1 Evidence for Epiphenomenalism

Let's begin with some unusual cases that illustrate how unconscious processes can drive quite complex behavior. Sleepwalking and other forms of *automatism* are unusual cases, but many people experience similar episodes in everyday life (Levy 2014). Most of us have experienced driving a car home from work on autopilot. You engage in a rather complex series of movements (accelerating, turning, breaking) and respond to information in the environment (stop signs, turn signals, pedestrians), despite being utterly unconscious of it all. As in many such cases, however, these behaviors are highly automated, stereotyped, or "overlearned" habits. Can unconscious processes drive behaviors among neurotypical individuals that aren't mere habits?

Reams of relevant studies can be found, particularly in the "situationist" literature in social psychology. For instance, in the famous bystander effect, study participants are much less likely to help someone in need—actually a "confederate" of the experimenters—if others nearby remain bystanders and don't jump to help or even investigate (Latané & Nida 1981). Lest we worry that such effects can only be generated in artificial lab settings, they have been found in field experiments as well. In one study, twice as many shoppers in a mall helped someone make change for a dollar when the opportunity arose in front of a store emitting pleasing aromas—e.g., from fresh baked cookies—as opposed to clothing stores with more neutral odors (Baron 1997). Or just think of the many ways you unconsciously mimic others when interacting with them. You adjust your legs, scratch your head, and touch your hair after these actions are done by your interlocutor, especially when you like this person or seek to cooperate with them. If you haven't noticed this before, pay attention and you'll see it everywhere. Beware, though, for this can be problematic if, as a result, you avoid mimicry, since it appears to serve important social functions. A number of studies suggest that we trust, enjoy, and feel more rapport with others who, like chameleons, mimic us in social interactions (Duffy & Chartrand 2017). The power of the unconscious mind remains alive and well, even if the details of Sigmund Freud's theory of psychoanalysis have not stood the test of time.

These psychological experiments are just a fraction of the relevant literature. It's unclear how many of these studies can be replicated (Open Science Collaboration 2015). But they illustrate a rather widely accepted view in cognitive science: much human behavior is driven by unconscious mental processes (see, e.g., Bargh & Chartrand 1999; Damasio 1994; Doris 2015; Brownstein 2018). Neuroscience provides additional, and perhaps more concrete, evidence for epiphenomenalism in everyday life.

Here we turn to classic studies conducted on ordinary subjects by the neurophysiologist Benjamin Libet. Since the 1960s, Libet had been studying how conscious and unconscious mental states correlate with neural activity, using electroencephalography (EEG), which measures electrical activity in the cerebral cortex using electrodes affixed to the subject's scalp. It had already been established that EEG could detect activity in the motor cortex called "readiness potentials" (RPs), which appeared to represent the preparation to move a muscle, say in one's hand. Libet eventually wanted to determine whether unconscious activity in the motor cortex came before one's conscious decision to act.

Testing this hypothesis required a clever and elaborate experimental setup (see Figure 2.2). As Libet (1985) reports, he and his collaborators asked participants to sit and spontaneously flick the fingers or wrist of their right hand whenever they freely felt the "urge, desire, or decision" to do so. Each of half a dozen subjects did this over and over, yielding many trials. An electromyography (EMG) machine was also attached to participants' hands to detect the precise moment of muscle activation. Libet just needed a way to measure one's conscious experience of choice. Participants watched a clock-like "oscilloscope" that rotated a dot of light around one revolution every 2.56 seconds, and they had to remember where the dot was when they felt the will to act. Averaging many trials across many participants allowed Libet to find

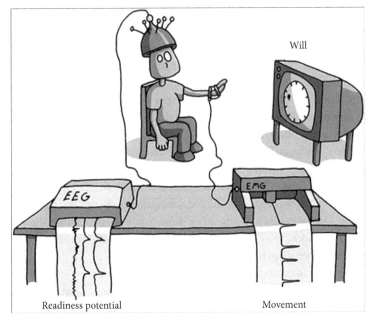

Figure 2.2 Libet's Experimental Setup
Participants note the time at which they become aware of the will to move; the EMG records their movement; the EEG records brain waves in the motor cortex.
Source: Image by Jolyon Troscianko, in Blackmore (2005).

the average amount of time before their movement when participants consciously felt the decision or will to act, which was about 200 milliseconds—a good while in neurophysiological terms. Yet the cerebral activity representing preparation to move (the RP) occurred about 350 milliseconds *before* the awareness of an urge or intention to move (see Figure 2.3).

So it appears unconscious brain activity can already initiate an action before the conscious choice to act. Assuming that causes must precede their effects, this appears to be evidence of epiphenomenalism. Even if one can consciously "veto" the initiated act, as Libet grants, these findings have shaken some beliefs in free will.

We shouldn't stake grand philosophical conclusions on one study, of course. But other researchers have replicated and extended such

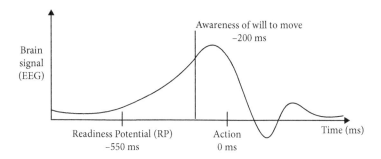

Figure 2.3 Summary of Libet's Brain Wave Data
Unconscious brain activity in the motor cortex (the RP) precedes conscious awareness of the will to move, suggesting that the conscious choice is not the primary cause of action.

findings. Further corroborating evidence has even been found by scientists who recorded neural activity in epilepsy patients using electrodes implanted directly into their brains (Fried et al. 2011). The activity in a small population of neurons in the motor cortex could predict participants' decision to tap their finger, up to 700 milliseconds prior to conscious awareness and with about 80% accuracy. Like Libet's study, however, this one has a key limitation. Participants were merely tasked with either moving or remaining at rest, and the unconscious brain activity might have merely reflected a readiness to perform *some* action, not an urge or intention to perform a *specific* action.

However, a more recent study had participants decide which of two specific actions to take: press a button on the left or on the right. The researchers used functional magnetic resonance imaging (fMRI) to detect brain activity, which was then decoded using statistical pattern recognition to predict subjects' thoughts and decisions (Soon et al. 2008; Wang et al. 2017). Notably, while conscious intentions were reported about 1,000 milliseconds before the button presses, researchers were able to predict above chance which button participants would press based on brain activity that occurred up to 10 seconds before the choice. Of course, at about 60% accuracy, the predictions were imperfect (see Soon et al. 2008, Supplementary Figure 6). A coin flip can predict a person's choice between two arbitrary options with 50% accuracy *10 years* in advance, or indeed as far back as one's heart desires

(Mele 2014b: 27). Still, this brain-imaging study does provide additional neuroscientific evidence of unconscious influences on choice. Thus, the case for epiphenomenalism might seem strong.

Criticisms of this conclusion abound, however. The two most powerful objections reinforce one another and question what exactly the studies show. First, suppose we grant that the early brain activity researchers measure does represent an unconscious intention that is sufficient on its own for action. There remains a concern about *external validity*, or whether the findings generalize to more ordinary contexts. These experiments involve highly artificial situations in which one is asked to make an arbitrary decision to move a body part for no particular reason. Indeed, subjects are meant to let the urge, desire, or intention spontaneously arise in themselves. Even if unconscious plans drive such voluntary actions, it doesn't follow that this is how it works in other more common circumstances, especially when one is weighing reasons for or against high-stakes decisions about, say, whistleblowing, theft, or divorce (Mele 2014a: 203).

Second, it's not clear that the early brain activity represents an unconscious choice or intention to move, rather than a mere *inclination* toward acting. Some recent work suggests that readiness potentials are more like random background activity in the motor cortex (Trevena & Miller 2010; Schurger et al. 2012). To be fair, as we've seen, support for epiphenomenalism comes from more than EEG studies of readiness potentials, including brain imaging and single-cell recording. Nevertheless, even supposing that the early brain activity does represent a psychological state that's relevant to the preparation for movement, it must represent an unconscious *decision* (or intention or plan) to act, not merely an *inclination* or urge to move (Mele 2014a: 202; Nahmias 2014: 14–16). Yet participants have no particular reason to move at any one moment, so it's unsurprising that prior to awareness we can observe the beginnings of an unconscious inclination. Participants are asked precisely to wait for an urge or intention to move, not to generate one consciously.

Even if all our actions were prompted first by unconscious inclinations, there are still many steps until we get to an intention, plan, decision, or choice to move. Consider a concrete, non-arbitrary example with great moral significance, such as the brave women who have spoken out about their powerful sexual abusers during the #MeToo movement. Defenders of free will can happily describe these cases as involving competing inclinations or desires that automatically come to mind, namely the impulse to remain silent versus the desire for justice. The question is whether the resulting choice (e.g., to speak out) is caused by the conscious intention to do so or instead *bypassed* by unconscious intentions that alone are sufficient for action. In other words, we acquire evidence for epiphenomenalism only if the following causal ordering of mental states is demonstrated (where → means "causes"):

Unconscious intention → Action & conscious intention

Yet the following interpretation of the results is consistent with the data:

Unconscious urge → Conscious intention → Action

Indeed, this latter interpretation is quite plausible given the situation participants are in. They are in effect waiting for an urge to guide their decision to move or press one button or the other.

In sum, the experiments in neuroscience alone don't strongly support epiphenomenalism. Notice that the first objection can be combined with the second one: the early brain activity represents merely an unconscious urge, *and* the experimental situation fails to represent most of the decision-making contexts of ordinary life. However, as we've seen, the studies in neuroscience do converge with numerous studies in psychology that suggest that unconscious factors influence many of our choices. As Neil Levy nicely puts it, objections to any particular study may win the battle but not the war (2007: 231). Thus, the empirical premise of the relevant argument against free will does have considerable support. To fully assess this argument, though, we need to determine whether its first premise is plausible. A single false or implausible premise makes for a faulty argument.

2.5.2 Is Consciousness Necessary?

Even if experiments do demonstrate that our actions are largely determined by unconscious influences, is free will undermined? The answer is complicated, and it requires careful analysis and re-examination of the empirical evidence. We'll see that free will can survive many unconscious influences, provided they do not significantly undermine choice, control, or coherence.

First, the connection between free will and conscious control is not a philosopher's fiction. Experimental surveys about various hypothetical cases suggest that most people don't regard an individual as having free will (or being morally responsible) if that person lacks consciousness control over their actions (e.g., Shepherd 2017). Such research suggests that consciousness is an essential part of our concept of free will (perhaps because awareness seems essential for control or coherence). Even if not definitive, there is a heavy explanatory burden on those who think free will is compatible with total epiphenomenalism.

Moreover, there are defensible rationales for why consciousness is relevant to free will. The most well-developed argument is that our actions are more controlled and reflective of our true selves when they are driven by factors of which we are consciously aware (Levy 2014). This argument turns on a prominent model of consciousness developed by the neuroscientist Bernard Baars (2002). On his *global workspace view*, conscious awareness arises when the mind's various subsystems make available their outputs to a domain-general "workspace" in which information can be integrated and used to influence one's behavior.

To illustrate, consider the well-trodden example of the *cocktail party effect*. Imagine you're at a party listening intently to a story being told by an important guest. While listening, you put out of consciousness many powerful stimuli in the background, such as music, laughter, and other conversations. Yet, if someone within earshot utters your name, it will pop out of the background and into your awareness, despite being no louder than other ambient sounds. How could this happen if you aren't paying attention to other conversations?

The answer seems to be that you are in a sense actually paying attention, just unconsciously. A saliency network in the brain, appears to be responsible for monitoring information in the environment and unconsciously evaluating whether it is significant enough to warrant attention and being thrust into consciousness (see, e.g., Corbetta & Shulman 2002; Kurzban et al. 2013). Like many other subsystems in the brain, however, the saliency network appears to perform a circumscribed task. Once its output is broadcast and consciously accessible, that information can be integrated into working memory with other information from various subsystems in order to consciously deliberate (e.g., consciously decide whether to abandon your present conversation for another). Thus, as Levy (2014) argues, consciously controlled actions are more likely to be guided by one's true beliefs and values that are responsive to reasons. More automatic and unconsciously driven actions are, in contrast, likely to be more impulsive and out of character—actions that usually cohere less with one's true self.

The global workspace view provides a useful model here, but it doesn't capture all the ways in which consciousness is and is not relevant to freedom and responsibility (King & Carruthers 2020). Although I won't fault you for stepping on my toe if you didn't realize it was in your way, other times I happily cast blame on others despite their being unaware of how their actions affect me. Forgetting an important anniversary or recklessly revealing confidential information with an off-hand remark isn't done consciously, but it can reveal the person to be careless or inconsiderate.

Indeed, the actions one takes without conscious deliberation are often more revealing of one's true feelings and cohere best with one's other attitudes. After a few beers among friends, what might have seemed like water under the bridge rises to the surface as animosity. The man who makes sexist remarks when hurried does so freely, even if he would rein such comments in when consciously monitoring himself. We take such automatic decisions as better reflections of the individual's true values and priorities. Philosophers have commonly taken their own unusually reflective mental lives as a model for all human agency, but we're learning that passive and spontaneous mental processes, such as mind-wandering, are commonplace and fundamental to human agency (Sripada & Taxali 2020). Indeed, despite being less controlled and conscious, such spontaneous thoughts are even more meaningful to us, as they apparently provide greater self-insight (Morewedge et al. 2014).

Unconscious processes aren't just simplistic reflexes either but can be highly sophisticated in their guidance of action. Think about the many complex choices that a skilled athlete or lawyer makes on the fly, on the basketball court or in the courtroom during cross-examination of a witness (Railton 2014; Brownstein 2018). Their choice of movements, words, and body language are strategic, yet little of it is conscious. When asked how they do it, most skilled individuals will say, "I don't know; I just do it." Yet we regard their feats as performed freely, and we don't withhold praise for their impressive achievements.

Although a number of philosophers agree that awareness is not always necessary for free will, we are left without much explanation about when and why. A mere sketch of a theory, which fits quite well with our ordinary practices and the global workspace view, is what I'll call the *corporate model of agency*. Like a corporation or other agency, the mind is a collection of parts that together act like a single entity. Corporations are composed of various people and their activities (the chief executive officer, managers, and other employees), whereas people are composed of mental states, processes, and capacities (from perception and memory to beliefs, desires, emotions, and personality traits). Many of these psychological processes are unconscious or only partially conscious, such as proprioception, peripheral vision, long-term memory, implicit associations, cognitive biases, and the subtle monitoring of body language. Some of these processes are automatic and impervious to conscious intervention, but others can be influenced by our conscious choices, even if indirectly. For example, you can invent a mnemonic device to lodge an anniversary into long-term memory or implement anonymous grading to avoid implicit biases. In this way, consciousness is like the CEO of a large organization that contains many workers and subgroups who individually carry out rather different tasks to help achieve an overarching goal. An executive doesn't control each task but does have some influence over many of them, either by setting policies or modifying the work employees generate. An executive's role is to oversee and partially direct the operations: to monitor the work done and to integrate it in a way that promotes various goals. Like an executive, your conscious mind has limited resources and is efficient if it attends only to some of the mental activity coming in, such as problems, errors, or more generally information that is surprising or unexpected.

Just as we sometimes identify corporations with their CEOs, we often think of ourselves as our conscious minds. But both are (understandable) mistakes. Jeff Bezos isn't Amazon, and your conscious mind isn't all there is to you. You and I are whole organisms, just as Amazon and Apple are whole organizations that extend well beyond their executives. We sometimes speak as if the CEOs are the singular essence of these massive organizations, but only because they play a privileged role in the direction of the agency. Similarly, we tend to identify ourselves with our awareness, perhaps because introspection suggests that our conscious minds play a special executive role in controlling and monitoring our own behavior.

While the global workspace view suggests that consciousness does have this special role, it can lead us toward a flawed model of agency, which I'll label the *executive model*. On this view, our free agency ultimately arises from the operations of our conscious, executive minds (compare the "searchlight view" articulated but rejected by Sher 2009; the view is arguably defended by Jones 2003; Kennett & Fine 2009; Harris 2012; Hirstein et al. 2018). However, just as organizations are more than their executives, we are more than our conscious thoughts and decisions. The executive may play a special role in steering the ship, and thus is sometimes a fitting focal point of control, agency, and responsibility for the group as a whole. But both our ordinary practices and the scientific evidence suggest that conscious control is only one part of the whole organism and how it regulates itself.

The analogy can be extended to freedom and responsibility as well. When does Amazon act freely, such that it can appropriately be held responsible for its actions? Certainly if Bezos orders workers to, say, build devices that spy on users without their consent. But Amazon isn't only responsible for actions directly ordered by its CEO. In an effort to further the company's growth and success, managers in research and development might order the construction of nefarious devices. Perhaps one will argue that we can "trace" Amazon's responsibility to something Bezos did, such as hire bad people, or something he didn't do, such as fail to ferret out bad apples and correct mistakes within the company (compare Smith 1983). However, since Amazon is more than its CEO, it will be held liable for what it does or fails to do, even if its CEO is unaware of it. If Amazon becomes a corrupt company, despite this not being traceable entirely to choices the CEO made or failed to make, Amazon would still be a company making choices and held accountable for them. Of course, there are limits. Imagine that an employee goes rogue and spies on customers in direct violation of the company's policies. We wouldn't be inclined to attribute this action to Amazon, presumably because the spying wouldn't be something it controlled or chose to enact (perhaps because the act doesn't cohere enough with Amazon as a whole to be reflective of it).

A similar approach to individual agency is appropriate. Awareness does play a privileged role in coordinating beliefs and values that reflect the whole agent, just as the choices of Bezos tend to be more reflective of Amazon's beliefs and values than the decisions of a low-level regional manager. But, like Amazon, an individual can make free choices, even if they aren't entirely under conscious, executive control (for theories amenable to this approach, see Arpaly 2002; Sher 2009; Doris 2015; Washington & Kelly 2016; Brownstein 2018). We needn't always trace an individual's free will (and responsibility) to conscious choices or some other special mental state. At a certain point, if enough lower level workers fail to obey the orders from above, their actions no longer are Amazon's. We have a mutiny. The analogous situation in an individual might be an alien hand or multiple personality. Importantly, though, a normal functioning mind, much like a corporation, operates largely through a complex orchestration of elements of which the conscious mind is not completely aware.

We can accordingly make sense of why awareness is not always required for acting freely. Although consciously controlled actions are often a good guide to one's attitudes, sometimes automatic processes are more revealing. Suppose that, at the cocktail party, Ned's gaze regularly shifts away from his interlocutor and he's keenly aware of any words floating around the room that are even remotely relevant to his recent work project. Ned is so easily distracted because he cares so little about other people's concerns and only wants to talk about himself and his work. As a result, Ned doesn't give his present interlocutor the attention and eye contact she deserves. These are actions, made freely, even if he isn't fully aware of them. Ned is a narcissist, and he is blameworthy for being inconsiderate. Even if this flaw is a blind spot of his, it reflects a coherence in his attitudes, both conscious and unconscious, that guide his behavior.

Of course, Ned and the rest of us didn't ultimately choose which collection of personality traits we started out with in childhood. Except in science fiction, none of us has control over our genotype and little control over our initial environment (just as a corporation, as a whole, lacks complete control over every element of its composition and environment). Nevertheless, we now have the ability to make choices in light of our preferences and deliberations—some of which are conscious, all of which are ours. A character from the television series *Fleabag* proclaims, "I'm not a bad guy! I just have a bad personality. It's not my fault" (Season 2, Episode 6). The quip works because it's a laughably poor rationale for abdicating autonomy or responsibility. Personality traits aren't choices, but what we do (or fail to do) with them or about them is a choice. Whether those choices are made with full conscious awareness isn't a litmus test for whether they are made freely.

The corporate model of agency suggests that awareness and conscious control are relevant to free will but not always necessary, and it goes some way toward explaining why. It should be unsurprising that corporations serve as a useful model for agents and agency, since corporations are agencies. Indeed, we presumably call corporations and other large organizations "agencies" because the individual mind is a model for *them*. Yet, when our topic is individual agency, and we need an example to help think through the case at hand, shifting to corporations and other agencies can inform our understanding of individual agents.

2.5.3 A Limited Threat

With the corporate model of agency in hand, let's reconsider the argument from epiphenomenalism. We have seen that the scientific evidence doesn't demonstrate that all of our actions are driven by unconscious choices. Most of our daily lives do not resemble that of Ken

Parks or other sleepwalkers who engage in out-of-character and stereotyped actions with no conscious guidance. Indeed, the global workspace theory suggests that awareness helps coordinate actions so that they are more reflective of one's overall set of beliefs and values. In artificial contexts, when you have no particular reason to move your hand, the conscious intention to do so may arise from an unconscious urge that bubbles up, but this is appropriate for such situations and poses no threat to free action generally. In other circumstances, free choice requires some awareness of the reasons for it, but Libet-style experiments hardly generalize to ordinary circumstances of important choices made for particular reasons.

Overall, the science does suggest that conscious, reflective choice plays less of a role in controlling our actions than we tend to think. Sleepwalking and other cases of automatism do suggest that people can engage in surprisingly complex behavior in the absence of consciousness. And experiments, primarily in social psychology, suggest that much ordinary behavior is automatic rather than consciously guided. However, many of these unconscious processes are habits or heuristics that have been automated by conscious deliberation in the past (Kennett & Fine 2009; Brownstein 2018). Like a corporation, most of your agency is carried out by processes that you don't directly control through conscious choice but rather guide indirectly. Moreover, the corporate model of agency suggests that having free will doesn't require that all of one's actions are traceable to some conscious choice. Rather, unconscious processes are a legitimate part of how free will is exercised in multifaceted organisms with limited attention spans. Indeed, actions driven by automatic and unconscious processes sometimes better express one's true self.

Now, there are many studies which purportedly demonstrate that much behavior is driven by automatic processes that are not responsive to genuine reasons or don't reflect one's values (Nelkin 2005; Doris 2015). For example, we apparently help others more after smelling cookies and rate résumés with stereotypically African American names lower than those with white-sounding names (Baron 1997; Bertrand & Mullainathan 2004). Some theorists have argued that most conscious deliberation is mere post hoc rationalization of gut feelings (e.g., Haidt 2001). We will return to this issue later (in Chapters 6 and 8), but for now we can note the limited threat it poses to free agency.

Psychological experiments do suggest that unconscious factors play a large role in human behavior, but not necessarily that these factors are arbitrary or non-reasons. The question is whether most of our behaviors are *substantially* influenced by *arbitrary reasons*. Often, however, these two conditions are not jointly satisfied. For example, when being helpful is morally optional, positive mood makes one substantially more inclined to help others. But "because I was in the mood" is a relevant reason to help someone make change for a dollar, even if it's no reason for being honest or respecting property rights (May 2018a: Ch. 9). In other studies, the issue is that the effects are small and isolated. For instance, although race is an arbitrary reason to devalue a job applicant, meta-analyses suggest that such implicit biases tend to exert only small influences on behavior and in particular circumstances—e.g., when rushed (see, e.g., Payne 2001; Greenwald et al. 2009; Oswald et al. 2013; Forscher et al. 2019). Even small, isolated effects on behavior are important when it comes to social justice, but the threat to free will is limited. At any rate, a dilemma arises: the purportedly problematic effects are either substantial or arbitrary but rarely both (Kumar & May 2019).

Ultimately, the extent of epiphenomenalism is often exaggerated, and it is a mistake to think that free will requires that conscious decisions influence every action one takes. Although consciousness plays a privileged role in the direction of a person's actions and the expression of their true selves, we are more than our conscious minds.

2.6 Conclusion

In this chapter, we've assessed several scientific threats to free will grounded in research on the human brain. Although neuroscience does not prove determinism or physicalism, it does provide evidence for some level of epiphenomenalism about conscious decisions. The case is particularly strong when combined with a plethora of findings in psychology. More often than we tend to realize, unconscious forces drive our choices. We thus retain varying degrees of free agency, even if *less* than we naïvely assume (Churchland 2006; Nahmias 2014). However, this shouldn't be shocking since we regularly mitigate blame of others because they were not fully in control, had few choices, or were acting out of character.

Indeed, Weinstein's unusual case was ultimately treated as one of slightly diminished self-control. He unquestionably killed his wife, but the issue is whether he did so freely, on account of an arachnoid cyst in his brain. We've seen that physicalism is no threat to free will, so it matters little that there is a neurobiological explanation for Weinstein's apparently uncharacteristic behavior. The act might have been out of character, which is a relevant factor in free choice, but that alone would not be sufficient for a significant reduction in blame for murder. Did Weinstein have diminished control? That is a difficult question to answer. The cyst was pressing on his frontal lobe, which does play a role in self-control, but so do many other brain areas (more on this in Chapter 5). Even if Weinstein had diminished control, he was clearly awake, aware of what he was doing, and had enough control to stage an accidental death or suicide. So it seems appropriate for prosecutors to charge him with murder, even if a lesser degree of murder.

Weinstein's case, then, is not so different from the neurotypical. Free will comes in degrees and varies across time, but less free doesn't mean unfree. This limited-free-will view provides an important foundation for the arguments and analysis in subsequent chapters. We will further examine agency and autonomy in neurotypical individuals and compare them to those with neurological disorders. Many of us start with the assumption that neurotypical individuals are categorically different from those with brain abnormalities and mental disorders. We will see they are more alike than unalike, which supports a continuum of human agency. We begin first, however, with the ethics of therapeutic brain manipulations and their potential threats to patient autonomy and identity.

3
Manipulating Brains

Neuroscience might not be the death of free will, but specific brain diseases and their treatments can compromise one's autonomy and even one's sense of self. The substance between our ears does have a special claim to being the primary seat of the self, even if the mind does spread out into the peripheral nervous system and beyond. Amputating your gangrened limb won't affect your personality quite like a lobotomy. Manipulating the brain thus raises ethical issues about fundamentally changing one's autonomy and identity.

The electrochemical properties of neurons allow them to be excited or inhibited with either electrical stimulation or the ingestion of drugs that alter brain chemistry. The primary purpose of direct brain interventions is to treat neurological disorders (though some individuals aim to *enhance* their cognitive capacities; see Chapter 7). Risks of adverse events from neuromodulation are concerning given the history of unethical medical procedures in neuroscience and the specter of eugenics. Although informed consent and patient autonomy are now standard, contemporary treatments in medicine are often overprescribed and their harms understudied.

If treatment risks changing one's identity, patients and physicians must understand what those changes entail. We'll see that continuity of memory and moral character are central to identity, yet the self is quite dynamic and flexible given the ubiquity of transformative experiences throughout human life. Ultimately, greater medical humility is warranted all around, especially in brain interventions. We begin with a fascinating case of brain stimulation treatment that sparks these interrelated issues of adverse side effects, patient autonomy, and personal identity.

3.1 A Parkinson's Patient

One of the most prevalent neurodegenerative disorders is Parkinson's disease, which primarily affects motor function. Rigid muscles, slowed movement, imbalance, and tremors can become so severe that ordinary activities are unmanageable. The Parkinson's Foundation reports that over 10 million people suffer from this disease globally. Motor symptoms result primarily from the death of dopamine-producing neurons in an area toward the top of the brainstem called the *substantia nigra*, which is part of a group of structures near the base of the brain known as the "basal ganglia." The substantia nigra is such a dopamine powerhouse that it has a distinctive black coloring from its high concentration of dopaminergic neurons (hence its Latin name meaning "black substance").

There is no known cure for Parkinson's, and treatment using pharmaceutical drugs, such as levodopa, is not effective for all symptoms, especially in the later stages of the disease. In 2002, the U.S. Food and Drug Administration approved deep brain stimulation (DBS) for Parkinson's (see Figure 3.1), and the devices have now been implanted in over 175,000 patients worldwide. The internet is chock full of videos showing patients whose motionless limbs start to tremble uncontrollably once their DBS is switched off.

Stimulation of the brain, of course, is not without its side effects. One Dutch man in his 60s, let's call him "Dimitry," had severe motor dysfunction that did not respond to drug therapies. So he elected to receive deep brain stimulation of his subthalamic nucleus (STN), which is part of the basal ganglia system. Three years later, Dimitry was experiencing full-blown megalomania and engaging in "chaotic" behavior that led to "serious financial debts" (Leentjens et al. 2004: 1397; see also Glannon 2009).

Since Dimitry's physicians deemed his judgment compromised in this state, they sought to eliminate the symptoms by reducing the voltage of the DBS system. Unfortunately, there was a sharp trade-off, where reducing the voltage enough to avoid mania left him bedridden, since the stimulation wasn't strong enough to control his severe motor dysfunction. An unfortunate dilemma emerged: either the patient would have to be placed in a nursing home without DBS or in a

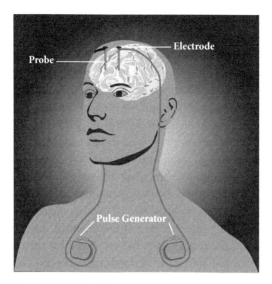

Figure 3.1 Deep Brain Stimulation

A pulse generator is implanted near the patient's collar bone, which is connected to electrodes that are surgically implanted into the patient's brain. A remote control can adjust the electrical impulses sent from the generator to specific areas of the brain that are under- or overactive.

Source: Public domain, image obtained from the National Institute of Mental Health library.

psychiatric ward with the brain stimulator. Dimitry had the capacity to make decisions about his care when the DBS was turned off, so in this state his physicians asked him to choose one of these options. The lesser evil, in the patient's considered judgment, was mania with motor control. The DBS system was thus reactivated and Dimitry was committed to a psychiatric ward.

3.2 What's the Problem?

The origin of manipulation by brain stimulation is often traced to the Spanish neurophysiologist José Delgado. In the 1960s, Delgado surgically implanted radio-controlled electrodes into a bull's brain. As the animal charged toward him, Delgado was able to stop the bull in its tracks with the mere push of a button. (The footage is readily available on the internet.) In his book *Physical Control of the Mind: Toward a Psychocivilized Society*, Delgado wrote that electrical brain stimulation "could possibly become a master control of human behavior by means of man-made plans and instruments" (1969: 88).

Direct manipulation of thoughts or desires certainly raises ethical questions, but Delgado recognized the great gulf between the neuroscience and the manipulation of human behavior. Are we any closer to this being a pressing ethical concern? Not only do we lack sufficient knowledge of the brain to manipulate the mind this way, it might be virtually impossible. Beliefs and desires don't stand alone in one's mind or in time; they are rationally connected to other mental states and responsive to ongoing information. A mad scientist might eventually be able to insert the thought that the local tyrant is trustworthy, but that belief won't last long if the lies and scandals continue. Similarly, an implanted desire for ice cream won't have much effect on someone who is a committed vegan. In short, there is a *holism* to the mind that constrains direct thought insertion and deletion through brain manipulation (Dennett 1978; Levy 2007: 161). So let's set aside this concern and focus instead on broader side effects of brain stimulation on one's personality.

Neurostimulation is now providing novel treatments for numerous brain disorders. DBS is only approved for movement disorders and epilepsy, but research underway is testing its ability to treat many other psychiatric conditions, including major depression, Tourette's syndrome, drug addiction, chronic pain, obsessive-compulsive disorder (OCD), dementia, and anorexia nervosa (Christen & Müller 2018). With such success in the treatment of Parkinson's, why be opposed to direct brain manipulation for other neurological disorders?

Brain interventions should not be deemed morally suspect just because they are neurobiological. Brain stimulation and antidepressant drugs alter the brain, but so does exercise, psychotherapy, and taking a relaxing leave of absence from a stressful job. Interventions on the body or one's circumstances should not be considered *less* morally problematic just because they only affect the brain indirectly. There is no deep metaphysical difference between the brain and the body (see the appendix to Chapter 1). Thus, as Neil Levy puts it, *"the mere fact that a technology is new and unprecedented, or that it involves direct interventions into the brain using new neuroscientific knowledge and techniques, does not give us reason to think that it raises new, or even— necessarily—especially great, problems"* (2007: 171). We should thus adopt a principle that counsels treating like cases alike when it comes to brain manipulation treatments (similar to, but distinct from, Levy's own parity principle):

> *Brain Intervention Parity Principle*: A neurobiological treatment does not raise special ethical issues just because it intervenes directly on the *brain* (as opposed to one's body or environment).

We already accept invasive interventions on the body, despite their potential for adverse side effects. When it comes to brain interventions, we could similarly calculate a *risk-benefit ratio* that allows one to accurately weigh the costs and benefits of treatment. In Dimitry's case, we would simply factor in potential changes to his personality as an adverse event rather than overinflating the risks of DBS treatment (Bluhm et al. 2020; Gilbert et al. 2021).

However, there might be principled reasons to be especially concerned about brain manipulation, not merely because it is neurobiological but because it leads to special adverse events. The driving question of this chapter will be the following: Do brain manipulation treatments raise special ethical problems? We explore three related answers tied to the brain's status as the seat of the self:

- special risks to patient *autonomy* through manipulation;
- significant changes in *personality* or *personal identity*; and
- unreliable *risk-benefit ratios*, given our particularly impoverished knowledge of the brain.

We'll see that the first two risks are easily overinflated while the last one is often underappreciated. Although our focus will be brain stimulation treatments, the ethical concerns arise for any form of direct neuromodulation, including drugs that alter brain chemistry and brain-computer interfaces.

3.3 Patient Autonomy

One potentially special adverse effect of brain modulation is a reduction in the patient's autonomy. Of course, brain interventions are often meant to restore psychological capacities relevant to autonomy, from executive function to motor control (Glannon 2019: Ch. 5). But some side effects can impair one's rationality and self-control. We saw in Dimitry's case that his DBS-induced mania seemed to impair his capacity to make decisions about his own care. The situation seems similar to cases of involuntary intoxication in the law, in which one is unaware that a substance one ingested impairs self-control (Klaming & Haselager 2013).

Impairments in autonomy don't always result from DBS and similar interventions, but might brain manipulation *as such* diminish one's autonomy? Manipulation of any form seems antithetical to freedom. While we blame cult leaders, we tend to pity their brainwashed followers as not fully in control of quitting their jobs and uprooting their families to the compound. A related ethical concern with direct brain manipulation, such as DBS, is that it undermines one's free will. Truly autonomous choice, it seems, must arise from one's "own mechanisms, which cannot be formed by pills, electronic stimulation of the brain or brainwashing" (Fischer & Ravizza 1998: 236). DBS patients can feel existential discomfort with their choices being influenced by an electrode in their brains. Some patients report feeling like "a robot," "a machine," or an "electric doll" (Schüpbach et al. 2006: 1813), perhaps due in part to a dualistic sense that the mind and brain are, or should be, fundamentally distinct (Shepard & May 2014). Yet one qualitative study of DBS patients reports that "in general, patients seemed to regard the device as something that had been integrated into their body" (Gilbert et al. 2017: 100).

Regardless of what patients believe, is their autonomy truly threatened by a treatment directly acting on brain mechanisms? The conception of free will from the previous chapter suggests otherwise. Brain stimulation and the manipulation of neurotransmitters are "merely" physical changes, and ones that operate below the level of one's conscious awareness. But neither of these is an inherent threat to freedom. Much of the psychological mechanisms that support free choice arise from unconscious physical processes in our brains. So, although there is a sense in which one's brain is being manipulated by direct brain interventions, it becomes part of one's capacities for agency, rather than bypassing them.

Even when brain interventions do impair autonomy, the patient's condition after treatment can be traced back to a free choice made earlier to accept the treatment. Compare *voluntary* intoxication: even if being drunk or high impairs self-control, one remains accountable for actions while in this state because we can, as philosophers say, "trace" one's present lack of control to a prior choice. Similarly, even if a brain implant or stimulation later impairs a patient's control—e.g., by inducing manic episodes as in Dimitry's case—the patient might be in control of this outcome given that it was a known side effect of the brain stimulation that was freely chosen (Glannon 2019: 202).

Of course, patients aren't always able to make a completely free choice to accept treatment in the first place. In 1874, at the Good Samaritan Hospital in Cincinnati, Dr. Roberts Barthalow treated Mary Rafferty, a patient with an open wound in her skull, apparently dying from brain cancer. Barthalow got Rafferty to agree to have her brain stimulated using his crude "electrotherapeutic" machine, which would administer current through electrodes stuck directly into her brain. Rafferty was subjected to multiple bouts of exploratory shocks that— after making her lips blue, her limbs flail about, and her mouth froth as she cried out—ultimately caused a seizure (Kean 2014: 232). Rafferty was not only subjected to gratuitous suffering, she also did not provide valid consent.

Nowadays informed consent is baked into experimental protocols and treatment procedures. Although brain stimulation is relatively new, pharmacological treatments for movement disorders run into similar side effects as DBS. Since Parkinson's slowly kills structures in the brain that produce dopamine, patients are often prescribed levodopa to increase production of the neurotransmitter. Excessive gambling and other behavioral addictions are possible side effects communicated to patients. Fortunately, both oral medication and brain stimulation treatments can be terminated, making them (relatively) reversible. Thus, if direct brain manipulation treatments do occasionally impair self-control, the effects on patient autonomy are not particular to such treatments.

3.4 Personal Identity

A more significant adverse event might be alterations in one's very personality or sense of self. Consider the famous case of Phineas Gage. In 1848, while working on a railroad in Vermont, an explosion catapulted a three-foot iron rod up through his left cheek and out the top of his head. Remarkably, he survived. But his personality reportedly changed so much that he was virtually unrecognizable as his former self, though the details aren't as well documented as we might have hoped (Macmillan 2000).

Brain stimulation is far from a rod tearing through one's frontal lobe, yet personality changes aren't uncommon. After 14 months of brain stimulation for Parkinson's, a 53-year-old woman told researchers: "I feel like I am who I am now. But it's not the *me* that went into the surgery that time" (Gilbert et al. 2017: 98). Alienation can be experienced by loved ones as well. This same patient reported that her children "said they don't recognize me" because "I am so impulsive and seem to change my mind all the time." In a similar report, the wife of a 48-year-old DBS patient reported being exasperated with her husband's new personality: "Now, he wants to live the life of a young man, go out, meet new people, all of that is intolerable! I would rather he be like he was before, always nice and docile!" (Schüpbach et al. 2006: 1812).

Now, it's possible that personality changes in patients aren't entirely due to brain stimulation generating new traits. They could result from the removal of psychiatric symptoms or the natural progression of the neurodegenerative disease (Gilbert et al. 2021: 6). Even Parkinson's disease, which is primarily a movement disorder, produces motivational and cognitive symptoms as it progressively impairs parts of the brain's motivational machinery. However, there remains an important sense in which brain manipulation results in personality changes, whether or not that's due to the removal of existing symptoms or the addition of new psychological traits. (Indeed, the line dividing the two is thin at best.) The reports of personality change could be rare flukes; more research is needed (Bluhm et al. 2020). But even rare adverse events enter into a risk-benefit analysis of treatment, especially if side effects are drastic enough to involve self-estrangement.

We now turn to such risks of alienation due to personality and identity change. Physicians and patients alike must understand the complexities of these peculiar risks to incorporate them into an informed risk-benefit analysis. What makes for a significant change in one's personality or identity?

3.4.1 Memory

Pause and think about your identity, broadly speaking—what makes you *you*. Personality traits are certainly important, but one unique aspect of yourself that provides continuity to your mental life is your memories. John Locke (1689/1975) famously argued that personal identity lies largely in memories of one's prior experiences and actions, which we would now call *episodic memory*. It remains common among philosophers and scientists to hitch identity to forms of memory. The Nobel Prize–winning neuroscientist Eric Kandel goes so far as to call memory "the storehouse of the self" (2018: Ch. 5).

Ethical concerns about identity change are often expressed in terms of memory. As biotechnology rapidly advanced at the dawn of this century, the President's Council on Bioethics (2003) in the United States raised worries about manipulating patients' identities. The head of the Council at the time was the physician and bioethicist Leon Kass, who arguably had a profound impact on federal policy in the United States. (Perhaps most notably the Bush administration ushered in a ban on federal funding of research using new embryonic stem cell lines.) Regarding biochemical means of memory manipulation, Kass cautioned that "to deprive oneself of one's memory . . . is to deprive oneself of one's own life and identity" (2003: 27).

Yet many people remain the same while forgetting important events in their lives. It is not uncommon to wish that painful memories could be expunged after a traumatic experience, such as sexual assault, violent conflict, or even heartbreak (the latter of which is creatively depicted in the film *Eternal Sunshine of the Spotless*

Mind). Researchers are actively exploring whether post-traumatic stress disorder (PTSD) can be treated by dampening dreadful memories with psychedelic drugs. Taking MDMA (ecstasy) while processing traumatic memories in psychotherapy has been shown to alleviate symptoms of PTSD by weakening the emotional significance of the traumatic memories, not eliminating them entirely (Mitchell et al. 2021). In general, patients are unlikely to experience significant changes in identity or personality as a result of losing (or acquiring) a relatively small set of memories.

Systematic impairments in memory are another matter. A core symptom of Alzheimer's dementia is significant memory loss, particularly the formation of new long-term memories. Early on, the disease chiefly affects cells in the *hippocampus*, a pair of seahorse-shaped structures deep in the temporal lobes that are central to the formation of new episodic memories. (Hippokampoi were the fish-tailed horses that pulled Poseidon's chariot in Greek mythology.) Alzheimer's patients commonly can't recall events from the previous day or from the previous moment if their attention has been sufficiently diverted from the present task or topic. Such impairments often render patients unable to live independently or care for themselves.

Some theorists have argued that many Alzheimer's patients lack a sufficient sense of identity to make autonomous decisions. The eminent legal philosopher Ronald Dworkin argues that patients with advanced Alzheimer's are "ignorant of the self . . . because they have no sense of a whole life, a past joined to a future, that could be the object of any evaluation or concern as a whole" (1993: 230). Treating such patients ethically becomes particularly difficult if their present desires conflict with prior plans and values.

Patients with Alzheimer's do often experience a significant change in their values in addition to their cognitive capacities. The philosopher Agnieszka Jaworska (1999) provides an instructive example based on a real patient, which we can paraphrase as follows:

> Mr. Burke's religious convictions meant he would never want to give up on his life. Once in the throes of Alzheimer's, however, his beloved wife passes and the dementia makes impossible the activities he most enjoys. Eventually he says repeatedly and sincerely that he

doesn't want to go on and that any life-sustaining treatment should be withdrawn.

Should Mr. Burke's children and physicians honor his present wishes to die with dignity or his past resolve to press on? Dworkin argues that we should respect the patient's *prior* decision, for only it was made with a cohesive enough identity to support autonomous choice.

Perhaps the bar for agency shouldn't be so high. Jaworska (1999) argues that patients with dementia retain enough autonomy for us to respect their present wishes. Memory does allow one's values to maintain greater coherence, especially over the long-term, but Jaworska maintains that one can express values and concerns in a relatively brief period of time.

Of course, brain interventions are meant to treat neurodegenerative diseases, not mimic them. Indeed, researchers are exploring whether DBS can improve the symptoms of Alzheimer's. So brain stimulation and drug therapies will not typically lead to drastic memory loss or impairments in the formation of new memories. But the debate about agency in dementia illuminates which psychological capacities are central to the self. Dworkin says continuity of values are key, which requires memory, while Jaworska thinks that present values matter enough to ground autonomy. Both seem to identify one's *values* as fundamental to agency, autonomy, and ultimately one's sense of self. Recent research suggests that this is exactly right: memory, while important, is only part of a more complex picture.

3.4.2 The Moral Self

Recall Gage's accident. Afterward, he reportedly became more impulsive, vulgar, rash, and even childish. Perhaps changes in moral character explain why he seemed like such a different person. In that case, contrary to the Lockean tradition, certain character traits are more central to how we conceptualize a person's identity.

One way to demonstrate this is to ask family and friends to evaluate how patients experiencing mental deterioration have changed over time. In one study, researchers compared responses from the friends and family of patients suffering from either one of three neurodegenerative diseases (Strohminger & Nichols 2015). The first was Alzheimer's, which leads primarily to memory loss, although numerous other cognitive impairments develop. The second was frontotemporal dementia (FTD), the leading form of dementia in people under the age of 65. As the name suggests, this disease causes neurons in the frontal and temporal lobes to die, which results in numerous changes in the patient's personality traits. Unlike Alzheimer's, patients with FTD regularly experience reduced impulse control and changes in their moral character. Patients can begin shoplifting, develop addictions and unhealthy habits, or become callous toward loved ones (Kandel 2018: Ch. 5). The last neurodegenerative disease, amyotrophic lateral sclerosis (ALS), served as a control condition, for it primarily impairs bodily movement. Friends and family in the study were asked to rate perceived changes in the patient's personality, moral traits, memory loss, and even identity (with questions like "Regardless of the severity of the illness, how much do you sense that the patient is still the same person underneath?").

Which neurodegenerative disorder would lead to more dramatic changes in how family and friends perceive the patient's identity? And which psychological alterations would explain the perceived changes in identity? The results supported the *essential-moral-self hypothesis*, which predicts that "moral capacities are the most central part of [perceived] identity" (Strohminger & Nichols 2015: 1469). Patients with FTD exhibited greater identity disruption than those with Alzheimer's or ALS. Moreover, across all three diseases, deviations in a person's moral traits—e.g., honesty, integrity, loyalty, and compassion—led to the greatest perceived changes in identity. Indeed, with the exception of deficits in speech (aphasia), moral traits were the only factor that were significantly correlated with perceived shifts in the loved one's identity.

The effect of morality on identity has been widely replicated in other contexts using different methods. However, it looks as though the perceived changes are a matter of *similarity*, not strict identity (Starmans & Bloom 2018; Schwenkler et al. 2022). In other words, if FTD causes your once compassionate aunt to become callous, you might regard her as very *different* but still your aunt. In philosophical parlance, Auntie is *numerically* identical to her previous self (one in the same individual), even if *qualitatively* distinct (dissimilar). The distinction cuts the other way as well: multiple copies of this book are qualitatively identical (similar) but numerically distinct (they are strictly two books, not one). Of course, both numerical and qualitative changes in identity matter to patients and their loved ones, so either is important when assessing risk-benefit ratios.

Many forms of neuromodulation would directly alter not just memory but also one's personality and values. In one case, DBS caused a 60-year-old Dutch man to develop a novel obsession with the music of Johnny Cash (Mantione et al. 2014). This was a change in the patient's aesthetic rather than moral values, which is arguably innocuous, but brain manipulation can cause patients to become impulsive, hypersexual, and apathetic about long-held passions in life or work. Such changes can be significant enough to cause marital strife. A study of 29 patients who underwent DBS for Parkinson's found that about 70% experienced relationship difficulties, some of which led to divorce (Schüpbach et al. 2006). Even if a patient's personality change is generally positive, it might be perceived as alienating to the patient or their family. Regarding the use of antidepressants that increase serotonin levels in the brain, Carl Elliott writes: "It would be worrying if Prozac altered my personality, even if it gave me a better personality, simply because it isn't *my* personality. This kind of personality change seems to defy an ethics of authenticity" (1998: 182).

Nevertheless, changes in value aren't all bad. Often they reveal one's *true self*. Appeals to authenticity found in prescriptions like "be yourself" span generations, from the ancients and the existentialists to romantic comedies. Insofar as pharmaceuticals or brain stimulation can alter one's values, it might do so in a way that actually enhances authenticity, whether we conceive of authenticity as self-discovery or self-creation (DeGrazia 2000; Nyholm & O'Neill 2016; Gilbert et al. 2017). One patient who received DBS for OCD happily reports

> that heavy load that I carried, that got lighter, that got less. I needed less time to pause at things, and think about things, so it took less time. Well, I was . . . yes, really changed 360 degrees. (de Haan et al. 2017)

Despite a substantial psychological change, this patient appears to see it as a positive, authentic development.

Studies have shown, however, that our attitudes about a person's true self are biased by our own values. Ample research shows that people across cultures tend to believe that most humans are fundamentally good (De Freitas et al. 2018). For this reason, we tend to impose our own conception of "good" on what represents a person's true self. If DBS, Prozac, or brain injury turns your callous uncle into a saint, loved ones will be inclined to see the "new" man as his true self who was always there, deep down. Not so if the moral changes go from good to bad. The brain stimulation that yields a newly callous aunt might be regarded as concealing her true self, who deep down is kind and considerate.

These biases in our judgments of authenticity come into stark relief on controversial moral issues, where people disagree about what it means to be fundamentally good. Consider an evangelical pastor, such as Ted Haggard or Mark Pierpont, who openly condemns homosexuality but privately engages in sexual activity with other men. Which part represents his true self? When study participants evaluate hypothetical versions of such cases, their responses depend on their own moral and political values. Compared to participants who identify as conservative, liberals were more inclined to regard the pastor's homosexual desires as reflective of his true self masked by his religious commitments (Newman et al. 2014). Because we assume that people tend to be fundamentally good, our conception of people's true selves is shaped by our own conceptions of which traits are good or acceptable.

So patients, physicians, and loved ones might have different assessments of whether a treatment has revealed a patient's true self or masked it. Imagine a patient considering DBS for treatment of anorexia nervosa. Such patients have been known to shift between mindsets, sometimes disavowing their intense fear of gaining weight while at other times identifying with their extremely low body mass index, despite knowledge of its serious health risks. If DBS allows a patient to lose her obsession with thinness and desire to continue treatment, does that reveal her true self? Physicians and family might be inclined to say yes, given that they don't value being dangerously underweight. Yet, as bioethicist Hannah Maslen and her co-authors caution, "physicians should not make the substantive claim that only a patient's desire to continue treatment is authentic" (Maslen et al. 2015: 227).

In sum, perhaps the greatest threat to one's sense of self is changes in one's values, even if the threat is to qualitative, not numerical, identity. Complicating matters further, our judgments about a person's true self are influenced by our own values. Morality, it seems, pervades human thinking, through and through. To respect the parity principle, however, we should ask: Are brain manipulation treatments likely to pose *special* threats to personality and identity, so understood? It is to this question that we now turn.

3.4.3 The Dynamic Self

Profound changes to one's sense of identity might seem particularly problematic if the self is normally static or relatively fixed. Yet the self is rather dynamic given that people regularly experience radical, sometimes abrupt, transformations in ordinary life in the absence of direct brain interventions.

The philosopher Laurie Paul (2014) naturally calls these "transformative experiences" and argues that they are ubiquitous. Parents, for example, commonly report having been fundamentally changed by having a child. They acquire novel experiences—from unconditional love to postpartum depression—that they couldn't understand or describe before having them. Such *epistemically transformative* experiences provide one with new information, such as what it's like to be a parent, not unlike a previously colorblind person who sees the color red for the first time (a scenario familiar from famous thought experiments). Becoming a parent is also *personally transformative* in that it yields novel priorities and preferences. New parents might find themselves enjoying children's books, strolls through the park, and group naps, all while their passions for clubs, concerts, or globetrotting fade away.

Transformative experiences aren't limited to child-rearing. You probably already had one as a teenager, when you went through puberty. In addition to underarm hair and other bodily transformations, puberty alters our brains considerably to sprout new sexual interests, social angst, and an unmistakable dip in risk aversion. Other common experiences are less saturated in sex hormones but no less transformative, such as traveling abroad, enduring bootcamp, battling severe illness, and having a mystical experience through religious ceremony or psychedelics.

Transformative experiences aren't just for the youth, as the notorious midlife crisis demonstrates. The brilliant developmental psychologist Alison Gopnik (2015) beautifully recounts her transformation at age 50. After a divorce, an empty nest, and a lifetime of heterosexual proclivities, she fell in love with a woman—and eventually suffered profound heartbreak. Unable to work in the throes of grief, Gopnik writes:

Suddenly, I had no idea who I was at all. . . . Everything that had defined me was gone. I was no longer a scientist or a philosopher or a wife or a mother or a lover.

Gopnik traversed her crisis in part by researching the Buddhist influences on David Hume (1739/2000), the great Scottish philosopher who argued that the self is nothing but a bundle of experiences. She found herself at ease with the obliteration of her former self, for the self is nothing but the experiences you create (on the Buddhist view of no-self and its relation to cognitive science, see Chadha & Nichols 2021).

We needn't go as far as Hume or the Buddhists and declare that the self is an illusion. But scientific theorizing and ordinary experience both suggest that the self is rather dynamic and flexible. Although your personality and moral traits are no doubt central to your identity, you can persist despite radical changes in them. Recall the corporate model of agency we developed in Chapter 2. The precise conditions on the identity of a corporation are nearly impossible to pin down, but it's clear that the CEO is not the only source of an organization's agency, nor are the workers who carry out most of its tasks. Employees, leadership, even the company ethos come and go while the corporation persists. Similarly, a person's identity is intimately tied to her psychological traits, including her memories and moral character, but the person can sustain quite radical transformations in those traits.

Of course, there are limits. A person's sense of self might not survive frequent and persistent transformative experiences. As Derek Parfit (1971) has argued following Locke, changes in personality, memory, and other psychological traits must enjoy some *continuity*. The kinds of transformations that individuals with neurodegenerative disorders experience can be rather frequent. Alzheimer's patients often exhibit dramatic fluctuations in their symptoms throughout the day (Palop et al. 2006). Recognizing a loved one in the morning doesn't guarantee recognition in the afternoon. However, the psychological changes that result from prominent brain interventions like DBS are not frequent and are, importantly, somewhat reversible. They more closely resemble the transformative experiences most people occasionally have throughout life. So concerns about identity transformation, although real, shouldn't be overblown or elevated to the level of science fiction. Transformative experiences are a natural part of neurotypical life.

Such experiences can be common and natural while being a threat to the self. They are often painful, and thus deserve to be factored into a risk-benefit ratio. But our main question is whether direct brain interventions pose *special* threats to the self. It doesn't seem that they do once we recognize the ubiquity of transformative experiences in everyday life. As the bioethicist Françoise Baylis puts it, if brain stimulation threatens personal identity, then so does "every other life event or experience integrated into an identity-constituting narrative including graduation, promotion, job loss, marriage, birth of a child, tsunami, divorce, death of a loved one, earthquake and so on" (2013: 523).

Moreover, neurological disorders themselves, which direct brain interventions are meant to treat, often lead to substantial changes in personality, including moral character. In his memoir *Lucky Man*, the renowned actor Michael J. Fox describes his experience with Parkinson's as unequivocally transformative, yet he regards it emphatically as a blessing that made him a better person:

> If you were to rush into this room right now and announce that . . . the ten years since my diagnosis could be magically taken away, traded in for ten more years as the person I was before—I would, without a moment's hesitation, tell you to take a hike. (Fox 2002: 6)

Of course, not all patients would, or should, regard their neurological condition as a gift. The point for our purposes is that, in the risk-benefit ratio for brain treatments, the risk of personality changes might be a wash. The question is not whether a particular brain intervention would be transformative, but whether it would be a more positive development for the patient than forgoing treatment. Indeed, in the treatment of psychiatric disorders, changes in personality may be desirable.

3.5 Unreliable Risk-Benefit Ratios

So far we've focused on the risks of brain interventions, but they should also be carefully weighed against likely benefits or lack thereof. In his memoir *Deep in the Brain: Living with Parkinson's Disease* (2009), the sociologist Helmut Dubiel describes being "dissatisfied with the overall outcome of the [DBS] procedure" (93). The operation improved his tremors and dyskenesias, but he also experienced awkward gait, loss of taste and smell, and speech disturbance, which resulted in a sense of alienation and ultimately major depression. Although he can reduce the intensity of the brain stimulation on the fly, which allows him to speak more clearly, he then faces a trade-off between, quite simply, talking and walking. At times Dubiel feels that "the upshot of this major and extremely expensive surgery had been to replace one set of grave symptoms with another" (93).

Whether the adverse events concern movement, identity, or mood, the risk-benefit ratio must contend with our limited knowledge of the brain. Even when medicine is evidence based, the sheer size of the enterprise and human fallibility can produce great uncertainty and variable results. The likely effectiveness of treatments and the severity of adverse events can vary as widely as human bodies do. Assessing and navigating the risk-benefit ratios of treatment isn't just an exercise in prudence on the part of patients; it's an ethical issue for healthcare professionals. Physicians must take seriously potential side effects and avoid overselling the powers of treatment.

3.5.1 Medical Hubris

Neurosurgery's checkered history provides a relevant backdrop. The Portuguese neurologist António Egas Moniz first developed lobotomy as a treatment for psychiatric disorders in the 1930s, which earned him a Nobel Prize. But the procedure became oversold and overused in the hands of the infamous Walter Freeman. Typically used to treat schizophrenia, Freeman's version severed the frontal lobe from the rest of the brain using an instrument resembling an icepick that bore a hole in the skull near the patient's tear ducts. From 1930 to 1960, the overzealous neurologist performed over 3,000 lobotomies on adults and children as young as 12 years old, with inconsistent outcomes. Freeman even lobotomized John F. Kennedy's sister, Rosemary, at age 23, leaving her with severe cognitive disabilities that required her to be institutionalized (Caruso & Sheehan 2017). The classic 1975 film *One Flew Over the Cuckoo's Nest* ably depicted the growing discomfort with neurosurgery for psychiatric disorders. Modern ablation techniques are now more precise and respectable treatments for certain disorders, such as OCD and schizophrenia, though the damage to brain tissue is completely irreversible, unlike DBS which is at least partly reversible (Pugh 2019).

Discussions of curing the mentally ill inevitably grapple with the shadow of eugenics. The term "eugenics" was coined in the late 19th century by Sir Francis Galton, a cousin of Charles Darwin. It merged together Greek words to mean "good in birth" (Selgelid 2014), and eventually a movement developed to enhance the human species, primarily by preventing the propagation of undesirable genes. Although associated with Nazi Germany, many countries adopted forms of eugenics under the guise of sound science, such as forcibly sterilizing citizens who were deemed intellectually disabled. In Virginia, the Eugenical Sterilization Act rendered infertile more than 7,000 people in the state between 1924 and 1979. One of those Virginians was Janet Ingram, who was deemed "feebleminded" and sterilized in her teens while rotating through foster homes (Gliha 2014).

The coercion characteristic of eugenics is now decried in medicine. Nevertheless, concerns about paternalism and overtreatment remain, as many medical interventions are either ineffective or harmful (or both). Severe limitations or adverse effects are sometimes only discovered after untold numbers of patients have been harmed. Birth defects befell children whose mothers took Accutane (isotretinoin) during pregnancy. After being on the market over 50 years, the analgesic Darvocet (propoxyphene) was withdrawn because it increased the risk of stroke and heart attacks. Even when drugs remain on the market, overuse can wreak havoc on patients and their communities, as demonstrated by the opioid crisis. These are just a fraction of the many examples in which previously unknown harms surface. Researchers can't anticipate all possible side effects, of course, but compared to the search for more treatments the "hunt for harms" is rather hollow, as the philosopher of science Jacob Stegenga (2018) puts it.

Modern medicine has certainly produced some *magic bullets*, as Stegenga dubs them. These interventions precisely, reliably, and substantially target ailments, with minor if any side effects. Magic bullets include antibiotics like penicillin, vaccines for deadly and debilitating diseases such as polio and measles, and some forms of surgery.

But magic bullets are not the norm, at least because many studies overestimate effect sizes and produce false positive results that can't be replicated. Teams of scientists, such as the Cochrane Collaboration, attempt to provide systematic reviews of medical research, including meta-analyses. Such efforts are limited, however, by the quality of the studies being conducted. One prominent scientist at Stanford University famously argued that most published scientific findings are false (Ioannidis 2005). A precise estimate is difficult to formulate with any confidence, but it's increasingly clear that not all biomedical research is gold. As the chief editor of the prestigious medical journal *The Lancet* put it (Horton 2015: 1380):

> Afflicted by studies with small sample sizes, tiny effects, invalid exploratory analyses, and flagrant conflicts of interest, together with an obsession for pursuing fashionable trends of dubious importance, science has taken a turn towards darkness.

Research on brain stimulation treatments are no exception, of course; methodological concerns are predictably present there as well (Christen & Müller 2018). Indeed, all scientists are human, so no corner of the scientific enterprise is immune to significant and persistent fallibility (May 2021; more on this in Chapter 8).

A number of factors are responsible for the proliferation of ineffective or harmful medical interventions, including methodological flaws and researchers' own biases. Money exerts a particularly powerful influence in many areas of science, especially when findings have direct commercial applications. Companies often have a vested interest in producing results—e.g., that a new drug reduces nausea in cancer patients. Companies also have an interest in finding null results—e.g., that a brain implant doesn't increase the risk of stroke. Inevitably, researchers are often funded (or otherwise influenced) by the companies whose profit rests on particular results. Such *conflicts of interest* introduce bias into the truth-seeking aims of science. As a result, it is common that industry-funded research tends to produce markedly different results from government-funded work on the same topic (Wilholt 2009). Whether consciously or not, researchers tend to adopt certain experimental protocols or interpretations of data that support a desired hypothesis. Perhaps the most infamous example is the tobacco industry's influence on the study of smoking's adverse health effects in the mid-20th century (Oreskes & Conway 2010).

Publicly funded research can exhibit bias too, such as the tendency to avoid null results. Consider the considerable decline in positive results reported in randomized controlled trials of cardiovascular interventions after the year 2000. Why the drop? The National Institutes of Health began requiring that the detailed plans of the studies they funded had to be *preregistered*—that is, publicly documented before acquiring data and reporting results. Remarkably, while 57% of the pre-2000 trials reported an effect of the study's intervention, only 8% of those published afterward did (see Figure 3.2). As the authors of the analysis explain, "Prior to 2000, investigators had a greater opportunity to measure a range of variables and to select the most successful outcomes when reporting their results" (Kaplan & Irvin 2015: 8).

Studies of psychiatric interventions are no exception. Consider antidepressants, such as selective serotonin reuptake inhibitors (SSRIs), which are widely prescribed drugs. Clinical trials of their effectiveness are commonly based on the Hamilton Rating Scale for Depression (HAMD). Antidepressants are regularly regarded

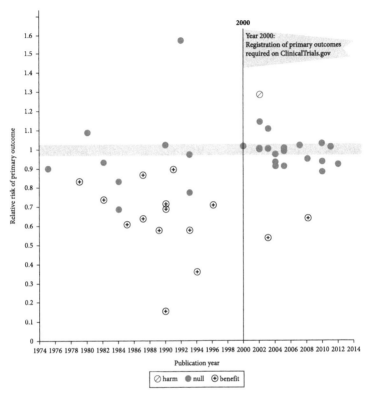

Figure 3.2 Null Results After Preregistration
Primary results of large clinical trials of pharmaceutical and dietary supplement interventions for cardiovascular disease.

Source: Kaplan and Irvin (2015). Reprinted under Creative Commons license Public Domain Dedication, CC0 1.0.

as effective if they can yield as little as a 3-point reduction on this 52-point scale. Yet 10 points on the HAMD concern insomnia and fidgeting, which are not central symptoms of depression. Thus, as Stegenga (2018: 116) puts it:

> A small improvement in sleep or a decrease in fidgeting caused by an intervention would warrant approval as an effective antidepressant,

despite the fact that the intervention might not mitigate any of the fundamental symptoms of depression, such as low mood, anhedonia, and feelings of worthlessness, guilt, and hopelessness.

In combination with industry influence and other biases, it's perhaps no surprise that, after decades of study, antidepressant medications seem to yield at best meager improvements in depression for some patients (Cipriani et al. 2018). Yet, as millions of patients' brains are flooded with serotonin over the long-term, known and unknown side effects run amok.

Conflicts of interest and other influences on the scientific process generally make it challenging to calculate a proper risk-benefit ratio. Both sides of the ratio can become unduly skewed in favor of treatment, based on

(a) *overestimates* of the effectiveness of interventions and
(b) *underestimates* of their harms.

In light of such fallibility, how does one treat patients ethically, especially in the context of novel brain interventions?

Although biases might skew risk-benefit ratios toward overtreatment, none of the forgoing examples justify the conclusion that modern medicine is worthless. Stegenga (2018) goes so far as to defend a thesis of *medical nihilism*, which states that we ought to doubt the effectiveness of most medical interventions. A more modest conclusion is what we might dub *medical humility*: risk-benefit analyses should factor in the tendency to overestimate the effectiveness and underestimate the adverse effects of most medical interventions. Adopting medical humility protects against a hubris that leads to the overtreatment of patients with drugs or technologies that are insufficiently safe or effective. Stegenga calls for a turn toward *gentle medicine*, in which physicians, patients, researchers, and policymakers all pursue less aggressive medical interventions, where feasible. A thesis as bold as medical nihilism isn't required to support gentler medicine that rightly denounces indiscriminate enthusiasm for all medical treatments.

3.5.2 Neurobiological Ignorance

The risks of medical interventions should be weighed carefully against their likely benefits, but that alone does not raise a special ethical problem with direct brain manipulation. Does the concern about medical humility run afoul of the parity principle?

Perhaps not, since some special concerns about direct brain manipulation arise from our particularly impoverished understanding of the neurobiological mechanisms. Our knowledge of how the brain works is so limited at present that the risk of adverse effects might be amplified compared to treatments of bodily ailments (Wolpe 2002). Failure to understand the underlying biological basis of disease makes effective treatment more difficult, though not impossible (Stegenga 2018).

Brain science has uncovered mechanisms in psychopathology, to be sure. We have learned, for instance, that several neurodegenerative disorders—e.g., Parkinson's, Alzheimer's, Creutzfeldt-Jakob disease, and fatal familial insomnia—involve misfolding proteins in the brain (Kandel 2018). Yet we remain largely ignorant of how cellular mechanisms give rise to mental and behavioral pathologies or precisely why certain treatments are effective. Electroconvulsive therapy can effectively treat major depression, but it is not known precisely why the seizure-inducing treatment works when it does. Scientists do not even know whether DBS is effective in Parkinson's because it excites or inhibits neuronal activity in the targeted region. Part of the problem is that, even when brain interventions target a small area of the brain, it nevertheless contains a large swath of neurons that project to, and receive input from, many other regions.

An impoverished understanding of the biological basis of neurological disorders hampers our ability to minimize side effects as well. Even basic motor control cannot be easily disentangled from motivation and learning more broadly. In one DBS case, a Parkinson's patient with no prior history of gambling began doing so obsessively, leading to debts so large that he lost both his house and his marriage (Smeding et al. 2007). The basal ganglia is a set of structures deep in the brain that help control movements and regulate learning as part of the reward system (more on this in Chapter 5). So it isn't surprising that stimulating nodes in this network would cause some patients to have symptoms associated with mania—such as increases in energy, insomnia, racing thoughts, sexual drive, and risk-taking, all of which can lead to reckless behavior.

A gentle approach to the treatment of brain disorders does not prohibit any direct intervention. Provided the patient is aware of unexpected complications (and has decisional capacity), substantial risks of treatment can be acceptable if inaction might be worse (Schermer 2011). The symptoms of many neurological disorders can become debilitating, even life-threatening. The Centers for Disease Control and Prevention reports that over 47,000 Americans died by suicide in 2019, making it the 10th leading cause of death. The risk is higher for those with depression compared to the general population. Some brain interventions for depression are noninvasive, such as pharmaceuticals and transcranial magnetic stimulation, though they remain insufficiently effective for many patients. More invasive treatments, such as DBS, are likely warranted when all other avenues of treatment have failed, particularly if the interventions can be proven effective. There have been some promising results from personalized DBS that delivers stimulation only when brain activity in patients indicates that they are slipping into a depressive state (Scangos et al. 2021). The results, however, are very preliminary and require much further study. Nevertheless, research in the near-term might produce sufficiently effective DBS for severe psychiatric disorders that are resistant to less invasive treatments.

The benefits of treatment, of course, are only one side of the risk-benefit ratio. Brain manipulation treatments carry risks of various adverse events, beyond effects on patient autonomy and identity. For example, although DBS has been remarkably effective in treating many movement disorders, it does carry the risk of hemorrhaging and infection from surgery, as well as psychiatric consequences, such as depression, anxiety, irritability, impulsivity, aggression, impaired cognition, hypersexuality, and hypomania (Davis et al. 2017; Christen & Müller 2018). DBS devices can be turned off, but we've seen that long-term changes in personality and relationships can remain. Such events are not always undone once the brain stimulator is switched off.

In the end, medical humility must reckon with patient autonomy. Physicians, researchers, and policymakers should exercise due diligence in not overselling the benefits of neuromodulation or underestimating its harms, but informed patients are the ultimate arbiters of risk management. Neurobiological interventions remain an ethical option if they provide a reasonable chance of preserving a patient's life or substantially mitigating unbearable suffering. Nevertheless, some special risks remain present with brain manipulation until our knowledge of brain mechanisms drastically improves.

3.6 Conclusion

There is great hope—even quantifiable in terms of research funding—that brain interventions will help patients with Alzheimer's, depression, OCD, and other neurological conditions. Existing treatments and those under development range from neurosurgery and brain stimulation to pharmaceutical drugs, including psychedelics.

Such brain interventions might rarely undermine a patient's autonomy or morph them into a new person. But the risks of adverse events should be taken seriously, especially given our limited understanding of the brain and its status as the seat of the self. Medical hubris in brain manipulation not only risks familiar side effects, such as infection, but also major depression, self-estrangement, and other psychiatric symptoms. Physicians must be cautious not to oversell the benefits of treatment relative to the costs or to impose their own values on patients.

Let's return to the specific case of Dimitry, the Dutch Parkinson patient. The discussion in this chapter suggests that he should be allowed to choose deep brain stimulation, even if it causes manic episodes. When the DBS device is switched off, he surely has the freedom to choose whether he prefers mania to immobility. Undergoing DBS is a transformative experience for this patient, though not unlike the decision to become a parent or a soldier, which radically alters one's preferences and values. Although one's moral character is integral to one's identity, the self is dynamic enough to persist through quite drastic changes in values, especially if they arise from a prior free choice to go through that transformation. Dimitry may become a different person (qualitatively if not numerically), but he freely chose that path. Our approaches to autonomous medical decision-making should respect patient autonomy by acknowledging not only a diversity of values and preferences across patients but also within individual patients across time. What one person considers an undesirable disability might be another person's valued identity.

One might worry that patients with mental disorders, in particular, simply aren't fit to make decisions about their own care. After all, aren't they excused from blame for immoral behavior caused by their symptoms? Can't they be found not guilty by reason of insanity in a court of law? In the next chapter, we'll continue to see that agency comes in many forms and thus that there is no such simple connection between agency and psychopathology.

PART III
CARE

4
Mental Disorder

So far we have primarily examined agency and autonomy in neurotypical individuals. In the previous chapter, we considered brain interventions to treat neurological disorders. But the risk of immoral behavior fell primarily on physicians and researchers, who might mistreat patients, oversell the power of interventions, or understate their risks.

In this chapter, we turn to the moral behavior of patients themselves who suffer from mental maladies. These patients might have neurological disorders, such as Alzheimer's, or psychiatric conditions, such as schizophrenia, major depression, and obsessive-compulsive disorder (OCD). Does having a mental disorder make one less responsible, even for heinous crimes? On the standard naïve view, the mentally ill are often regarded as clear examples of individuals lacking full-fledged freedom and responsibility. Our evolving understanding of the brain and human agency, however, reveals that there is more agency in mental disorders than it might seem at first blush. Psychopathology affects agency in such a variety of ways that it's difficult to draw an inference about one's moral responsibility merely from the fact that one has a mental disorder. Symptoms only sometimes reduce one's agency and sometimes enhance it. This nuanced view paves the way for a cognitive continuum on which all people lie, which can help reduce the stigma we commonly attach to mental disorders.

4.1 Two Homicides in Texas

In the summer of 2001, in a small town outside of Houston, Texas, Andrea Yates drowned each of her five young children in a bathtub, one by one. Yates's psychiatrist had recently taken her off of Haloperidol, an anti-psychotic medication. In previous years, she had attempted to take her own life and was treated for major depressive disorder. During her trial, Yates pleaded not guilty by reason of insanity, and the jury ultimately agreed. Her lawyer proclaimed the verdict a "watershed event in the treatment of mental illness," presumably because it promoted the idea that having a mental disorder can compromise one's free will and thus reduce one's culpability, even for terrible acts (Newman 2006).

Some vehemently resist such conclusions, however. Just over 10 years later in Texas, Eddie Ray Routh was convicted of killing two men at a shooting range, one of whom was celebrated sniper Chris Kyle. A former marine, Routh had been diagnosed with post-traumatic stress disorder (PTSD) and schizophrenia. His counsel sought the insanity defense but failed to convince the jury that Routh did not know his actions were wrong. The district attorney, Alan Nash, won the jury over, stating, "I am tired of the proposition that if you have a mental illness, you can't be held responsible for what you do" (Dart 2015).

The debate here is about legal responsibility, but the question presumably is not merely one about legal standards. Criminal liability in such cases rests, at least in part, on the more fundamental question of whether the defendant is *morally* responsible. A verdict of "not guilty by reason of insanity" is chiefly based on the M'Naughten Rule, which states that a defendant is "insane" if, at the time of the crime, she suffered from a mental disorder that prevented her from (a) knowing what she was doing, or (b) knowing that what she was doing is wrong. At any rate, our focus will be on the core question of moral responsibility, which can then inform separate discussions about legal liability and public health policy.

The standard approach to moral responsibility is to consider people with some category of psychopathology and determine whether the individuals are (or could be) responsible for any action at all. However, we'll see that different disorders operate quite differently. Even within a given disorder, its symptoms don't always have a singular effect on capacities relevant to responsibility. An alternative approach maintains that there is no generally supported inference from an individual's having a mental disorder to any claims about that person's responsibility. We begin by comparing these two theories before discussing their ethical implications.

4.2 Two Theories

4.2.1 The Naïve View

Mental disorders might always affect responsibility to a small extent, whether by influencing one's choices or one's control over outcomes. Decision-making is a mental phenomenon, after all, and mental illness can certainly affect relevant mental states and processes. Severe depression, for instance, affects one's attention (e.g., drawing it toward negative thoughts) and preferences (e.g., reduced interest in social activities). But these psychological effects can impact one's life to some degree without significantly mitigating blame, similar to one's mood, personality traits, or extenuating circumstances. For example, while some emotions may hinder self-control, a neurotypical adult is normally still fully blameworthy for abusing a child during a fit of rage. What interests many philosophers and policymakers is: When does a factor, like psychopathology, affect one's capacities and abilities to a sufficiently high degree that it *mitigates* or *eliminates* responsibility?

Merely labeling a mental condition a "disorder" strikes many people as at least typically mitigating some forms of responsibility. Psychiatrists will often describe mental disorders to their patients in the same ways as non-mental illnesses, such as diabetes, precisely because it suggests the disorder is out of one's control (Arpaly 2005). Experimental studies suggest that ordinary people also tend to attribute (slightly) less free will and moral responsibility to hypothetical criminal offenders described as having a history of mental disorder, compared to offenders described as having a criminal history or no history at all (e.g., Berryessa 2018; Monahan & Hood 1976). Researchers find such reductions in our attitudes of blame when defendants are described as having a history of psychiatric treatment or as having certain psychopathologies—e.g., autism, frontotemporal dementia, or attention-deficit/hyperactivity disorder (ADHD).

Philosophers also commonly treat the possession of a mental disorder as an excusing condition. Galen Strawson, for example, identifies as paradigm constraints on one's freedom the manifestation of mental disorders, including "kleptomaniac impulses, obsessional neuroses, desires that are experienced as alien, post-hypnotic commands, threats, instances of force majeure, and so on" (1994: 222; quoted in Meynen 2010). Similarly, when discussing cases in which individuals are simply exempt from being held accountable for their actions, R. J. Wallace includes as "accepted exemptions" cases of "insanity or mental illness" (1994: 165), along with addiction, psychopathy, posthypnotic suggestion, and the like. Daniel Levy (2003) even names more specific disorders—e.g., PTSD, Tourette's, schizophrenia, bipolar disorder, and OCD—and considers them all "maladies" of free will.

It can certainly be tempting to think that mental disorders always or nearly always excuse. Shouldn't the mentally ill be treated, not blamed or punished? This leads us to the following:

The Naïve View: Having a mental disorder itself implies something about one's freedom or moral responsibility (and thus blameworthiness or praiseworthiness).

Why might someone adopt such a view? It is rarely given an explicit defense, but let's consider a few potential arguments.

1. The Argument From Pathology. One might argue that mental disorders are *pathological*, almost by definition, and so actions influenced by them inherit the property of being pathological or disordered. One might argue that, like children and nonhuman animals, those with mental disorders are not appropriate targets of the "reactive attitudes," such as resentment, that underwrite praise and blame. At least for some disorders with more pronounced and serious effects, a kind of "deep-rooted psychological abnormality" (Strawson 1962: 11) might warrant taking a wholly "objective attitude" toward the individual, as a thing to be controlled or managed, rather than held responsible.

However, even if an action is in some sense pathological, that doesn't imply that one is thereby excused. Consider Tourette's syndrome. Many people assume tics are entirely unintentional or involuntary and thus clear candidates for excusable actions not performed of the patient's own free will. But patients with this syndrome often report acting voluntarily; it's just increasingly *difficult* to overcome the impulse (Schroeder 2005). While those with Tourette's syndrome may sometimes lack responsibility for their tics, this case illustrates that matters are often more complicated than they seem. At any rate, we'll see below that there appear to be cases in which one is still responsible for an action despite it being the result of a mental disorder.

2. The Argument From Ultimacy. A second rationale for the naïve view is the idea that one isn't responsible for actions resulting from psychiatric disorders because one isn't *ultimately responsible* for having the disorder itself. This thought is reminiscent of "sourcehood" principles according to which one is responsible for an action only if one is responsible for what led to it, including one's genes and environment (Strawson 1994).

A problem for this rationale is that it overgeneralizes to ordinary actions that don't arise from the symptoms of a mental disorder. Ultimately, no one is responsible for the sources of their actions if we trace the causal chain far enough back. So it's difficult to see how this kind of rationale could be applicable only to mental disorders. We'd be left with an uninformative general skepticism—no one is responsible for anything—which is a far cry from the naïve view. Our question is whether there is a general relationship between moral responsibility and psychopathology that is grounded in facts internal to both these concepts, not reliant upon a controversial position held for reasons that have nothing to do with the specifics of mental illness.

3. The Argument From Control. Finally, mental disorders might seem to involve irresistible impulses that preclude proper control over one's conduct (Wallace 1994: 169). Many psychopathologies do involve powerful anxieties, phobias, urges, delusions, and other automatic thoughts and feelings that can hinder self-control (Sripada 2022a). This argument for the naïve view is more difficult to dismiss, for it identifies a core aspect of agency that is clearly relevant to freedom and responsibility. But do mental disorders always or necessarily impair agency? Below we'll attempt to answer that question. First let's understand what an alternative to the Naïve view might look like.

4.2.2 More Nuanced Approaches

Other ethicists have developed more nuanced accounts. David Shoemaker, for example, denies that mental disorders necessarily excuse, but thinks this is because the concept of responsibility itself is nuanced. He contends that there are senses of "responsibility," only some of which apply to those with particular disorders, but which sense corresponds to which disorder varies. For example, he maintains that one form of responsibility (attributability) is mitigated in clinically depressed individuals, while a distinct form of responsibility (accountability) is reduced for some autistic individuals (Shoemaker 2015: 143–147). So, for particular kinds of responsibility, Shoemaker still seems to maintain a version of the naïve view.

Can we get even more nuanced? Nomy Arpaly argues that "while many mental disorders do seem to provide exempting, excusing, or mitigating conditions, some do not, and with others things are complicated" (2005: 291). However, even this approach maintains that some disorders categorically excuse. Carl Elliott (1996), for example, doesn't contend that all mental disorders bear the same relationship to responsibility, yet he still argues roughly that psychopaths and those with compulsive disorders categorically aren't responsible, while people with personality disorders are (more on psychopathy in Chapter 6). A number of theorists have made such friendly amendments to the standard approach (e.g., Feinberg 1970; Meynen 2010; Kozuch & McKenna 2015; Hirstein et al. 2018). But can we go even further?

An unqualified rejection of the naïve view would deny that any mental disorder bears a simple relationship to agency and responsibility. That would yield:

The Nuanced View: There is no general relationship between moral responsibility and psychopathology.

One's moral responsibility on this view is not influenced by the mere possession or type of psychopathology but the specific way symptoms arise in an individual (see Morse 2006a; Pickard 2015; King & May 2018). We ought, in other words, to evaluate responsibility on a case-by-case basis, not based on categories of mental disorder. The relevant phenomena to focus on are symptoms, such as impulsivity, delusions, hallucinations, anxiety, psychological incoherence, melancholy, diminished motivation, memory loss, blunted emotions, mania, difficulty focusing, loss of consciousness, powerful urges, and so on. In the rest of this chapter, we evaluate this nuanced view and unpack its implications.

4.3 The Need for Nuance

There are two main lines of support for the nuanced approach to the relationship between moral responsibility and psychopathology. First, we'll see that sometimes symptoms can *increase* rather than reduce responsibility for one's choices. Second, although symptoms can also diminish agency, this occurs only in *some* circumstances and only *sometimes* to a degree that reduces responsibility. Either way, psychopathology is too heterogeneous for it to permit a simple connection to moral responsibility.

4.3.1 Symptoms (Sometimes) Enhance Agency

The naïve view says that, in general, mental illness excuses relevant behavior or significantly mitigates blame (and praise). This view is initially suspect given that some symptoms are capable of *enhancing* one's responsibility.

First we need to consider how psychiatric symptoms can affect one's responsibility. It's controversial whether freedom and responsibility require choice, control, or coherence, but certainly it requires some such aspects of agency (see Chapter 2). When individuals are responsible for an action it is due to features of their agency or its exercise, and we often associate mental disorders with deficits in agency. Yet what disrupts a person's mental life in some circumstances can turn out to be beneficial in others.

Consider just a sampling of examples. Individuals on the autism spectrum often have restricted interests that lead to an intense focus on numbers, objects, and dates, but this trait is quite beneficial in Silicon Valley and other contexts in which mathematical acuity, innovation, and pattern recognition are rewarded (Silberman 2015). As Temple Grandin puts it in her landmark book *Thinking in Pictures*, "the first stone spear . . . was probably invented by an Aspie who chipped away at rocks while the other people socialized around the campfire" (Grandin 1995/2006: 122). Creativity is a form of agency that also flourishes in some patients with Alzheimer's and frontotemporal dementia who garner well-deserved praise for their art (Kandel 2018: Ch. 6). Depressed people tend to more accurately judge the degree of control they have over their circumstances, while neurotypical individuals tend to overestimate (Alloy & Abramson 1979; Ackermann & DeRubeis 1991). Even anxiety, which is typically unpleasant, can alert one to relevant information and reduce uncertainty about potential threats to oneself or others (Kurth 2018). Delusions and memory loss likewise serve an important function by making sense of peculiar experiences. The early effects of dementia can free one from haunting memories of abuse (Earp et al. 2014), and delusional beliefs can help patients cope with psychological trauma and low self-esteem (Bortolotti 2015), not unlike the rationalizations frequently found among neurotypical individuals (see Chapter 8).

Some of a mental disorder's symptoms may even enhance certain capacities, such that, surprisingly, one becomes "hyper-responsible," as Stephen Morse (2006a) puts it. Here we may find parallels with the enhanced responsibilities of those possessing advanced skills or knowledge (Vincent 2013), as when we hold only physicians accountable for being unwilling to provide medical assistance to a passenger on an airplane. Enhanced capabilities might merely increase the number or kinds of responsibilities, rather than degrees of responsibility itself (Glannon 2011: 120). Nevertheless, enhanced responsibility can result from an increase in mental capacity, whether from higher education or psychopathology.

Conditions that increase attention are natural candidates for enhanced agency. Consider, for example, disorders involving episodes of hypomania, such as bipolar disorder (Arpaly 2005: 290; Morse 2006a; Vincent 2013). Unlike mania, episodes of hypomania don't severely disrupt one's life, but in either case patients often experience symptoms that enhance agency. According to the *Diagnostic and Statistical Manual of Mental Disorders* (DSM), manic patients need much less sleep (e.g., "feels rested after only 3 hours of sleep"), have a "flight of ideas," and exhibit increased "goal-directed activity" (American Psychiatric Association: 124). Some of these symptoms read as desired effects of cognitive enhancers, like amphetamine or modafinil (see Chapter 7), even if they can be rather disruptive in certain contexts or when combined with other typical symptoms, such as risky behavior.

Another disorder that might lead to symptoms that enhance agency is OCD. Patients' obsessive thoughts are often tied to a specific anxiety or source of distress, such as uncleanliness (e.g., excessively washing hands) or danger (e.g., repeatedly locking a door). Those with scrupulosity, in particular, are especially concerned to behave morally or piously, such as obsessively checking food for poisons or ridding one's mind for adulterous thoughts (Summers & Sinnott-Armstrong 2015). Such hyper-awareness and sensitivity to morally relevant considerations may, in certain circumstances, enhance capacities relevant to freedom and responsibility. For example, suppose your friend Otto, who is known to obsessively check that he has locked doors, leaves your door unlocked after feeding your cat while you're vacationing in Milan. If a gang of raccoons ransacks your house, you might hold Otto more responsible given his hyper-awareness of whether doors are locked. Similarly, while we might mildly praise Olive for mindlessly locking the office door and preventing a robbery, we'd likely praise Otto even more if it resulted from his heightened concern for safety.

Of course, patients often don't have knowledge of, or control over, when they will have any purportedly enhanced capacities. So it may seem inappropriate to hold them more accountable (Turner 2010), at least in many circumstances. That is precisely what the nuanced view would predict, since it maintains that there is no necessary connection between possession of a mental disorder and responsibility, whether reduced or enhanced. It's not the possession of psychopathology as such that enhances one's responsibility; it's the specifics of certain *symptoms* and *circumstances*, which only sometimes affect one's agency.

Now, the term "symptom" is often used to refer to only the *undesirable* effects of an underlying disorder. But a broader meaning includes any phenomena that are characteristic, indicative, or symptomatic of a condition, which includes unproblematic or even desirable effects. After all, underlying dysfunction can remain while undesirable symptoms of a disorder are not manifest. In Alzheimer's, for example, neurodegeneration typically begins long before the patient notices any symptoms, such as confusion or forgetfulness (Palop et al. 2006). It is the broader sense of "symptom" that is relevant to assessing whether an underlying disorder affects whether praise or blame is warranted in a given case.

4.3.2 Symptoms (Sometimes) Diminish Agency

Of course, the symptoms of mental illness can also diminish one's agency and thus moral responsibility. Symptoms plausibly excuse bad behavior if they yield an action that entirely *bypasses* one's agency, such that an outcome is the result of no action at all or an entirely unintentional one. Take narcolepsy, which is characterized by abnormal sleepiness during the day or lapses into sleep and is often accompanied by cataplexy, or sudden muscle weakness that can make patients collapse. Suppose Nate's narcolepsy makes him prone to sudden, unpredictable cataplexy, and during one such episode, drops the priceless vase he was carrying. Ordinarily, one might be blameworthy for dropping a vase. But it seems the mental disorder provides a ready, and full, excuse.

Now it might be argued that such excuses are quite limited. Once one becomes aware that one has a disorder, one has a responsibility to manage its effects. Suppose that a patient with schizophrenia responds well to treatment with an anti-psychotic medication, such as loxapine. When she discontinues use, she typically has haunting hallucinations that cause her to attack those around her, misperceiving them as imminent threats. In such cases, where symptoms are expected and their effects can be mitigated, one might be responsible for harm caused to others, even if due to hallucinations, because the patient knows such situations can be prevented by staying on the medication. In such cases, we might attribute responsibility for an outcome that resulted from diminished agential capacities by transferring forward the prior responsibility one has for not allowing those capacities to diminish in the first place (Summers & Sinnott-Armstrong 2015).

However, this oversimplifies the notion of tracing responsibility for acts to some prior opportunity to prevent them. Such scenarios are not common, as symptoms often first present without warning or can't be managed anyhow. Moreover, even when one can knowingly manage symptoms, it remains controversial how best to trace responsibility for outcomes to prior failures to take suitable precautions (King 2014).

Of course, even if symptoms of narcolepsy sometimes excuse the actions (or inactions) they cause, we cannot necessarily generalize to other situations and other psychopathologies. Like nearly all mental disorders, narcolepsy exists on a spectrum with more or less severe symptoms that vary with the circumstances. Although narcolepsy brings to mind sudden loss of consciousness, some patients merely experience intense sleepiness or the need to nap multiple times a day. Nate's narcolepsy only excuses his dropping of the vase so completely because the condition is *directly relevant* to the action in a way that does not hold true of every mental disorder. Contrast someone suffering from OCD who experiences intrusive and unwanted thoughts that cause anxiety. In many cases, an episode of such intrusion will have little bearing on their ability to carry a vase. And so their mental disorder will not significantly affect their responsibility for dropping the vase, should they drop it. Thus, it seems that one's disorder must not only compromise a capacity relevant to agency, but it also must be relevant to the act in question (Feinberg 1970: 273).

Suppose, for example, that a man with ADHD assaults an individual at a sporting event after an angry confrontation that escalated from a disrespectful gesture into violence. ADHD involves difficulties in paying attention, staying focused, and organizing one's life for success in school or work. Given the nature of this disorder, it is unlikely that it played a crucial role in generating an aggressive action, especially one that might typically arise in anyone without ADHD, as it simply involves relatively normal emotional reactions to a show of disrespect.

Now, ADHD can involve increased impulsivity, in which case the symptoms of the disorder could play a crucial role in an act of aggression. A similar analysis seems appropriate for conduct disorders affecting impulsivity, such as kleptomania, which can obviously play a key role in an act of stealing. Even if it's controversial whether kleptomania should excuse or mitigate responsibility, this is a case where the disorder clearly influences a particular act, such that someone in similar circumstances but without kleptomania is unlikely to steal. In the same vein, however, kleptomania would appear irrelevant to a case of acting out of aggression—indeed, irrelevant to most of the actions one performs.

It might be uncharitable to interpret the naïve approach as saying that anyone with a psychiatric disorder is thereby excused from all of their actions, including those not influenced by the disorder's symptoms. However, an even more charitable version of the view is problematic, for there are cases in which actions are directly affected by a mental disorder without yielding mitigation or excuse.

Part of the reason psychopathology only sometimes excuses lies in the notion of capacity. By definition, mental disorders affect mental capacities, and some of these capacities are integral to freedom and responsibility. However, diminished capacity does not entail *lack* of capacity (Glannon 2011: Ch. 3). Many disorders, such as autism, involve a varied spectrum. Some patients on the autism spectrum may appropriately be described as having an *inability* to pick up on nonverbal social cues or navigate the social world successfully. Others, however, have only minor difficulties in this respect (Grandin 1995/2006; Silberman 2015). Indeed, many disorders—from depression to bipolar disorder—present along a continuum. The upshot is that, for many disorders, being diagnosed does not necessarily affect one's responsibility and certainly not in the same way as others in the diagnosed class. Sometimes the symptoms will be so slight they hardly diminish a relevant agential capacity.

Now, a proponent of the naïve view might emphasize that mental disorders can excuse even when they don't entirely bypass one's agency; the disorder just needs to compromise agency to a significant degree. Consider, for example, the famous case of *Clark v. Arizona* (48 U.S. 735 2006; discussed in Morse 2011). The defense argued that Clark, who suffered from paranoid schizophrenia, did not kill a police officer intentionally because he thought the officer was a space alien. Now the U.S. Supreme Court thought Clark still knew that resorting to murder was wrong, but other delusions or hallucinations might lead one to do something that, from the patient's perspective, should be counted as morally permissible (Broome et al. 2010: 183). Suppose, for example, that a patient throws his roommate's prized vase in the trash while hallucinating that it's a rotten watermelon, the source of a foul smell saturating the kitchen.

In such cases, however, we see that mitigated blame rests not on one's having a disorder but on one's agency in the particular circumstances being substantially compromised by one's psychiatric symptoms. Often one can have a mental disorder that doesn't substantially diminish one's agency to warrant a significant reduction in blame. ADHD, for example, does not appear to disrupt one's general capacity to form intentions and act on them. When someone with this disorder acts, their agency is not always significantly diminished. One's ability to focus may be limited, but that doesn't distinguish ADHD from more ordinary, even if transient, conditions like being extremely tired or distressed due to unusual demands at work.

4.3.3 Psychopathology Is Heterogeneous

The general issue here is that mental disorders are not a homogenous class. An initial complication is that many disorders occur with others (comorbidity), such that in any particular case there may be multiple disorders at work. Another complication is that different disorders affect different psychological capacities and the ways they affect those capacities can vary widely. So there are many ways in which mental disorders might (or might not) significantly affect the exercise of one's agency.

Let's draw two cross-cutting distinctions that can be applied to categorize how disorders might present themselves. First, symptoms of a disorder can be episodic or static. *Episodic symptoms* present themselves in (more or less) discrete instances. Narcolepsy, again, is a good example, as the associated loss of consciousness comes in discreet instances. Though a patient with narcolepsy is always possessed of their condition, it is only episodically activated, as it were. Similarly, while there is currently no cure for Alzheimer's, patients can within the same day go from experiencing relative clarity of mind to confusion, despite unchanged neurodegeneration (Palop et al. 2006). Other examples might include dissociative identity disorder, PTSD, bipolar disorder, specific delusions, and various phobias—each of which can manifest in discrete episodes, sometimes in response to specific triggers. In contrast, some symptoms are more *static*, like those of autism, depression, dementia, anti-social personality disorder, and generalized anxiety disorder. The ways in which each manifest is more likely to persist over time, with no clear boundaries. Perhaps their effects can wax and wane, but we wouldn't naturally carve them up into discrete episodes.

The second distinction concerns the degree to which a disorder's symptoms impinge on one's agency. Narcolepsy, for example, has quite *global* effects: loss of consciousness can undermine the affected patient's abilities across the board. In contrast, certain disorders may only be relevant to a subset of agential abilities, yielding more *local* effects. For instance, kleptomania, as a compulsion, presents as strong urges to steal, but it leaves other elements of an agent's psychology relatively untouched. Specific or "simple" phobias are another kind of example, as they are tied to certain cues, such as spiders, heights, or blood. Similarly, while some delusions can be more systematic (as in forms of schizophrenia), others are rather specific and relatively circumscribed, as when patients with Capgras delusions take a familiar person to be an imposter (Bortolotti 2015).

These distinctions cross-cut, so either element of each can pair with either element of the other (see Table 4.1). Narcolepsy can be an episodic, global condition, whereas severe schizophrenia has global effects on agency but is often more static (though it too can manifest in discrete episodes). Anxiety disorders may have localized

Table 4.1 Pathological Effects on Agency

	Episodic	Static
Local	e.g. phobias	e.g. anxiety disorders
Global	e.g. narcolepsy	e.g. schizophrenia

symptoms, despite being relatively static conditions, while some episodic conditions, like specific phobias, will similarly only present locally.

Drawing these distinctions further motivates the nuanced account. Mental illness can indeed excuse actions, provided the symptoms significantly undermine some feature of one's agency that generated the act in question. However, the diversity of ways in which the symptoms of mental disorders affect action makes psychopathology an extremely heterogeneous class. Many disorders have local, rather than global, effects on specific agential capacities, sometimes in fairly discrete episodes that leave the rest of one's life relatively isolated from the disorder's effects.

Even disorders such as schizophrenia, which might seem to lend the most support to the naïve view, don't support the general inference. Consider this excerpt from the TED talk "A Tale of Mental Illness" by Elyn Saks, a distinguished professor at the University of Southern California, who suffers from chronic schizophrenia herself:

> Everyone has seen a street person, unkempt, probably ill-fed, standing outside of an office building muttering to himself or shouting. This person is likely to have some form of schizophrenia. But schizophrenia presents itself across a wide array of socioeconomic status, and there are people with the illness who are full-time professionals with major responsibilities.

Saks goes on to describe particular psychotic episodes in which she experienced a "shattered" mind, rife with delusions, hallucinations, and incoherent "word salad." Such episodes substantially diminish core aspects of her agency, and the symptoms directly impact her behavior. Most other times, however, she manages her symptoms well, through three primary methods: excellent treatment, loving friends and family, and a supportive work environment. Saks's case ably illustrates how a diagnosis of psychopathology, even one with widespread effects on agency that operates across time, is not enough to draw an inference about the patient's responsibility, either in general or at any particular time.

Diagnostic categories often obscure the diversity within and between them. After decades of attempts to find biomarkers for conditions like autism and ADHD, researchers have come up short, partly because there is little neurological unity to these broad psychiatric categories (Uddin et al. 2017). Some researchers already caution that standard psychiatric categories are unlikely to group patients together in the most informative way for discovering facts about mental illness (e.g., Tabb 2015; Arpaly 2022). In response to such issues, the National Institute of Mental Health now employs a set of criteria for assessing research projects that departs from diagnostic categories. These Research Domain Criteria encourage researchers to frame their projects as addressing particular psychological phenomena rather than specific disorders. A study of anxiety, for instance, may include patients exhibiting rather different kinds of disorders identified in the DSM—not just generalized anxiety disorder, but OCD, PTSD, and so on. A large consortium of researchers has followed a similar path by developing a classification scheme for mental disorders that is dimensional rather than categorical (Kotov et al. 2017; Krueger et al. 2018). Even if diagnostic categories remain useful in certain contexts (e.g., in having clear categories for clinical treatment), psychopathology is heterogenous any way you slice it.

In sum, psychopathologies do not categorically justify inferring anything about patients' responsibility across all contexts. Focusing on specific symptoms highlights how they can vary widely across patients. Many (if not all) disorders lie on a spectrum. Like traits on the autism spectrum, symptoms of depression, anxiety, delusions, and phobias range in their severity and frequency. At many points on the continuum, one's agential capacities are diminished to some degree but not severely diminished. The suggestion is not that psychiatric patients are *always* (or nearly always) blameworthy, even for acts substantially influenced by their symptoms (compare Szasz 1961/1974; Foucault 1988). The nuanced account precisely shirks any such general claims about moral responsibility and psychopathology. Sometimes one is responsible despite a mental illness, sometimes not. We should instead identify the particular circumstances in which a reduction of blame (or praise) is warranted.

4.4 Ethical Implications

Adopting the nuanced view of psychopathology and moral responsibility forces us to broaden our conception of agency and responsibility. We've seen that all neurological conditions present on a spectrum, and, more importantly, their symptoms fluctuate throughout the day. In other words, psychiatric symptoms are *graduated* and *fluid*, like agency generally. We'll now see how the neurotypical and atypical are more alike than unalike, which can empower patients with the autonomy necessary to improve their symptoms while promoting compassion for all.

4.4.1 Neurodiversity

A broader conception of human agency has radical implications. Once we recognize this continuum *within* the category of any one neurological condition, we see continuity with those *outside* of it. Thus, a corollary of the nuanced view is the following:

> *Cognitive Continuity*: Neurotypical individuals and people with psychopathologies are more alike psychologically than they are unalike; their psychological differences are primarily a matter of degree, not kind.

Cognitive continuity helps explain why the case-by-case (or rather action-by-action) approach prescribed by the nuanced view is the same approach we take to assessing responsibility for neurotypical individuals. We recognize that individuals sometimes make impaired decisions while grappling with a divorce, bereaving the death of a loved one, or operating on little sleep due to a colicky newborn. Thus, while we should readily admit that some symptoms of psychiatric disorders do diminish one's agency, that is not categorically different from neurotypical mental life.

Cognitive continuity is related to, but arguably distinct from, a "neurodiversity" approach to mental illness. The concept of neurodiversity arose in the context of autism (Singer 1999; Silberman 2015), primarily as a movement among members of that community. For example, in a powerful video posted on YouTube in 2007 titled "In My Language," Mel Baggs urges viewers to see their autistic way of being as legitimate, even if abnormal. The video is intended to be a "strong statement on the existence and value of many different kinds of thinking and interaction in the world, where how close you can appear to a specific one of them determines whether you are seen as a real person."

Could this approach be extended beyond autism? At its core, neurodiversity "recognizes that many people have a combination of neurological and psychological abilities and disabilities," as bioethicist Walter Glannon puts it (2007: 1). This of course is essentially the cognitive continuity idea that we derived from the nuanced approach to *all* mental disorders. So the nuanced view suggests that we can extend something like a neurodiversity approach to other psychiatric disorders, provided we isolate continuity from other claims commonly associated with the neurodiversity movement.

4.4.2 Disability

Many proponents of neurodiversity in autism also reject a dominant approach to disorder and disability (Leadbitter et al. 2021). The standard *medical model* views disability as undesirable itself and the appropriate target of treatment. The *social model*, in contrast, holds that the disadvantages arise solely from "society's failure to provide appropriate services and adequately ensure the needs of disabled people are fully taken into account in its social organization" (Oliver 1996: 32). The primary target of treatment, then, is society, not the individual.

To further illustrate, let's turn our attention away from psychiatric disorders and toward treatment of neurological conditions that affect the senses. Deaf people have a discernible community that involves a shared history and language. Members of the community often welcome being identified as "Deaf" (*identity-first language*) rather than a person who suffers from deafness (*person-first language*). In contrast, individuals who don't identify with their condition often prefer to be described as someone who suffers from it—e.g., someone "with paraplegia" or "with schizophrenia," as opposed to being a "paraplegic" or "schizophrenic."

The social model of disability provides one rationale for why some Deaf people aren't interested in "curing" their disability. Disadvantages that arise from the inability to hear might simply arise from conditions in society that only favor more common human bodies. Deaf people can function well in societies with the right accommodations, such as closed captioning, telecommunications relay services, and a lack of stigma among people who can hear. The social model ultimately draws our attention to prejudice against all people with disabilities (*abilism*). Even just investing in and promoting the elimination of certain disabilities might be ethically fraught. The Deaf community, for example, could one day vanish with the proliferation of cochlear implants (Sparrow 2005), which convert ambient sounds into electronic signals that stimulate the auditory nerve that travels into the brain.

Some people in the Deaf community view their condition as such a central and valuable part of their identity that they prefer to have children who share it. One couple, Sharon Duchesneau and Candy McCullough, went so far to use only a sperm donor who was also Deaf (Mundy 2002). Although they regarded any resulting children as a blessing, they were delighted with the outcome: both their daughter and son, born five years apart, are congenitally Deaf. Such parental choices might seem reckless, even selfish, but we should pause and reflect on those reactions. Our ability to understand what it's like to be on the other side of a transformative experience is limited, and personal values easily influence our own descriptions of other people (see Chapter 3).

The medical and social models might not exhaust the available approaches to disability (Barnes 2016), but they provide a useful contrast for understanding different attitudes toward physical and mental impairments. A social model of disability could be applied to some mental disorders. Advocates of neurodiversity describe autism as a difference not necessarily a deficit. Of course, virtually all mental disorders present on a wide spectrum, and some individuals with autism view it as a deficit, even if also a difference to be respected not denigrated (Kapp et al. 2013). Whether a social model could be extended to many other disorders is a further question. Consider patients grappling with major depression, anxiety, or personality disorders, for instance. Many of these patients adamantly seek cures for what they regard as a deficit, even if at the same time sympathy and societal accommodation are always welcome.

So it looks like conceptions of disability are distinct from the cognitive continuity thesis, which is our focus. Proponents of neurodiversity could conceivably adopt a medical model of mental disorder. But do we then lose the reduction in stigma? The social model certainly makes stigma inappropriate. If disability is a problem with society, not the individual, then stigmatizing disabled individuals is certainly inappropriate. Society ought to change. We'll now see, however, that recognizing cognitive continuity might be sufficient to reduce stigma.

4.4.3 Stigma

Stigmatizing mental illness has obvious ethical implications. It harms patients through marginalization, cutting them off from many of the interactions with others that humans so often crave and need to thrive, such as love and friendship. Fear of stigma can even make one less inclined to seek mental health services and to pursue gainful employment or independent living (Rüsch et al. 2005).

Regarding patients as having reduced agency might seem more compassionate and destigmatizing, for it reduces responsibility and blame. We might say "It's not her fault" or "He should be treated, not chastised." Yet we run the risk of exacerbating stigma if we deny that patients have agency and responsibility. As Jeanette Kennett (2007: 103) puts it, patients might reason:

> It is hard to construct a rich positive sense of self as we become increasingly invisible to others, as they refuse eye contact, turn away at our approach, end conversations abruptly, and show less and less interest in what we say and do.

A *vicious loop* can then develop whereby treating patients as exempted from responsibility promotes social exclusion, which erodes one's agency, which promotes further social exclusion, and so on. Thus, the removal of responsibility can be a double-edged sword: reducing blame while reinforcing stigma (Haslam & Kvaale 2015; Wiesjahn et al. 2016).

Some ethicists have argued that withholding responsibility does not make stigma inevitable. One can still build meaningful relationships with mentally ill individuals (Kennett 2007; Shoemaker 2022). Although your grandmother is in the early stages of Alzheimer's and your uncle has schizophrenia, you can still share a laugh, empathize, and bond with them. However, many other valuable interactions—and forms of effective treatment—rest on the presumption of autonomy. Being responsible, even to a modest degree, allows the possibility of praise and discourages a passive attitude toward one's condition that can impede improvement. Some theorists have explicitly defended therapies that encourage such patients to "take responsibility" for their behavior, including the aim of achieving mental health (e.g. Bjorklund 2004; Pickard 2011).

Recognizing a cognitive continuum among the neurotypical and atypical can help reduce stigma by treating mental illnesses as in some ways analogous to physical illness. We are all subject to both mental and physical illness, whether chronically or acutely, and their effects can sometimes diminish our agency. Some people do grapple chronically with anxiety, depression, or schizophrenia, for example, in the way that a person can always have diabetes. But other individuals only temporarily or occasionally experience symptoms of anxiety, depression, phobias, and other psychic troubles that can come and go, depending on one's life circumstances and quality of treatment. Sometimes the symptoms of psychopathology naturally ebb and flow or respond to treatment, much in the way that one occasionally gets the flu or is prone to migraines that later diminish in frequency with preventive measures. The more we see psychopathology as lying on a continuum, the more it can be seen as similar to other forms of illness that afflict us all, not just a select few who have a deep debilitating dysfunction in body or mind. Thus, less stigma and more compassion seem to follow easily from recognition of cognitive continuity (more on this in Chapter 10).

4.4.4 Blame

By recognizing how the neurotypical and atypical are more psychologically alike than different, we can reduce stigma by humanizing and empowering psychiatric patients. Blame can be painful for the blameworthy, to be sure, but it expresses a respect for them as a fellow person who can be held accountable. That said, blame isn't always appropriate—for the neurotypical or not. How can moral responsibility be widespread and yet blame inappropriate?

Part of the answer lies in recognizing that there can be *responsibility without blame*, as the philosopher Hanna Pickard (2011) puts it. The two categories often go together: blame seems appropriate if someone is responsible for a wrongdoing. Yet being responsible isn't sufficient for blame. Suppose your friend is responsible for breaking her promise to water your plants during your travels. Nevertheless, her wedding is no time to air your grievances (King 2020). Further imagine she apologizes—thereby taking responsibility—and reveals that the plants slipped her mind because the stress of wedding planning prevented her from sleeping well at night. She offers this as an explanation, not a justification or excuse. Despite her being responsible, blame seems inappropriate well beyond the wedding day.

Similar to a haggard friend, we naturally mitigate blame upon realizing the great challenges that people face when in the grips of a mental disorder. Symptoms can occur so frequently and incessantly—e.g., intrusive thoughts, paralyzing fear, crushing sadness—that it's difficult to maintain employment or keep promises to friends. These psychiatric symptoms should certainly be recognized as restricting the ability to control one's actions or to regulate one's impulses, not merely a matter of unusually strong preferences to, say, avoid heights, repeatedly check locks, or stay in bed all day (Sripada 2022a). Patients often experience spontaneous impulses extended over such long intervals of time that their capacity to regulate them inevitably fails. Even an all-star basketball player will inevitably miss some shots while attempting them over and over. Nevertheless, throughout all this, one can enjoy a great deal of agency and responsibility.

Put in this light, psychiatric symptoms seem continuous with the psychic troubles of the neurotypical. In both cases, agency varies dynamically over time but a sufficient level of responsibility remains constant. While regarding others as responsible agents, we attenuate our blame of them upon learning that their control or judgment have been compromised by challenging circumstances or even personality type. Your partner might not be clinically depressed, but you don't blame him for neglecting your needs over the past few months, because you know he has been grieving his beloved mother's death. Your friend might not have social anxiety disorder, but your awareness of her introversion prevents you from chastising her for being unwilling to socialize more than once a week. And you let your supervisor off the hook for being a mediocre mentor once you realize she has been engrossed in a legal battle all year with her abusive ex-husband. The range of examples is as varied as the vagaries of life.

What distinguishes psychopathology from these more "ordinary" mental obstacles is largely a matter of frequency, persistence, and severity. As many of us know all too well, death, divorce, and destitution alone can cause severe anxiety and depression; they aren't considered pathological because over time they naturally wane. After an economic downturn, depression and anxiety typically fade over time as a neurotypical person returns to baseline. But the psychic struggles during that period are no less real, and the respite at baseline is ultimately temporary, as life continues to throw up challenge after challenge. There are differences between typical and atypical minds, but there are parallels as well (see Table 4.2).

We needn't adopt a detailed theory of free will or moral responsibility to see the parallels between mitigated blame among neurotypical and atypical individuals. Why don't you fully blame your grieving spouse for neglecting your emotional needs? It might

Table 4.2 Nonpathological Effects on Agency

	Episodic	Static
Local	e.g. family emergency, distraction	e.g. work burnout, physical injury
Global	e.g. sleep deprivation	e.g. stress, grief, divorce

be because his persistently negative, self-loathing thoughts dominate his deliberations, impairing his ability to respond appropriately to relevant reasons for attending to important matters. Or perhaps it's because depression masks his true desires or values: he really does care about you, despite the apparent neglect (Arpaly 2022). Whether the problem is control, coherence, choice, or some combination of these (see Chapter 2), mitigated blame is often tied to effects on such agential capacities. But, again, there is a reduction in blame without an elimination of agency or responsibility.

In sum, rejection of the naïve view does not require ignoring that mental disorders can impair one's agency. Indeed, part of the point is that the neurotypical and psychopathological are more alike in this way than they are unalike. That's not to deny some important differences, and it's certainly not to deny the need for compassion and treatment, in both cases. Put in this perspective, the nuanced view seems far from revisionary. Although humans often delight in judging others and punishing wrongdoers, in ordinary life we frequently see mitigation of blame, even if full exculpation is rare.

None of this implies that pathological symptoms or behavior are desirable or morally acceptable, just as we needn't accept all physical illness as desirable. Migraines are a pain, as is depression. On the nuanced account it's entirely possible for a psychopathology (e.g., antisocial personality disorder) to be morally problematic and give rise to behaviors one should be held accountable for, to some degree (see Chapter 6). In practice, mitigation of blame just comes so cheaply that we should expect to often see it as warranted, even when one remains accountable.

4.5 Conclusion

We began with disputes over whether having a mental illness does or does not categorically exculpate one for inappropriate behavior. Underlying this dispute is a naïve view on which there is a straightforward connection between psychopathology and moral responsibility. We have seen, however, that these matters of responsibility are rather complicated. Although particular symptoms of mental illness can sometimes impose limits on one's agential capacities, other times it seems one's capacities either remain or aren't diminished enough to warrant a reduction in responsibility.

Let's return to the cases of Andrea Yates and Eddie Ray Routh. It's plausible that symptoms from the defendants' mental disorders did contribute to their criminal acts. Yates's psychiatrist warned about her having a fifth child, given that Yates attempted suicide soon after having her fourth. So it seems her postpartum depression and various delusions plausibly contributed to the choice to end her children's lives just months after the birth of her fifth. Similarly, Routh's PTSD plausibly contributed to his homicides, as his attack was on two military veterans at a shooting range. However, arguably these disorders do not typically yield actions that bypass one's agency entirely. Whether Yates and Routh should be judged "not guilty by reason of insanity" is a legal question. Should they be blamed or held accountable to some degree? A more nuanced approach allows us to answer "Yes" even if some reduction in blame is warranted.

Arguably, a nuanced approach is already dominant in legal and medical settings. Despite public discourse on such high-profile cases, the law generally operates with something like the nuanced view. Lawyers can't simply establish that their clients have a mental disorder. They must show that the relevant symptoms of the disorder causally contributed to the act in question and compromised some psychological capacity relevant to the elements of legal liability, such as negating the requisite mens rea or voluntary act (Morse 2011; Sifferd 2022). Similarly, the competence of patients to make an informative and autonomous decision is not determined simply by categorizing them as having a mental disorder. Rather, doctors and caregivers evaluate the specific case at hand, quite independently of how the patient fits into psychiatric categories (see, e.g., Appelbaum 2007).

When mitigated blame (or praise) is warranted, any differences with neurotypical agency might be a matter of degree, not kind. The nuanced view paints the neurotypical and disordered as more psychologically alike than unalike. This motivates something like a neurodiversity approach not only to autism but also to psychopathology generally: agency often arises in many different types of mental lives, including those that are atypical. Thus, perhaps we should accord more autonomy to those suffering from mental illness and recognize the limits of autonomy among the neurotypical. When evaluating the appropriateness of blame or praise, we do better to focus on the particular symptoms and circumstances of the individual in question, rather than on whether they are best thought of as neurotypical or disordered. The key is to recognize that most (adult) human beings are appropriate targets of praise and blame, but their agency can be diminished to various degrees in some contexts. As a result, we should often accord both more agency and less stigma to those grappling with mental disorders.

Now, some forms of mental affliction might seem to categorically excuse. Psychopathy or anti-social personality disorder, for example, might prevent a proper understanding of right and wrong (see Chapter 6). Another potential exception to the nuanced view is addiction or substance use disorder, which is now commonly treated by clinicians and researchers as a brain disease, akin to diabetes. Don't addicts experience a chronic loss of control that makes them categorically less responsible for their consumption of drugs or alcohol? In the next chapter, we attempt to answer this question by examining the neurobiology of addiction.

5
Addiction

The previous chapter focused on paradigm mental disorders, such as depression and schizophrenia. One might concede that there is often agency in such cases, but aren't there others in which one's self-control is categorically impaired by brain dysfunction?

Addiction, or substance use disorder, stands out as a potential exception. It is now commonly regarded as a chronic brain disease that greatly inhibits self-control with respect to using drugs (including alcohol). Shouldn't addicts be treated rather than held accountable for their drug abuse? Continuing with our nuanced approach, we see in this chapter that the situation is not so simple. Although addiction is certainly a disorder of some sort, it's not clearly a brain disease that precludes control. The brain mechanisms involved in addiction are similar to those involved in more ordinary failures of self-control. The difference is one of degree rather than kind. Our discussion begins with the case of an opioid addict who is punished for relapsing.

5.1 Reprimand for Relapse

Julie Eldred began using Oxycontin in her teens. The prescription opioid provided a euphoria that dampened her social anxieties and kept episodes of depression at bay. Eventually Julie progressed to using heroin regularly, occasionally stealing from others to pay for the drugs. In 2016, at age 28, she was convicted of larceny for taking over $250 in jewelry from the home of a person for whom she provided dog-walking services. The judge ruled that Julie could avoid jail time if she attended outpatient services and remained drug free for a year. Within 12 days, however, she tested positive for fentanyl, a synthetic opioid 50 times more powerful than heroin. As a result, she spent 10 days in jail—the time it took for a spot to become available at an inpatient treatment center (*Commonwealth v. Eldred*, 101 N.E.3d 2018; Lam 2018).

Julie and her lawyer, Lisa Newman-Polk, objected that the relapse did not constitute a willful violation of the probation terms. Relapse is a symptom of Julie's substance use disorder, so she is unable to remain drug free. Newman-Polk stated that her client "did not 'choose' to relapse any more than a person who has hypertension chooses to have high blood pressure" (Ewing 2017). In an interview with the Institute for Innovation in Prosecution, Julie similarly explains: "In the beginning, I guess when I was 14 or 15, yeah, it was a choice to pick it up. But the way it chemically made me feel, and emotionally made me feel, I don't know if I ever really did have a choice in the matter" (IIP John Jay 2021). In the 1960s, the U.S. Supreme Court rejected a similar compulsion argument for a defendant's addiction to alcohol (*Powell v. Texas* 1968). The verdict in Julie's case was no different. The Massachusetts Supreme Court considered her appeal in 2018 but ruled unanimously in favor of the judge's initial decision.

Julie's case exemplifies the heated debate over whether substance use disorder is a *brain disease* and whether addicts really have *control* over their powerful urges to use. The two issues are often entangled, but throughout this chapter we'll try our best to separate them, since addiction could be a disease even if it doesn't impair self-control. Julie's case also illustrates that we won't be focusing on responsibility for actions carried out while under the influence of drugs or alcohol, which one can experience without being addicted. Our concern is with addiction specifically and whether it impairs one's ability to refrain from using or procuring the means to use.

5.2 What Is Addiction?

Addiction used to be treated as a moral failing, simple as that. People who drink, smoke, or shoot up to excess were thought to simply have bad habits on account of weak wills, not unlike the chronic nail-biter or nose-picker. Since the early 20th century, however, scientists and health professionals have moved away from moralization and increasingly conceptualized addiction in medical terms.

5.2.1 The Brain Disease Model

The latest version of the *Diagnostic and Statistical Manual of Mental Disorders* (DSM-5) includes addiction, just not under that label. *Substance use disorder* involves repeated use of drugs or alcohol despite the damaging effects on one's health, work, relationships, and other aspects of life (American Psychiatric Association 2013). The DSM captures a fairly natural conception of addiction without treating it as a monolith. Like other disorders, substance abuse is complex, varied, and lies on a spectrum. One can abuse substances as different as alcohol, heroin, cocaine, prescription opioids, and cigarettes. One's dependency on such substances can vary greatly in strength. Some people find it impossible to quit drinking several beers each evening, while others can't do without drinking vodka throughout the day.

What's also rather uncontroversial are some key stages and elements of addiction (Koob & Volkow 2010). It often starts with *initial use* of the drug for the pleasure of the high or the pain it numbs, which is felt rather strongly and often helps one cope with other mental or physical health issues. As with any intensely pleasurable experiences, users become motivated to seek them out again. With repeated use over time (*binging*), one begins to develop increased *tolerance*, in which a larger amount of the drug is required in order to achieve the same physiological effects. But we aren't necessarily to addiction or substance use disorder yet (see Table 5.1).

Arguably more central to addiction is physical and psychological *dependence* on the drug to feel normal. Users experience intense *cravings*, particularly in response to thoughts or perceptions of things

Table 5.1 Some Key Elements of Addiction

Pre-Addiction Stage	initial use, increased use/binging, increased tolerance
Addiction Stage	dependence, cravings, withdrawal, remission, relapse

Note: These are some common stages of addiction but needn't occur in this particular order or occur at all for every individual.

associated with using, such as paraphernalia, locations where one normally uses, and certain times of day. The constant cravings and dependence often cause problems with work, school, relationships, and the law—either during active use or after long periods of abstinence (*remission*). However, quitting at this point yields unpleasant *withdrawal* symptoms, which vary depending on the substance of abuse but can include irritability, anxiety, depression, muscle aches, trembling, and insomnia. Powerful cravings persist even after making it through withdrawal, which makes it difficult to avoid using again after some period of abstinence (*relapse*).

Some agencies and health professionals go further and describe addiction, at least in its more extreme forms, as a disease with other specific characteristics. In the United States, the National Institute on Drug Abuse (NIDA) defines addiction as "a chronic, relapsing disorder characterized by compulsive drug seeking and use despite adverse consequences" (NIDA 2020: 4). The Institute further describes addiction as a "brain disease" that "is a lot like other diseases, such as heart disease" (4), though unlike heart disease "impairment in self-control is the hallmark of addiction" (6).

The disease model has many proponents among current health professionals. It gained prominence in the 1990s, following an explosion of neurobiological research on addiction. In a well-known article, "Addiction Is a Brain Disease, and It Matters" published in *Science*, the former head of NIDA, Alan Leshner, proclaimed:

> A metaphorical switch in the brain seems to be thrown as a result of prolonged drug use. Initially, drug use is a voluntary behavior, but when that switch is thrown, the individual moves into the state of addiction, characterized by compulsive drug seeking and use. (Leshner 1997: 46)

Two other notable titans also hold leadership positions at the National Institutes of Health. Nora Volkow (pronounced "Vul-kahv") is the current director of NIDA, while George Koob directs a parallel organization, the National Institute on Alcohol Abuse and Alcoholism (NIAAA). The two have co-authored explanations and vigorous defenses of the brain disease model (e.g., Koob & Volkow 2010; Volkow & Koob 2015).

Put simply, the *brain disease model* asserts that addiction is a brain disease that involves compulsive drug use. Unpacking it further reveals three key elements that are rarely disentangled:

1. **Disease**: Addiction is a *disease* because it involves damage or at least *dysfunction* in the user's body. (This presumably goes beyond a mere syndrome or disorder, as in "behavioral addictions" to gambling, pornography, social media, and the like.)
2. **Brain**: Addiction fundamentally involves dysfunction in *brain circuits* caused by the substances of abuse. So *treatment* is appropriate, and the primary target should be the patient's brain—e.g., medications that alter neurotransmitters to reduce cravings. (Social and economic conditions are comparatively less important and at best secondary targets.)
3. **Compulsion**: The neural dysfunction in addiction yields *irresistible* cravings that result in compulsive use and substantially diminished control.

There are several approaches to addiction, but our focus will be on this brain disease model, partly because our interest is primarily in neuroscience but also because it's arguably the dominant view among health professionals. Both philosophers and scientists have leveled criticisms against it, but they're often not clear about which element of the model is targeted. We'll canvas objections to each of the three elements and evaluate whether some can be modified or jettisoned while the model otherwise remains intact. To do so, we'll have to understand the neurobiology of addiction.

5.2.2 Dopamine and Reward

Neuroscience is quite useful for the topic of addiction, not because it can tell us whether drugs of abuse alter the brain. Of course they do. Despite many headlines to the effect of "X actually changes the brain!," such findings are not newsworthy; they're *neuroredundancy*, to use a term coined by Sally Satel and Scott Lilienfeld to denote things we already knew prior to the neurobiological data (2013: 22). Even Descartes and other die-hard dualists admit that any change in mental states results in a change in brain states (see the appendix to Chapter 1). Neurobiology helps instead to uncover *how*, not whether, drugs affect the brain. Descending into the mind's hardware allows us to acquire important evidence about whether drugs of addiction affect the brain much differently than other forms of motivation and habit formation.

The general consensus is that dopamine in the reward system of the brain is central to addiction. Many drugs of abuse increase the release of dopamine either directly or indirectly, with the end effect of *reinforcing* drug intake. Cocaine, a stimulant, allows dopamine to remain longer in the synapses where it has been released by blocking transporters that normally clear it away. Alcohol and heroin, in contrast, are "downers" that suppress the central nervous system by directly increasing rather different neurotransmitters (GABA and opioids), yet they both also increase dopamine. Indeed, although different drugs have quite distinct effects on brain chemistry, there is some evidence that all or most drugs increase dopamine to some extent. This "dopamine hypothesis" has been criticized, but it's the dominant view among neuroscientists.

Dopamine is important because it regulates motivation and learning in the brain's reward system. In the 1950s, scientists found that most rats would press a lever hundreds of times per hour when it triggered electrical stimulation of a particular pathway in the brain (Olds & Milner 1954). This "mesolimbic" dopamine pathway is situated near the middle of the limbic system and carries dopamine from the ventral tegmental area of the brainstem to the nucleus accumbens of the limbic system (see Figure 5.1). The mesolimbic pathway primarily triggers motivation to act based on expectations of reward. The pathway works with many areas of the cortex to recognize, anticipate, and predict positive experiences, from tasty foods to academic achievements that promote the long-term goal of earning a degree.

It used to be thought that dopamine was the neurotransmitter responsible for pleasure. But we now know that's not quite right and that it's rather misleading when it comes to addiction. Dopamine is often correlated with pleasure because we typically enjoy getting what we want. Imagine a child who eats a donut for the first time and loves the

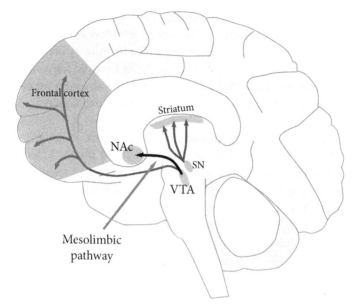

Figure 5.1 Three Dopamine Pathways
The **mesolimbic pathway** carries dopamine for reinforcement from the ventral tegmental area (VTA) in the brainstem to the nucleus accumbens (NAc) of the limbic system. Projections from the VTA also ascend into the frontal cortex via the **mesocorticolimbic pathway**. These can be contrasted with other dopamine pathways, such as the **nigrostriatal pathway** involved in motor function, which carries dopamine from the substantia nigra (SN) to the striatum.

delectable mixture of sugar and fried dough. Her brain is awash in dopamine. The next time she's near the donut shop—or come Saturday morning when her family last visited the shop—the child will yearn for another treat and voice her desire, "Can we get donuts again?!" Her brain just spiked in dopamine, but not because she ate another pillowy pastry. The spike occurs (and then fades) before she even eats, and even if her request is denied. Moreover, people don't always find pleasure in what they desperately seek out. The child might wolf down three donuts but soon feel sick. As the saying goes, "Be careful what you wish for."

Wanting and liking are not only distinct concepts but also supported by distinct brain chemicals. Dopamine in the mesolimbic pathway is primarily responsible for the *motivation* to get something one wants, not for pleasure, which is the function of opioids (Berridge & Robinson 2016). Wanting and liking can be decoupled in ordinary life, but the brain often adjusts motivation accordingly. As the child learns not to overeat delicious treats, her mesolimbic pathway no longer becomes awash in dopamine at the thought of downing three donuts in one sitting.

In addiction, however, the decoupling can persist. Prolonged use of addictive substances changes how the reward system functions such that users want the drug even after they come to see it as destroying their lives. During his decades of addiction, the philosopher Owen Flanagan describes a recurring theme of self-loathing, viewing himself as "a wretched, worsening train wreck of a person" who was "contaminating, possibly ruining" the lives of those he loved (2011: 278). Yet Flanagan continued to consume alcohol and benzodiazepines daily. Since drugs of abuse appear to increase dopamine themselves, ingestion *always* teaches the user (unconsciously) that the drug is rewarding, thereby generating motivation to procure it.

Addictive substances don't just manipulate desire when they are ingested. Over time, consumption of drugs or alcohol change the brain's reward system so that it becomes particularly sensitive to cues that make the substances salient (Koob & Volkow 2010; Berridge & Robinson 2016). One change involves *suppression* of this pathway's normal function. After repeated use of a drug that introduces large amounts of dopamine, the mesolimbic pathway suppresses dopamine's normal stimulation (among that of other neurotransmitters, of course, depending on the particular drug of abuse). It's as if the brain is saying, "OK, we're getting plenty of this stuff from outside, so we can slow down its effect here." Previously, dopamine in the reward pathway was functioning normally, but repeated hits of the drug begin to decrease the number of dopamine receptors or otherwise impede dopamine's normal effects. This *down-regulation* is meant to bring brain chemistry back to equilibrium, with the expectation that drug use will continue. The user then requires the drug to feel normal. That's the mechanism behind dependence. Now, to go beyond normal—to feel high—the user must ingest larger and larger doses. That's tolerance. Abstinence then leads to withdrawal symptoms because the user's brain has been rewired to dampen down the effects of dopamine (among other neurotransmitters) in order to compensate for what the drug is contributing. Once drug use stops, an addict's brain is still wired to down-regulate dopamine functioning—until withdrawal wanes, when the brain adjusts back to normal.

This isn't the whole story, at least because key elements of addiction persist after successfully going through withdrawal. Even after completing rehab, for example, addicts regularly crave the drug intensely and often relapse. So which changes in the brain are responsible for these key elements of addiction? According to the prominent theory of *incentive salience*, craving and relapse are effects of the drug shaping the mesolimbic dopamine pathway to become *hyperactive* in response to drug cues (Berridge & Robinson 2016). To understand how this occurs, we must recognize that dopamine regulates desire largely by functioning as a learning signal. A hit of dopamine paired with an experience teaches you, even if unconsciously, that the experience is rewarding. That experience can even make you sensitive to any cues associated with the reward or incentive, and dopamine can spike just from the *anticipation* of getting it (Schultz et al. 1997). It's as if dopamine's role here is to tell you, "Hey, stop whatever you're doing and pay attention; something rewarding is available!" Repeated drug use makes the reward pathway inordinately sensitive to anything related to what produced so much dopamine in the past. When an addict in remission drives by the place where she used to purchase opioids, her mesolimbic pathway becomes excited and inundated with dopamine, which generates intense cravings.

It bears emphasis that this description of the neurobiology of addiction is enormously oversimplified, and the current science is certainly incomplete. We're zooming in on the role of dopamine in the mesolimbic pathway, primarily because most drugs of abuse seem to cause rather long-term, even if reversible, changes there. Some research suggests that other brain areas can become impaired as well, including portions of the frontal lobe (Koob & Volkow 2010). Nevertheless, most researchers agree that addiction centrally involves rewiring of dopamine pathways in the brain.

These neurobiological effects of drug use at least *seem* to support the disease model. After all, addictive substances appear to cause long-lasting changes in the brain that might appropriately be described as *dysfunctional*, perhaps even damaged. These changes directly lead to cravings that drive addicts to use, even if they don't much like or value using. Addicts don't appear to be hedonists seeking out pleasure but rather patients *compelled* to use by a brain circuit that becomes hyperactive just by seeing or thinking about anything associated with the drug of abuse. Similar to a hyperactive thyroid that produces too much thyroxine, appropriate treatment should target the *dysfunctional brain circuits*. For example, medications, brain stimulation, and other neurobiological interventions could dampen cravings by making the reward pathway less sensitive to drug cues.

That's the model. Let's scrutinize it, working through each element as introduced above. We start with claims about compulsion, then consider how central the brain is to addiction and whether addiction is a disease of some sort.

5.3 Loss of Control in Addiction?

The idea that addiction involves irresistible urges is not new. William James, a forefather of psychology, wrote that cravings in severe addiction are "of a strength of which normal persons can form no conception" (1890: 543). People in the grips of serious alcoholism, according to James, make truthful statements like:

> Were a keg of rum in one corner of a room and were a cannon constantly discharging balls between me and it, I could not refrain from passing before that cannon in order to get the rum.

James relied on the experience and testimony of those suffering from addiction. The disease model purports to provide objective neurobiological evidence that addictive substances impair control by creating dysfunctional brain circuits. Like James's characterization, the modern idea is not merely that resisting the temptation to use is difficult but *practically impossible*. The bioethicist Louis Charland, for example, asserts that drug-induced changes in the reward pathway "usually nullify any semblance of voluntary choice" (Charland 2002: 41).

5.3.1 Hijacking vs. Resisting

To illustrate how drugs can lead to compulsive use, some scientists and policymakers use the metaphor of the drugs "hijacking" the brain's reward system (e.g., Hyman 2005). The hijacking that's relevant to compulsion doesn't primarily concern tolerance and withdrawal. Withdrawal is unpleasant but certainly bearable (Pickard & Pearce 2013: 171). Many addicts get clean, which requires going through withdrawal either on their own or in a rehab facility. If brain dysfunction in addiction causes loss of control, it arguably arises from intense cravings, which can persist even after withdrawal, during long periods of abstinence. So, if there is hijacking it would presumably be the sensitization, not suppression, of the mesolimbic dopamine pathway.

One glaring problem with the compulsion claim is that drug use is often demonstrably *resistible*, even in severe cases of addiction. Some users deliberately go through withdrawal to reduce their tolerance and once again experience a high from smaller, cheaper doses. Others temporarily halt use to achieve or maintain other goals, such as gainful employment or relationship repair (Heyman 2009; Hart 2013). Such deliberate abstinence has also been demonstrated in controlled studies. Participants addicted to cocaine and other drugs will regularly turn down a free dose in favor of a small monetary reward (e.g., Higgins et al. 1994). The use of such incentives to reward abstinence forms the basis of rather successful treatment programs known as "contingency management" (Stitzer & Petry 2006). That is a marked contrast with other brain disorders. "Imagine," as Satel and Lilienfeld put it, "promising a reward to people with Alzheimer's if they can keep their dementia from worsening" (2013: 63).

Of course, exertions of self-control among addicts are often temporary. Flanagan writes of his struggles with substance abuse:

> Even at the end there was some control that came in the form of maintenance so that I could minimally do my job. Very minimally. After class I could drink vodka, which I preferred to beer. This pathetically degraded self-control was pretty much all the control I had left and then only sometimes. (Flanagan 2011: 277)

Resisting temptation is exhausting. Loss of control might be inevitable, just as strained muscles will eventually give out and overworked athletes are bound to make mistakes (Levy 2007: 213; Sripada 2018).

Nevertheless, loss of control can't always be inevitable, since many users who constantly battle cravings manage to quit, as Flanagan eventually did. Some even experience "spontaneous remission," in which they recover in the absence of any treatment (Walters 2000). Most addicts appear to eventually "mature out" by the age of 30 (Winick 1962; Blanco et al. 2013). Getting married and becoming a parent, for example, are both associated with reductions in cocaine and heroin use (Heinz et al. 2009). So it's not as though loss of control is inevitable or that self-control is confined to unusual, rare, or contrived circumstances.

To be clear, other elements of the disease model can explain spontaneous recovery and maturing out. Our bodies regularly recover from infectious diseases over time without treatment (Kennett 2013). Recovery in addiction, however, requires control over cravings. Thus, the compulsion claim within the disease model remains difficult to square with common forms of recovery, deliberate abstinence, and other successful executions of self-control by individuals in the throes of addiction. In light of such evidence, Hanna Pickard concludes: "however hard it is for addicts to control their use, and however important it is for others to recognize and respect this struggle, addicts are not in fact compelled to use but have choice over their consumption in many circumstances" (2017: 171).

5.3.2 A Difference in Degree

Perhaps the compulsion claim could be weakened. The National Institute on Drug Abuse does say that its use of the term "addiction" is restricted to *severe* forms of substance use disorder (NIDA 2020: 4; Volkow & Koob 2015). Intense cravings are more difficult to resist than moderate ones, particularly if they persistently dominate an addict's mental life (Sripada 2018). A hyperactive mesolimbic dopamine pathway can affect both the intensity and frequency of cravings. If sufficiently sensitized, this brain circuit could yield significantly diminished control in severe cases.

However, it's difficult to cleave cases into distinct categories when they lie on a continuum. The difference between mild and extreme dependence is one of *degree*, not kind. The neuroscientist Marc Lewis (who has personally struggled with addiction) makes the point well with a metaphor: "Big, strong horses might seem qualitatively distinct from small, weak horses. But they're not. They're just bigger and stronger" (2017: 168). Arbitrarily restricting the term "addiction" to extreme cases courts confusion, since we normally apply the term more broadly. Better instead to adopt a more nuanced approach to substance use disorder, as with other mental disorders (see Chapter 4). Then we can include all relevant cases, provided we recognize the great heterogeneity among them.

Whether extreme or mild, cravings don't force an addict to use like a mindless robot. A hyperactive dopamine pathway works by representing the drug as *rewarding*, which leads to a kind of reasoning. Consider how the legendary musician, Eric Clapton, described his cravings as a kind of rationalization:

> My selective memory of what drinking was like told me that standing at the bar in a pub, on a summer's evening with a long, tall glass of lager and lime was heaven, and I chose not to remember the nights on which I had sat with a bottle of vodka, a gram of coke and a shotgun, contemplating suicide. (Clapton 2007: 215)

Similar narratives are given by those whose drug of choice soothes anxieties. Although Flanagan describes using alcohol and benzodiazepines as often feeling automatic and "unstoppable," the substances provided a deeply satisfying reward: "*I felt release from being scared and anxious*" (Flanagan 2011: 275). Rather than irresistible compulsion, it seems addiction "enslaves by appeal, rather than by brute force" as Gary Watson once put it (1999: 11).

There is not only a continuum within the category of substance use disorder but also a continuity with those outside of it. The mesolimbic dopamine pathway becomes hyperactive in addiction—that is, active to a greater degree than in normal life—but that doesn't necessarily amount to this pathway being damaged or fundamentally rewired. Cravings look like the kinds of rationalizations that fuel all manner of temptations (May 2018a: Ch. 7; Sripada 2022b; more on this in Chapter 8). As Neil Levy puts it, neuroscience suggests that the loss of control in addiction "is a more dramatic version of the kind of loss to which we are all subject, when we find ourselves giving in to temptation" (2007: 215; see also Watson 1999; Clarke-Doane & Tabb 2022). It seems addiction is no exception to the cognitive continuity we see across other mental disorders: the neurotypical and atypical are more alike psychologically than they might seem at first blush (Chapter 4). Similar to other circumstances in life, addiction's relation to agency is nuanced.

5.4 Is Addiction a Brain Disease?

We've landed on the idea that addiction can constrain self-control, but only sometimes and to varying degrees. This more nuanced conception of agency in addiction might be compatible with viewing it as a brain disease. Although proponents of that model often insist that addicts lose control and that relapse is inevitable, such claims aren't necessary. Calling something a "disease" doesn't mean that those afflicted can't control it. People can deliberately infect themselves with influenza. And having the flu doesn't mean patients can't control whether they get better or contract it again. Imagine someone who doesn't bother to wash his hands, exercise, eat well, or get vaccinated. Once ill, he chooses not to rest, drink fluids, or take his medication properly. These are free choices amid disease, which suggests the two can come apart.

Regardless of whether addiction impairs self-control, the disease label could be justified by dysfunction in the mesolimbic dopamine pathway (Holton & Berridge 2013; Berridge 2017). Perhaps one could draw an analogy to a brain disease like Parkinson's (see Chapter 3). Similar to that movement disorder, addiction might involve dysfunction in brain circuits that only sometimes impair control to some degree, depending on the stage of the disease, the task at hand, the time of day, and many other features of the patient's mental health. Addicts don't choose to have cravings any more than a Parkinson's patient chooses to have tremors in her hand. But both individuals can exert varying degrees of control over how they respond to symptoms. Such a nuanced conception of control would still allow the disease model to say that addicts need treatment for brain dysfunction.

Let's now turn to these other elements of the brain disease model, which are more central to it anyhow. Setting aside compulsion, there remain two key claims: (1) addiction principally involves *dysfunction*, and (2) it's in the *brain*. We will evaluate each in turn.

5.4.1 Dysfunction vs. Normality

Is addiction appropriately characterized as dysfunction in a bodily system? Repeated ingestion of addictive substances does seem to cause long-term (even if reversible) changes in the brain, particularly the mesolimbic dopamine pathway.

However, drugs don't appear to damage this pathway so much as inflate or suppress its normal responses. Tolerance and withdrawal appear to be mechanisms of *homeostasis* (specifically through allostasis)—the body's ongoing attempt to maintain stable internal states despite changes introduced from the environment outside of the body. The brain responds this way whenever an unusually high amount of any substance is regularly introduced into the body. And craving seems to result from the normal mechanism of reward learning, which is not so much hijacked in addiction as it is ramped up. The mesolimbic dopamine pathway becomes more sensitive than normal to reward cues. Thus, drug-induced changes in the brain might be different only in degree from normal physiological processes.

Indeed, the neuroscience might support our tendency to apply the term "addiction" to habits that don't rise to the level of problematic substance use. Even if you've never been addicted to illegal drugs or alcohol, chances are you consider yourself addicted on some level to caffeine from coffee (or tea or energy drinks). When you first had coffee, you felt the high, including a spike in energy and motivation. Now you need many more cups of java to feel such effects (tolerance). Despite having little sleep one night, a couple of cups could perk you up, but not anymore. Now you've grown to simply depend on coffee to function normally (dependence), especially in the morning and after the post-lunch slump. Even with a good night's rest, an absence of coffee can leave you feeling sluggish and irritable with a characteristic headache (withdrawal). Even if you've never experienced a day without coffee, you surely yearn for a caffeinated beverage at the usual times, and when it's unavailable your mind becomes preoccupied by thoughts of how to procure some (craving). The cravings are even more palpable if you try to quit, which makes relapse more likely. The influential food writer Michael Pollan (2021) describes this process by going through it himself (in his delightful book *This Is Your Mind on Plants*).

Of course, saying you're "addicted" to caffeine can feel a bit inappropriate. It doesn't count as substance use disorder, because physical dependence on caffeine doesn't tend to cause serious problems in life. But the physiological differences between caffeine and cocaine dependence seem to be one of degree, not kind. Each involves normal brain mechanisms of neuroplasticity that arise from homeostasis, reward learning, and other vital processes, just in response to more or less extreme parameters (Lewis 2015). Recognizing the parallels doesn't belie the extreme differences in degree or make it inappropriate to treat substance use disorder but not caffeine addiction. We can recognize that mustangs and ponies are both horses without forgetting that one is considerably more unruly than the other.

Whether regular coffee drinkers are truly addicted might be beside the point if the neural changes in drug addiction are just more extreme versions of normal neural changes. Lewis, a staunch critic of the disease model, goes so far to say that the "kind of brain changes seen in addiction also show up when people become absorbed in a sport, join a political movement, or become obsessed with their sweetheart or their kids" (2015: 26; see Burkett & Young 2012).

One might reply that normal mechanisms become dysfunctional when taken to extremes. Cravings are a normal motivational mechanism, but the extremes to which they are taken in severe addiction might be more akin to craving food after weeks of starvation (Berridge 2017: 32). However, although starvation is terrible, it's not a disease. A normal mechanism of the brain is merely operating in unusual conditions. Similarly, ordinary choice and addiction might be explained by the same brain mechanisms, just as "the diurnal cool breezes at evening and the once in a lifetime hurricane are explained by the same physical principles" (Heyman 2009: vii).

We should all agree that severe forms of addiction cause dysfunction of some sort, either in one's body or circumstances. The question is whether that dysfunction is appropriately labeled a "disease." Settling that question depends on whether the dysfunction is primarily physiological, rather than, say, social or economic. So let's consider whether the dysfunction lies fundamentally in brain circuits or elsewhere.

5.4.2 Beyond Brain Dysfunction

Even if addictive substances do cause dysfunction, it might not lie primarily in the drug's effects on the brain. Neural dysfunction could be necessary for addiction, but not sufficient. In that case, it seems inappropriate to say that addiction is a disease (Levy 2013) or at the very least it wouldn't be a *brain* disease.

Leshner (1997) used the metaphor of addiction resulting from a switch being thrown in the brain. If there is such a switch, however, it isn't always thrown by drug use. Only about 10–25% of people become addicted after using alcohol, opioids, and other addictive substances (Grant & Dawson 1998; Schlag 2020). Perhaps that's not a problem for the disease model. Alzheimer's is no less a disease if it afflicts only a fraction of the population (Kennett 2013). Nevertheless, the brain disease model would only then apply to a rather restricted set of cases (Pickard 2022).

Low rates of addiction among those who have tried drugs also provide perspective on what *kind* of disease addiction could be in these special cases. It would be less like malaria and more like cystic fibrosis. Those who become addicted are susceptible not primarily because they came into contact with a substance, but rather because of their genes and other circumstances.

The low rates of addiction also suggest that the mere increase in dopamine can't be the only, or even the primary, explanation for addiction. Many of the standard medications used for the treatment of attention-deficit/hyperactivity disorder (ADHD), such as Ritalin and Adderall, are similar to methamphetamine and likewise increase dopamine directly. Yet these stimulants are rarely abused by patients and aren't associated with other substance abuse (Hechtman & Greenfield 2003; cited in Hart 2013: 91). Other factors must be necessary for the addiction "switch" to be thrown.

There is ample evidence that environmental conditions contribute greatly to addiction, even when chemical dependence is held constant. When lab rats addicted to morphine are given an opportunity to drink regular water or water laced with the narcotic, they initially seem to compulsively consume the latter. However, it's no surprise that the animals in such studies regularly prefer to get high, since they're typically kept alone in boring cages. Like humans, rats are deeply curious and social creatures. In the 1970s, Bruce Alexander and his collaborators suspected that rats would actually prefer regular water to morphine if alternative sources of enjoyment were available. In several experiments, the researchers found that rats addicted to morphine tend to prefer regular over morphine-laced water while living in a large open box with other rats, but not when isolated in a standard laboratory cage (Alexander et al. 1978). An attempt to exactly replicate this famous "Rat Park" study failed to reproduce the same results (Petrie 1996). However, many other subsequent experiments have demonstrated that "environmental enrichment" makes rats less inclined to use a range of drugs, including heroin and methamphetamine (e.g., Sikora et al. 2018).

Environmental factors are paramount for sobriety in humans too. While fighting in the Vietnam War, many American soldiers used heroin, and nearly 20% became addicted. A leading psychiatric researcher, Lee Robbins, studied hundreds of Vietnam veterans for several years upon their return to the United States in 1974 (Robins et al. 2010). She and her team found that remarkably few of the vets became readdicted in the years following their return home—only 2% after three years. It's not that heroin wasn't available; half of the soldiers who were addicted overseas had used the drug again in America. What's more, recovery was common regardless of whether a vet had received prior treatment for addiction in Vietnam. The findings suggest that living in stressful conditions (like war) is a powerful cause of addiction and that a more hospitable environment facilitates recovery.

Of course, genuine diseases can be responsive to changes in environment too. Travelers can be at greater risk of contracting an infectious disease in one country compared to when they return home. Similarly, the symptoms of a chronic disease like celiac can subside in gluten-free environments. But the brain disease model describes addiction as a chronic illness that persists even in favorable circumstances. That's certainly not what was observed in either the Vietnam vets or the rodents in Rat Park.

Another key cause of addiction is the presence of other mental disorders. Substance abuse often serves as a form of self-medication by combating symptoms like anxiety and depression. Users also struggle with personality disorders, such as borderline and anti-social personality disorders, that come with symptoms such as impulsivity that make it difficult to resist *all* impulses, including drug cravings. For decades, clinicians have been aware that personality disorders frequently occur with substance use disorder—that is, they are *co-occurring* or "comorbid." Although the prevalence of personality disorder is low in the general population (about 10–15%), one systematic review estimates that among patients being treated for substance use disorder the rate is 57% (Parmar & Kaloiya 2018). Moreover, personality disorder predicts a worse response to addiction treatment. As one philosopher-psychiatrist duo put it: "The stereotype of addiction as a chronic disorder, with little hope of recovery . . . is [only] an accurate picture for psychiatric patients" (Pickard & Pearce 2013: 166).

Of course, brain dysfunction might underly mental disorders. The problem of co-occurrence is that other mental disorders contribute heavily to addiction *above and beyond* drug consumption and its effects on dopamine and reward pathways—beyond the supposed "chemical hook" of drugs, as the journalist Johann Hari (2015) has put it. Opponents of the brain disease model object to its claim that the addict is "someone whose mind (read: brain) has been altered fundamentally *by drugs*" (Leshner 1997: 46; emphasis added).

The same goes for environmental causes of addiction. They also ultimately affect neurobiological processes. A hostile environment contributes to addiction by producing activity in the brain that the user experiences as stress. But stress, trauma, and other such psychological ailments are distinct from the supposed chemical hook of drugs. What the Vietnam vets and the rodents in Rat Park suggest is that there are factors *other than the drug's specific effects on the brain* that contribute significantly to addiction. Of course, addictive substances have some effects directly related to these other factors. Drugs can produce pleasurable effects that reduce the stresses of war, socioeconomic hardship, and so on. The point is that individuals without these other problems are much less likely to become addicted or to relapse once addicted, *despite also taking drugs* with their characteristic effects on the brain. The objection to the brain disease model here is that, even if addiction involves dysfunction, it is not *only* or primarily *drug-induced* brain dysfunction. Compare: poverty has detrimental effects on the brain, but it would be misleading to call poverty a brain disease.

5.5 Addiction as a Disorder

Each element of the brain disease model faces formidable objections (see Table 5.2). Might it nevertheless be useful for reducing the suffering experienced by addicts? Perhaps the disease label can be morally, even if not scientifically, motivated. Before turning to an alternative model, let's consider whether conceptualizing addiction as a brain disease is all that beneficial.

5.5.1 Is the Disease Label Helpful?

Proponents of the brain disease model sometimes acknowledge its limitations but stress its benefits, such as reducing stigma and promoting more effective treatments (e.g., Volkow & Koob 2015; Berridge 2017). We certainly shouldn't ignore the immense suffering that substance abuse can cause users and their loved ones. Drug overdoses are now the leading cause of death among Americans under the age of 50 (Katz 2017). In 2021, the United States reached a tragic milestone of over 100,000 overdose deaths in a 12-month period (CDC 2021). Such harms of addiction plague many countries, yet the condition is highly stigmatized throughout the world, which is a barrier for addicts to obtain treatment, housing, employment, benefits, and thus recovery.

Table 5.2 Claims and Criticisms of the Brain Disease Model

Element	Thesis	Objections
Disease	Addiction involves physiological dysfunction akin to disease.	Addiction involves normal brain mechanisms (e.g., homeostasis, reinforcement learning) that are responding to unusually strong rewards.
Brain	The dysfunction is primarily in brain circuits that addictive substances manipulate, and treatment should target them.	Factors other than drug use contribute greatly to addiction (stressful conditions, lack of social support, financial instability, other mental disorders).
Compulsion	Addiction yields irresistible cravings to use.	Many addicts exhibit control over use even without treatment (through deliberate abstinence, spontaneous remission, maturing out, etc.).

Perhaps a brain disease model can help address the opioid crisis and other tragedies of addiction. As U.S. Surgeon General admiral Vivek Murthy put it in the *New England Journal of Medicine*: "We can use our position as leaders in society to help change how our country sees addiction—not as a personal failing but as a chronic disease of the brain that requires compassion and care" (2016: 2415).

This *moral argument* might seem fallacious on its face, since a scientific theory isn't true because it reduces suffering. But the argument might not be for the truth of the disease *model* but the usefulness of the disease *label* (Pickard 2022). Advocates of "harm reduction" strategies—such as needle exchange programs and supervised injection sites—might urge us to focus most on what helps mitigate suffering. The hope, it seems, is that labeling addiction a "disease" will help to achieve *three noble goals*:

a) reduce stigma,
b) improve treatment, and
c) reform drug laws and policies.

The disease label might seem well-suited to achieve these goals, since it implies that addiction is a disease in need of treatment, not a choice deserving punishment. Yet, even if we're happy to turn from truth to utility, the disease label arguably frustrates more than it facilitates these laudable goals.

First, calling something a "disease" doesn't necessarily protect against stigma. Plenty of diseases are stigmatized, such as leprosy and sexually transmitted diseases, particularly HIV (Pickard 2022). Studies do suggest that the medicalization of mental disorders generally reduces the public's propensity to blame patients, but biomedical labels also stoke more fear of patients, including addicts, as dangerous and unpredictable (e.g., Kelly et al. 2021).

Second, the disease label is disempowering. Describing substance abuse as a brain disease has been shown to reduce attitudes of blame toward addicts, but such biomedical descriptions also make addicts and clinicians less optimistic about the prospects of recovery (Kelly et al. 2021). Addicts need to be encouraged and empowered, not deflated. A defeatist attitude is counterproductive, a self-fulfilling prophecy. Yet the focus on irresistible cravings and analogies to chronic illnesses like heart disease suggests that overcoming addiction is nearly impossible. Recovery clearly requires agency, which conflicts with the language of disease and compulsion (Pickard & Pearce 2013; Lewis 2015). The idea isn't that addicts should simply stop using through sheer force of will, which would be like asking someone with depression to just stop being sad. Rather, patients can be empowered to exercise agency over their circumstances, habits, and overall mental health—not unlike neurotypical individuals (recall Chapter 2, Sec. 2.4). One can choose to see a therapist, take medication, exercise, take up productive hobbies, join a support group, continue to attend meetings, cut ties with enablers, read self-help books, and so on.

Third, the disease label might also support harmful drug policy by neglecting other causes. Brain chemistry becomes the primary focus of attention and funding, both of which are finite resources (Satel & Lilienfeld 2013). Of course, identifying a condition as a disease is compatible with studying or treating its social and economic causes. Researchers actively investigate potential environmental causes of cancer, heart disease, and Parkinson's, from pollutants to poverty.

However, when one looks at the present state of addiction research, social and economic factors seem to stand in the shadow of the brain's limelight (Grifell & Hart 2018). Prioritizing neurobiology in this way is a rather intentional effect of the brain disease model.

The issue becomes one of social justice, as addicts' economic hardships, social support networks, and general mental health are not prioritized. The neuroscientist Carl Hart goes so far to say that the brain disease model "contributes to unrealistic, costly, and harmful drug policies" (Grifell & Hart 2018: 160). As an African American who grew up in the projects of Miami, Hart argues that the brain disease model does little for his community, which is governed by a system that has "an irrational focus on eliminating certain drugs" that ultimately promotes "a vicious cycle of incarceration and isolation from mainstream society" (2013: 329). Combating cravings and withdrawal symptoms might be pointless in any community without addressing other social and economic factors, including unemployment, discrimination, alienation, and trauma.

The potentially harmful consequences of the disease model are compounded by its need to focus narrowly on more severe cases. The label "disease" is most appropriate at the extremes of addiction when prolonged drug use leads to brain and bodily changes so extreme that restoration to normal is possible only with medical intervention. However, the three noble goals include milder forms of substance abuse as well. The injured athlete who abuses prescription opioids or the bank teller with an increasingly expensive cocaine habit also don't deserve stigma or excessive punishment.

5.5.2 Disease vs. Disorder

If addiction isn't a brain disease, then what is it? Let's start by peeling away the elements of the disease model to see what's left. Suppose we drop the claim that addicts lose control and that their condition is primarily a matter of drug-induced brain dysfunction. Now we're left with the core of the disease model, its most essential element that cannot be jettisoned: conceptualization of the phenomenon as a *disease*. That claim too is subject to criticism, as we've seen. However, a slight modification might be viable. Simply opt for the label *disorder*, as it is in the DSM, without defining addiction as a chronic disease that nullifies self-control (see, e.g., Heyman 2009; Wakefield 2020).

The distinction between disease and disorder is subtle but important. Consider Alzheimer's (discussed in Chapter 3), which is clearly a brain disease. There is a categorical difference between those with Alzheimer's and those without it. Neurotypical individuals don't have a mild form of Alzheimer's, and they aren't in any sense exposed to the disease. In contrast, the "disorder" label, which focuses on symptoms not underlying disease, embraces heterogeneity within the category and continuity with those outside of it. Unlike your friend with generalized anxiety disorder, the troublesome anxiety you tend to experience in life might not be sufficient for a diagnosis, but your symptoms are different in degree, not kind. Similarly, being severely addicted to cocaine is importantly different from milder dependence—or even casual use that one can more easily curb—but a disorder model allows us to view these scenarios as lying on the same spectrum.

A disorder model also helps explain the similarities between substance abuse and so-called *behavioral addictions*. Some people seem to become addicted to gambling, sex, pornography, gaming, social media, and even fasting—all without ingesting any drugs that increase dopamine. Some research does suggest that behavioral addictions involve similar brain changes to those observed in regular users of cocaine, alcohol, and other drugs of abuse (Brewer & Potenza 2008). That's predictable. Persistent gambling and heroin abuse have much in common. Both involve powerful reinforcement learning, which results in a myopic focus on one form of reward to the exclusion of others. Both are surely disorders in the sense that they cause the patient significant and persistent distress. Yet gambling doesn't involve ingesting a drug that artificially manipulates dopamine. There are "no chemical hooks on a craps table," as Hari (2015) puts it. Addiction does have a genetic basis to be sure, but so does OCD and other psychiatric conditions that we label as disorders, not diseases. The disorder model allows us to emphasize similarities among these various conditions.

The disorder model doesn't preclude brain-based treatments, such as pharmaceuticals and even deep brain stimulation (discussed in

Chapter 3). Recent clinical trials suggest that psychedelics are a promising treatment for addiction (Koslowski et al. 2021). A disorder model is free to incorporate such brain-based treatments without focusing on them to the exclusion of social and economic factors or other features of one's mental health. Indeed, psychedelics don't target dopamine and aren't used in isolation; rather, they are augmented with therapy in order to provide insight into one's circumstances and how one responds to them (more on this in Chapter 7).

Importantly, a disorder model is compatible with the three noble goals. Theorists often assume that without conceptualizing addiction as a brain disease we're left with the old, moralized approach in which efforts to curb addiction trade only in blame and punishment. But this is a false dichotomy; there is a middle path (Hart 2013; Satel & Lilienfeld 2013; Pickard 2022). On the disorder model, addicts deserve treatment and compassion, just as everyone does, but also agency and empowerment. The approach would be similar to that of other psychiatric categories, such as depression, generalized anxiety, borderline personality disorder, and phobias. We can recognize patients suffering from mental disorders as having agency while directing more compassion and support toward them than judgment and blame (see Chapter 4). The key is to again follow Pickard and *distinguish responsibility from blame* (recall Chapter 4, Sec. 4.4). Addicts can be responsible for the choice to use—or to procure the means to using—without it being appropriate to chastise, punish, or admonish them. Blaming is a choice too, on the part of clinicians, friends, family, and lawmakers (Pickard 2017; Heyman 2009: 20).

Yet there are ample reasons to curb blame toward addicts. Many clinicians, users, and loved ones report that compassion, support, and the expectation of responsibility promote recovery while anger and blame promote relapse. One rather successful treatment for addiction and other psychiatric disorders is membership in "therapeutic communities" in which both clinicians and patients work together to hold members accountable while being careful to withhold judgment—responsibility without blame (Pickard & Pearce 2013; Pickard 2017). With responsibility comes agency, control, and support, not ridicule: *You've got this*; not *you're helpless*.

5.6 Conclusion

Let's return to Julie Eldred, who was judged to have willfully violated her parole by using opioids again. Our analysis of addiction suggests that it's generally appropriate to hold addicts like Julie accountable for relapse. Addiction is probably not best construed as a brain disease that abolishes self-control. Abstaining is extremely difficult, to be sure. In more advanced stages of substance use disorder, it might make sense to speak of episodes in which one "loses control," because that is certainly how users can feel. However, it appears that addicts are able to control their drug use to varying degrees. Of course, Julie deserves compassion and understanding, but such attitudes are compatible with responsibility and accountability. Perhaps, as the National Association of Drug Court Professionals has maintained, a judge's ability to impose consequences for relapses is integral to the long process of overcoming addiction.

Despite widespread acceptance of the brain disease model, different strands of converging research suggest that addiction results from factors other than drug-induced changes in the brain. As Julie tells it, her drug use was fueled in part by the desire to cope with anxiety and depression. These prior conditions can be appropriately conceptualized as mental disorders, but they are not brain diseases, or at least not *drug-induced* brain diseases. Failure to give such other factors their due could yield ineffective treatments and unsound drug policies.

In the end, even if the disease label isn't harmful, it seems superfluous. All of the research and arguments we've encountered are compatible with conceptualizing addiction as a *disorder*, similar to major depression or generalized anxiety disorder. As we saw in the previous chapter, being diagnosed with a mental disorder doesn't necessarily preclude agency, responsibility, and accountability, which can often be decoupled from blame and judgment. In some cases, it might be inappropriate to hold an addict responsible for relapsing or even for an unconscionable crime. But the excuse will lie in some particular features of the individual and their circumstances, not the mere fact that they have been diagnosed with substance use disorder.

In the next chapter, we turn our attention to moral character. But we continue to blur the boundaries between normal and abnormal brain function by discussing psychopathy and the role of reason and emotion in moral judgment.

PART IV
CHARACTER

6
Moral Judgment

So far we have focused mostly on autonomy and responsibility. We now turn to distinct but related questions about moral character. Even if free will is an illusion, human beings would still make moral judgments that either guide or fail to guide their behavior. Saints are saintly and jerks are insufferable, regardless of whether it's of their own free will. Our questions now are: How do we know right from wrong? How can we become morally better?

Neuroscience helps answer such questions. By uncovering the psychological processes that underly our moral beliefs and decisions, we better understand when it all goes well or poorly. A scientific understanding of moral knowledge can then aid the development of safe artificial intelligence, such as autonomous vehicles. We can even draw conclusions about whether we should trust our gut feelings in ethics and politics. These investigations set us up in the next chapter to ask whether and how to enhance ourselves morally. Compare the question of how best to improve a vehicle's fuel efficiency. To answer that question, it's wise to pop open the hood and make sure you know how it works. In this chapter, we look under the skull and examine how moral attitudes are formed, in both neurotypical and pathological cases. We begin with a particularly disturbing case of the latter.

6.1 Dugan's Defense

In 1983, 10-year-old Jeanine Nicarico was home alone sick with the flu. At the same time, Brian Dugan was trolling the Chicago suburb for homes to burglarize. He broke into the Nicarico residence, kidnapped Jeanine and later sexually assaulted and beat her to death. This wasn't the first (or last) time Dugan engaged in abduction, sexual violence, or murder. He was eventually imprisoned for other crimes to which he confessed, including the killing of Jeanine. Remarkably, this particular confession ultimately exonerated two other men who were wrongfully convicted of Jeanine's murder, adding another unethical dimension to this tragic case.

Dugan is a bona fide psychopath. He describes himself as such and displays the characteristic traits. He is manipulative, prone to impulsive violence, and lacks genuine empathy and remorse. Dugan's brain scans also indicate the characteristic neurological profile of this personality disorder, namely abnormal function in brain regions that are activated when ordinary people think about moral statements and dilemmas. Defense lawyers argued that Dugan should be spared the death penalty because he wasn't fully in control of his actions. Nevertheless, Dugan was sentenced to death in 2009, though he is now serving life in prison because Illinois abolished capital punishment in 2011.

Psychopathy (sometimes called *sociopathy*) is a personality disorder, though it's not listed in the *Diagnostic and Statistical Manual of Mental Disorders* (DSM). The condition is similar to, but more narrow than, anti-social personality disorder, which does appear in the DSM. Psychopaths are not just callous and anti-social but also tend to lack moral conscience. Among other vices, they are characteristically shameless, remorseless, and exhibit a superficial charm that allows them to manipulate others who are often ultimately left battered or destitute. They represent only about 1% of the general population but make up approximately 25% of the prison population (Hare 1993). People often associate the term "psychopath" with serial killers like Ted Bundy, but such extreme cases don't represent the norm. Often psychopaths are simply indifferent to harming others and to the consequences that follow.

Diminished control was debated during Dugan's trial, but ethicists have tended to argue that if psychopaths aren't fully accountable it's because they don't properly understand right from wrong (e.g., Fine & Kennett 2004; Levy 2007; Shoemaker 2015). Recall the M'Naughten Rule for the insanity defense, which states that defendants aren't culpable if, due to a mental disorder, they either don't know what they're doing or don't know that it's wrong (Chapter 4). Some psychopaths do exhibit slight difficulties distinguishing moral rules from mere conventions (Aharoni et al. 2012). We can also see from interviews that some struggle to properly deploy moral concepts and reasons in conversation—e.g., misusing words like "guilt" and "feeling bad" about a crime (Hare 1993; Kennett & Fine 2008). Inmates with psychopathy also tend to give atypical responses to emotionally charged moral dilemmas (Koenigs et al. 2012).

Our primary question won't be whether psychopaths like Dugan should be deemed not guilty by reason of insanity. Instead, we'll use psychopathy as a springboard for exploring what normal versus abnormal moral judgment looks like in the brain. The chapter is broken up into two main parts. First, we'll examine both typical and atypical brains and compare the role of reason versus emotion in moral judgment. The neurobiological evidence suggests that the distinction is fraught. Second, we turn to the related issue of whether we can trust our gut feelings in ethics, particularly those that lead us to make moral judgments that privilege the needs of the few over the needs of the many. If we should distrust those intuitions, then perhaps we should accept utilitarianism, a rather counterintuitive moral theory that counsels us always to elevate the needs of the many over the needs of the few. Such an ambitious conclusion, as we'll see, isn't clearly forced upon us by the evidence. Finally, we'll return to Dugan's case and see that our investigation suggests that psychopaths might be morally incompetent, but only in extreme cases. As usual, mental capacities come in degrees that do not switch off or on with a psychiatric diagnosis.

6.2 Are Gut Feelings Necessary?

The psychological and neurological profile of psychopaths seems to suggest that emotions are necessary for normal, competent moral judgment. However, the neurobiology of morality increasingly belies any sharp distinction between emotion and reason. We'll examine both neurotypical moral judgment and how it deviates in abnormal brains.

6.2.1 The Moral Brain

Since the late 1990s, neuroscientists have studied how moral judgment works in the brains of typical adults. Moral judgments, compared to other kinds of judgments, tended to produce greater activity in a spatially distributed group of brain areas: the amygdala, the cingulate cortex, portions of the prefrontal cortex, and portions of the temporal lobe (see Figure 6.1). Other brain regions are not irrelevant to morality, but this same set consistently crops up in many other studies that use a diverse range of measures and methods, from neuroimaging to brain stimulation. Systematic reviews of the literature suggest that this network of areas represents a well-corroborated picture of at least some core forms of moral cognition (Moll et al. 2005; Greene 2009; Churchland 2011; Demaree-Cotton & Kahane 2018; May et al. 2022).

It turns out that in psychopaths these very same brain regions typically exhibit abnormal structure and function. Proper development of these structures is perhaps never fully achieved for individuals with psychopathy. Part of the explanation is genetic, such as mutations that disrupt neurotransmitters. But other important factors include adverse circumstances, including childhood trauma, neglect, and even

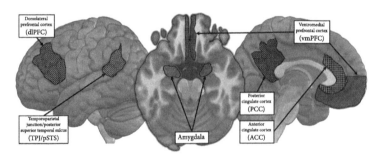

Figure 6.1 Key Brain Areas in Moral Cognition

Depicted are some key areas of the human brain commonly regarded as essential for moral judgment and behavior. We'll encounter many of these areas throughout the book. The left image views the outside of the brain from the side. The middle image is a view of the brain from below (inferior view). The image on the right shows the center of the brain viewed from the side (sagittal view).

Source: May et al. 2022. Reprinted with permission from MIT Press.

lead exposure (Blair 2007; Kiehl 2006; Kiehl & Sinnott-Armstrong 2013; Glenn & Raine 2014).

Let's examine these brain areas one by one and attempt to uncover the role they play in shaping evaluations of right and wrong. The first region is the *amygdala*, a pair of small almond-shaped nodes deep in the brain. These nodes, along with the limbic system of which they're a part, have classically been associated with emotion, particularly fear. But we now know the amygdala is involved more broadly in assessing the significance of an object or event—e.g., whether it's valuable or threatening. The amygdala is thus a region crucial for many processes of learning in light of rewards or punishments, and dysfunction early in development naturally leads to a host of cognitive and behavioral problems. Amygdala dysfunction might explain psychopaths' indifference to the suffering of others, as well as their difficulty learning from punishment.

Now consider the *ventromedial prefrontal cortex* (vmPFC), which is roughly the inner underside of the "prefrontal" cortex (the front of the frontal lobe). The frontal lobe generally subserves one's ability to plan and make complex choices, which reflects one's personality and character traits (recall the case of Phineas Gage in Chapter 3). These specific portions of the prefrontal cortex behind the eyes seem to integrate gut feelings that guide judgment and decision-making. Patients with vmPFC damage often develop what neurologist Antonio Damasio (1994) dubs "acquired sociopathy." This label is misleading, however, since the clinical profile is rather different from that of psychopathy. Far from callous or remorseless, adults who acquire damage to the vmPFC primarily suffer from poor decision-making that is not necessarily anti-social or harmful to others. Patients seem to retain many of their intellectual capacities; they even give typical responses about how one ought to make hypothetical choices (Saver & Damasio 1991).

The problem instead is a shortage of gut feelings that help guide decisions about what to do in the moment. Compared to neurotypical individuals, vmPFC patients typically have difficulty making a wide range of decisions, from how to rack up points in a card game to which variety of apples to purchase at the grocery store. Consider two patients as examples:

- **Elliot**, one of Damasio's (1994: Ch. 3) patients, had an orange-sized tumor that originated near his nasal cavity. Removal of the tumor also resulted in damage to his frontal lobe (primarily orbital and medial portions). After surgery, Elliot remained intelligent in many respects but struggled with planning and decision-making. He was eventually fired from his job because he could no longer stay on task and properly manage his time. His relationships suffered as well, from what some described as his foolish and irrational behavior, leading to multiple marriages and divorce.
- **Tammy Myers** presents a similar form of decision-making deficit. A terrible motorcycle accident resulted in damage to her orbitofrontal cortex, which overlaps with the vmPFC. Tammy reports that "she often spends all day on the sofa" not primarily because she is depressed but rather because even simple decisions about what to do next are agonizing (Eagleman 2015: 119).

These patients seem to struggle with decisions about what to do *oneself* in a *particular situation* (Kennett & Fine 2008). A patient might recognize that it's healthier to buy organic fruits, but what should *she* do right *now* when the opal apples, though sprayed with pesticides, taste divine? Without gut feelings, patients seem paralyzed by the many variables present in any particular decision. Presumably it was adaptive for humans to develop emotional heuristics that motivate swift action (Yikes, a snake, back away!) than to overanalyze the situation (Is this really a poisonous snake? Maybe I should examine it first . . .).

In contrast, the decision-making deficits in psychopathy take on an anti-social character, presumably due to the presence of other brain abnormalities. Dysfunction of the vmPFC might combine with amygdala dysfunction to explain why psychopaths struggle to make moral or prudent decisions in the moment. Consider one case in which a man later diagnosed with psychopathy broke into what he thought was an empty home but found an irate resident inside who wouldn't "shut up." Instead of fleeing, the burglar calmly beat the elderly man unconscious, then took a nap on the sofa, only to be woken up later by police (Hare 1993: 91). Taking a nap at the scene of the crime or abducting a child on a whim in broad daylight are not cherry-picked examples. Such imprudence and senseless aggression are common among psychopaths (Maibom 2005), given that their self-centered impulsivity is often short-sighted and reckless.

The third brain area of interest is near the *temporoparietal junction* (TPJ), where the rear end of the temporal lobe meets the parietal lobe. This region is known for its role in understanding the minds of others, such as a person's hopes, desires, or malicious intent (Decety & Lamm 2007; Young & Dungan 2012). This capacity for "theory of mind" is primarily subserved by overlapping brain areas variously identified by different markers (e.g., the posterior superior temporal sulcus, angular gyrus, and inferior parietal lobule).

In moral cognition, researchers have primarily studied how the TPJ is involved in reasoning about intent. We often evaluate the morality of an action by whether it caused harm, but the adage "No harm, no foul" only applies in limited circumstances. As with attempted murder, malicious intent can be enough to make an act morally objectionable (indeed criminal), even if it ultimately caused no harm. An absence of malicious intent, as in cases of accidental harm, is often enough to judge a culprit less harshly, even if the outcome is tragic, such as a heartbreaking loss of life. These judgments are correlated with greater activity in the TPJ (Young et al. 2007), and even modulated when that brain area is disrupted noninvasively through transcranial magnetic stimulation (Young et al. 2010).

Now psychopaths are notorious for being conning and manipulative, which requires knowing what other people think, feel, and desire. Dysfunction of the TPJ and nearby regions, however, might explain some deficits in theory of mind. One meta-analysis suggests that individuals with psychopathic tendencies struggle to identify sad and fearful facial expressions (Marsh & Blair 2008), presumably making it difficult to appreciate displays of distress in one's victims. Individuals with psychopathy also show a reduced appreciation of the moral significance of intentional versus accidental harms (Koenigs et al. 2012). So, despite being somewhat able to read the minds of others, it makes sense that the brains of psychopaths often exhibit deficits in the relevant region of the temporal lobe.

Finally, there is the anterior portion of the *cingulate cortex*, a surface layer of the brain tucked down in between the two hemispheres of the brain. (Imagine pushing a butter knife down into the middle of a ball of dough: the surface area surrounding the knife is akin to the cingulate.) The anterior portion plays a role in attention and performance monitoring, both of which are impaired in psychopathy. We've seen that psychopaths tend to be impulsive, irresponsible, and imprudent. Combined with callousness and grandiosity, it's no wonder that individuals with this personality disorder not only regularly break the law but frequently get caught.

Overall, it's clear that regions of the "moral brain" support recognizable elements of morality (Table 6.1). Although more research is needed, we're beginning to see how these areas work together to form neurotypical moral judgments (at least about harmful acts). In one set of studies, participants viewed short videos of intentional versus accidental harms while wearing an electroencephalography (EEG) cap that records brain waves at fine-grained timescales. In a mere 60 milliseconds,

Table 6.1 Functional Contributions of Brain Areas to Moral Cognition

Brain Area	Plausible Moral Functions
Temporal cortex (especially posterior portions: angular gyrus/temporoparietal junction/posterior superior temporal sulcus)	Understanding the thoughts, feelings, desires, and intentions of others (including any malicious intent behind an action).
Amygdala	Learning and evaluating whether stimuli are threatening or valuable, including assigning a valence (positive or negative) to intentions and actions. (E.g., harming others is negative, helping is positive.)
Prefrontal cortex (especially ventromedial and dorsolateral)	Integrating the actor's mental state and action with the consequences of the action and comparing this information to general moral rules or heuristics.
Cingulate cortex (especially anterior portions)	Detecting conflicts and errors in one's expectations about moral situations or dilemmas.

participants inferred the agent's mental states using posterior portions of the temporal cortex. Just a few hundred milliseconds later, the amygdala appears to mark the harmful intent as significant, which is then fed into areas of the prefrontal cortex, at which point a moral judgment is made (Decety & Cacioppo 2012; Yoder & Decety 2014). As neuroimaging researchers have likewise found, the amygdala seems to provide an assessment of the positive or negative value of the act in question, which the prefrontal cortex then integrates with information about harmful outcomes to make an overall moral evaluation, such as condemning an act of intentional harm for personal gain (Shenhav & Greene 2014; Hutcherson et al. 2015; Salzman & Fusi 2010).

Several caveats are in order. First, our model is based on research that primarily studies harm, not other moral values, such as loyalty and fairness (see Graham et al. 2013; Parkinson et al. 2011). So at most we can say that this network subserves at least one core form of moral judgment, though one that is commonplace across most societies (Barrett et al. 2016; McNamara et al. 2019).

Second, neuroimaging studies only provide correlations between moral judgment and brain areas (see the problem of "reverse inference" in Chapter 9). However, the model is also based on corroborating causal evidence, such as brain stimulation and patients with brain damage.

Finally, talk of the "moral brain" is merely a stylistic device. There doesn't appear to be a moral module in the human brain (contra Mikhail 2011). Rather, we see domain-general circuits that facilitate moral and prudential cognition and much more still (Moll et al. 2005; Greene 2009; Churchland 2011; Arvan 2020; May et al. 2022). The brain areas central to moral cognition deploy general reasoning capacities that are simply applied to ethical situations. Theory of mind, for example, appears to be a general capacity that can be deployed in areas well beyond ethics, such as figuring out how to intimidate an opponent on the football field or learning to dance with a partner.

6.2.2 Reason vs. Emotion?

Psychopaths appear to have some deficits in moral cognition, but are they ultimately emotional or rational deficits? The comparative role of reason versus emotion in ethics is a long-standing debate among philosophers and psychologists. Yet the neuroscience suggests that it must be refined.

The traditional sentimentalist view in ethics is associated with the likes of Adam Smith and David Hume, among others. They argued that moral beliefs are like judgments of beauty in that they require certain emotions (Gill 2007). You don't need any emotional reactions to the thought that "Tehran is the capital of Iran" in order to accept it, and the same goes for the mathematical thought that "to infer the length of a right triangle's hypotenuse from the length of its other sides, one ought to use the Pythagorean theorem." But it's hard to imagine truly believing that "Yosemite valley is breathtakingly beautiful" without at least being inclined to have that distinctive feeling of awe that it inspires. Similarly, without feelings of compassion or indignation, sentimentalists think it impossible to make genuine moral judgments about helping others in need or rectifying social injustices. Contemporary defenders of the psychological thesis of *sentimentalism* likewise contend that moral cognition requires emotional responses (see, e.g., Nichols 2004: 83; Prinz 2016: 46; D'Arms & Jacboson 2014: 254; Tappolet 2016: 79).

In contrast, philosophers like Plato and Kant treat reasoning or inference as central to moral judgment and knowledge. Proponents of *rationalism* maintain that moral judgment is ultimately "the culmination of a process of reasoning" (Maibom 2010: 999; see also Kennett 2006: 70; Sauer 2017; May 2018a: 7). Emotions in their view are either merely the natural consequences of reasoning or provide just one way of instigating or facilitating inference. Of course, that's not to say that moral evaluation is always rational or reasonable. Reasoning can be downright irrational while being part of our "rational capacities."

Imagine a company aims to build military androids or autonomous vehicles with knowledge of ethics, so that the artificial intelligence (AI) can properly navigate moral dilemmas and avoid atrocities. Rationalists would expect the AI to acquire moral judgment over time if placed in an environment rich with opportunities for learning based on general inferential capacities (including theory of mind, calculating outcomes, assigning value to actions, and the ability to categorize actions as consistent with or violating norms). Rather than model moral cognition on reasoning through a mathematical proof, modern rationalists take a page from advances in AI that use deep learning algorithms to model human cognition (Scheutz & Malle 2018; Haas 2020). If the AI cannot feel emotions, sentimentalists would regard the resulting "moral knowledge" as derivative at best. Although the AI might be able to understand morality in some sense, their predicament would be analogous to how a congenitally blind person can know that ripe bananas are yellow by relying on the visual experiences of others.

The neuroscience, however, increasingly questions the dichotomy between reason and emotion. Consider the patients with vmPFC damage. As Damasio emphasizes, these cases exemplify the entanglement of reason and emotion. When learning a new task or making a decision, patients seem to have an absence or attenuation of gut feelings (or *somatic markers*) that help one settle on decisions that feel right. Without such feelings, one's ability to choose among competing options is impaired, specifically the ability to unconsciously integrate values into an overall inference about what to do right now in these particular circumstances. Some lines of research suggest that the vmPFC in mammals facilitates certain forms of reinforcement and statistical learning that are largely unconscious (e.g., Hare et al. 2008; Woodward 2016) and can be applied to moral judgment and other domains. Reason and emotion are exceedingly difficult to distinguish in these processes of judgment and decision-making.

Psychopathy likewise demonstrates a blurring of the reason/emotion dichotomy. Psychopaths clearly don't have normal emotional responses to the harm and suffering of others. Many theorists have remarked that psychopaths seem to be in some sense rational, at least in their general understanding of the world and how to go about manipulating it. A common analysis is that psychopaths thus demonstrate the necessity of emotions for a genuine understanding of right from wrong (e.g., Haidt 2001; Nichols 2004; Prinz 2016). However, the psychopath's deficits in guilt and compassion are accompanied by numerous impairments in learning and reasoning. The personality disorder is marked by irresponsibility, poor attention span, delusions of grandeur, and difficulty learning from punishment (Maibom 2005; May 2018a). Such impairments affect learning and inference throughout life, which prevent psychopaths from internalizing habits and strategies for making decisions that are ethical or prudent. So both emotional and rational deficits are entangled in the abnormal moral thought and behavior of psychopaths, which often lead not only to violence and manipulation but also imprudence and imprisonment. What we're seeing is that purportedly emotional (or broadly "affective") capacities are intertwined with reasoning capacities, though they are often unconscious.

Apparently "emotional" processes appear to be entangled in reasoning generally, provided we conceive of reason properly. Although the paradigm of reasoning is *conscious* deliberation, we must resist the urge to identify reasoning with this narrow class of mental phenomena (May 2018a; May & Kumar 2018). Unconscious cognition, even if automatic, is also a form of reasoning that can involve sophisticated mechanisms of inference. Indeed, it might help to think of reasoning more in terms of *inference*, which isn't as closely associated with conscious deliberation. For example, over time I've come to infer that smoking causes cancer on the basis of my acceptance of the scientific consensus, and I conclude that I shouldn't smoke on the same grounds. I never sat down and consciously deliberated, with my head perched on my fist in front of a chalkboard with a list of reasons. Think of reasoning or inference, then, less as going through a mathematical proof and more like recognizing that the traffic you're stuck in will make you late for an appointment, or realizing that you technically violated the rules of a game, or figuring out how exactly to turn a key to open a stubborn lock.

A blurring of the reason/emotion dichotomy might seem to trivialize the debate between rationalists and sentimentalists, but the overall picture remains friendly to a traditional form of rationalism. The picture of the moral brain that emerges is arguably of a reasoning machine that blends inference and affect (or gut feelings), not the traditional sentimentalist thesis that moral judgment is driven ultimately by specific moral emotions such as anger, compassion, guilt, and disgust, conceived as distinct from learning and inference. Twinges of affect are necessary for all forms of cognition, from judgments about ethics to judgments about which apples to purchase at the market (Huebner 2015; Seligman et al. 2016). Indeed, a growing consensus in neurobiology is that "affect is a form of cognition" (Duncan & Barrett

2007). Even if, say, the amygdala gives rise to affect, such feelings facilitate inference generally.

Recall that moral cognition arises not from a module dedicated to it but from domain-general capacities. That may well support the traditional rationalist idea that moral cognition isn't special; it involves affect in just the way that other forms of inference do (May 2023). Compare the domain-general reasoning capacities in moral cognition to more domain-*specific* brain functions. Sometimes damage to a neural circuit seems to impair rather specific capacities, such as the ability to identify animate objects but not inanimate objects. For instance, just months after traumatic brain injury or stroke, some patients struggle to name fruits and vegetables but not animals (see patient P.S. in Caramazza & Shelton 1998: 3). We don't tend to find such domain-specific deficits in moral cognition. Damage to the vmPFC might seem to selectively disrupt the normal ability to condemn intentional harm (Koenigs et al. 2007). But a more complete picture of the evidence suggests that dysfunction in the vmPFC disrupts a more general-purpose learning mechanism and accordingly exhibits a wider range of deficits. Psychopaths and patients with "acquired sociopathy" don't just provide abnormal moral judgments; they exhibit deficits in prudence, learning from punishment, and even deciding what to eat for dinner.

So does the neuroscience support rationalism or sentimentalism or something in between? We shouldn't get hung up on the labels. What's clear is that something like "gut feelings" are essential to normal moral cognition. But these are twinges of positive or negative thought—so-called *affect*—that play a crucial role in all processes of learning and inference. The resulting picture of the moral brain seems to require a central role for reason, inference, and learning. It matters little whether we call this "rationalism" or "sentimentalism" or something else entirely.

6.3 Are Gut Feelings Always Reliable?

So far the neuroscience suggests that gut feelings (or twinges of "affect") are a key component of ordinary moral cognition, something that psychopaths lack. But don't gut feelings often lead us astray in ethics?

6.3.1 From Neural Is to Moral Ought

Some philosophers and scientists have used neuroscience to draw conclusions about the reliability of moral intuitions and ultimately about which moral views we should accept. Could research on how moral judgment *does* work tell us how it *ought* to work? Philosophers at least since Hume (1739/2000) have cautioned against cavalier attempts to bridge the *is-ought gap*, but there is a way. We simply have to use science to uncover the psychological processes that drive moral judgment *and* use ethical analysis to determine whether those processes are reliable guides. Bridging the gap requires some moral assumptions.

Compare the reliability of using a compass. Suppose you're far out on a hiking trail when you drop your phone off a towering cliff while taking a summit selfie. The phone, with its handy GPS, is now destroyed. You know that if you could just travel north, you'll get back to the trail head. So you whip out a compass, see which direction the needle points, and judge that it's the right direction to travel. Not so fast, says a fellow hiker who happens to be an orienteering enthusiast. The compass needle points toward *magnetic* north, not true north. The process by which you're orienting yourself on the trail is unreliable (you need to factor in the declination of your area and calculate true north). In this way, discovering the process or method one is using can undermine or "debunk" the resulting judgment or decision.

Similarly, if we discover that some of our moral beliefs are formed by questionable processes, then the beliefs are called into question, unless we can use a better method to support them. Such debunking arguments take roughly the following schematic form (Nichols 2014):

Debunking Argument Schema

1. Belief B is *mainly based on* psychological process P. [empirical premise]
2. P is an *unreliable* process. [normative premise]
3. So: B is unjustified.

Philosophers and scientists have used such arguments to debunk different sets of moral beliefs. Some debunkers argue that disgust is an unreliable basis for moral beliefs (e.g., Kelly 2011). Other debunkers contend that all, or nearly all, moral beliefs are suspect because they are all problematically influenced by evolutionary processes or other psychological biases (e.g., Joyce 2006; for review, see Kumar & May 2019). However, we'll focus on a class of commonsense moral beliefs that tend to privilege the needs of the *few* over the needs of the *many*. Attempts to debunk such beliefs have drawn specifically on brain-imaging research.

Debunking arguments can even be expanded to support particular ethical theories. Some moral theories seem objectionable because they lead to abhorrent moral verdicts. Recall that utilitarianism, a form of consequentialism, says that one ought to always produce the best outcomes, even if that occasionally requires acts that are normally prohibited, such as manipulative lying, discrimination, or even murder (see appendix to Chapter 1). Many such commonsense moral prohibitions seem to conflict with utilitarianism, and alternative theories like deontology can be easier to swallow. Both camps enjoy some level of abstract theoretical support, but utilitarianism might seem to lose in the end because it is too counterintuitive. But what if our deontological (or non-utilitarian) judgments are driven by unreliable psychological biases? Then they can't be relied upon to either reject utilitarianism or support alternative theories. That's exactly what one of the most famous ethicists on earth—Peter Singer—has long argued. Though he didn't always have hard data to back up his psychological claims, his former student, Joshua Greene, a philosopher turned neuroscientist, purports to have provided the evidence.

6.3.2 Sacrificial Moral Dilemmas

The relevant studies in moral neuroscience examine how we trade off different values in the context of moral dilemmas. In these *sacrificial dilemmas*, one must indicate whether it is morally appropriate to promote the greater good at the expense of inflicting harm on the few. Ethicists, such as Philippa Foot (1967), have illustrated these trade-offs using hypothetical scenarios involving runaway trolleys, which neuroscientists then adopted for studying moral judgment.

Consider one well-known pair of trolley cases. In the first, known as *Switch* (or Side Track), we imagine a man, call him "Sanjay," situated at a switch that can divert a trolley from its main track and onto a side track. Sanjay sees that there is a runaway trolley barreling down the tracks about to smash into five innocent people stuck on the main track. Although he can flip the switch to move the trolley onto a sidetrack, there is unfortunately one innocent person stuck there (for illustration, see Figure 6.2).

Should Sanjay let the trolley kill five people or intervene and sacrifice one instead? You might be uncertain about what will happen in either case. What if a superhero came and saved everyone? But just imagine it's all happened already (and, sadly, no superheroes came). Sanjay does throw the switch, the trolley is diverted, and the one person is killed while the five are saved. Was that morally acceptable? Large-scale studies suggest that the vast majority of people across many cultures and classes find such actions acceptable (e.g., Hauser et al. 2007; Pellizzoni et al. 2010; Mikhail 2011; Gold et al. 2014).

That's a relatively easy judgment to make. But is it always morally acceptable to sacrifice the few for the greater good? Contrast the Switch case with *Push*. Here we imagine again that the lives of five innocent people are threatened by a runaway trolley. Sanjay himself is too small to stop the train with his own wiry frame, but he can save the five innocents by physically pushing a large person off of the footbridge onto the tracks (Figure 6.3). Imagine he does this, the one man is killed, but the train grinds to a halt and the five people are thereby saved. Is Sanjay's

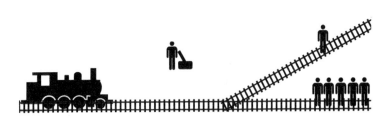

Figure 6.2 The Switch Dilemma
Should the protagonist flip the switch and save five innocent lives at the cost of one?
Source: May (2018a).

action morally acceptable? The vast majority of people around the world say "No!" presumably based in part on a gut reaction.

Sacrificial dilemmas demonstrate a classic conflict in ethics. We exhibit utilitarian (or, more broadly, consequentialist) concerns about promoting the best outcomes but also non-consequentialist concerns about upholding general rules or principles, such as those that prohibit treating others as if they were mere objects to be used as a means to one's ends. The trolley scenarios are rather peculiar, perhaps even difficult to entertain or take seriously. However, it's important to recognize that they are just one example of the vignettes researchers employ. Other more realistic dilemmas are used as well, such as a scenario in which one can encourage the use of a vaccine that will harm some citizens but save many others (see the "Vaccine Policy" case in the supplemental materials of Greene et al. 2001).

Greene and his collaborators suspected such moral conflicts arise from a general system, or rather two systems, in the human brain. According to a familiar *dual-process theory* of cognition, we have two fundamentally different modes of thought. One generates fast, automatic, intuitive judgments; the other produces slow, reflective, deliberations—thinking fast vs. thinking slow, as the Nobel Prize–winning scientist Daniel Kahneman (2011) puts it.

We can see these dual systems in action across all human cognition, from language to mathematics and even social norms. Consider, for example, a famous mathematical problem from the Cognitive Reflection Test (Frederick 2005):

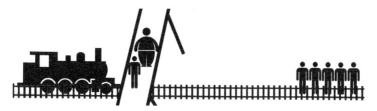

Figure 6.3 The Push Dilemma
Should the protagonist push the large man to save five innocent lives at the cost of one?.
Source: May (2018a).

A bat and a ball cost $1.10 in total. The bat costs $1.00 more than the ball. How much does the ball cost?

The intuitive answer is 10 cents, but some deliberation should yield 5 cents. (A dollar more than a 5-cent ball is $1.05, which sums to $1.10.) The same tension in thought arises in other domains as well, such as social norms related to naming (Thomson & Oppenheimer 2016):

Emily's father has three daughters. The first two are named April and May. What is the third daughter's name?

(Test yourself: Which is the automatic intuitive response, and which is the correct response you get upon reflection?) The phenomenon is not restricted to word problems either. Consider the well-known Stroop task in which one is instructed to report the *ink color* that a series of color-words are written in (e.g. "red" written in purple), rather than report the *meaning* of the word (Stroop 1935). Modern literate people are so habituated to reading words that they must deliberately override the automatic impulse when faced with this task, and thus they must slow down in order to avoid mistakes. These examples show that intuitive responses are not necessarily unlearned, innate intuitions but often based in large part on prior experience, habit, and cognitive automation, through both conscious and unconscious inference. Indeed, if one practices enough, the Stroop task and Cognitive Reflection Test become less arduous.

Now that we have some examples in hand, consider an analogy to illustrate dual-process theory. Sometimes your camera phone automatically implements flash, and so you can "think fast" by relying on its automatic heuristics like "In low light, the flash should be on." But if a flash doesn't suit your present artistic needs, you have to "think slow" and deliberately shut it off. "Flash on in low light" is a good rule of thumb, but it's not always appropriate. Sometimes you have to manually override the automatic settings to get the right result. Dual-process theory argues that our minds similarly contain two modes of thought in order to manage the trade-off between efficiency and flexibility (Greene 2014). Using automatic heuristics (thinking fast) is quick and efficient but less flexible. Controlled deliberation (thinking slow) is less efficient but more flexible.

Specific neural circuits appear to be dedicated to these two systems of thought. Although a number of brain areas are involved, two of the key players reside next to each other in the prefrontal cortex (Miller & Cohen 2001; McClure et al. & Cohen 2004). One of these, our friend the vmPFC, is linked to quick intuitive responses, such as the gut feelings we encountered above. Talk of gut feelings isn't wholly metaphorical. If you really focus on the idea of pushing someone to his death, it ignites a flash of anxiety or unease (at least among neurotypical people). That's very likely the vmPFC and amygdala working together to tell you something's not right. Such affective alarm bells aren't specific to ethics. Think about that flash of anxiety you get in your core—somewhere near your stomach and chest area—when you contemplate encountering a tarantula or your ex-boyfriend for that matter. The same brain system seems to give rise to more subtle gut reactions that help you decide which apples to buy at the farmer's market or whether to accept (or offer) a marriage proposal.

The other key brain region, the *dorsolateral prefrontal cortex* (dlPFC), is associated with slow deliberation and the regulation of automatic thoughts. In contrast with gut feelings, the dlPFC appears to support the kind of thinking required to give the correct answer to the bat and ball question, or to override the impulse to read a color word rather than name its ink color, or to consider how much suffering one action would cause compared to another. Like thinking fast, thinking slow is a domain-general function that can be applied to judgments or decisions about math problems, reading tasks, social norms, and much more.

The insight from Greene and his collaborators was that moral cognition likely exhibits the same dual-system conflict, particularly when we evaluate a moral dilemma. Moreover, they provide evidence that what underwrites this conflict is the usual cast of neural circuits in dual-process theory (Greene et al. 2001, 2004; but compare Kahane et al. 2012). When participants give automatic intuitive responses to an emotionally charged moral dilemma like Push (don't sacrifice the few for the greater good), neuroscientists observe elevated activity in the vmPFC, as well as the amygdala, posterior portions of the cingulate cortex, and posterior portions of the temporal lobe (roughly the TPJ). Heightened activation in the cingulate is unsurprising given that it's associated with, among other functions, resolving conflicts. When participants make colder judgments about a dilemma like Switch that doesn't require up close and personal harm, they exhibited greater activity in the dlPFC, as well as the inferior parietal lobe, which overlaps with the TPJ. For Greene, the key regions to contrast are two distinct portions of the prefrontal cortex: the vmPFC (thinking fast) and the dlPFC (thinking slow).

Greene and his collaborators argue that these two key brain areas (and modes of cognition) are tied to specific moral values. The dlPFC preferentially supports characteristically utilitarian judgments (sacrifice one to save five), while the vmPFC tends to underwrite non-utilitarian moral judgments (don't push!). Greene (2014) does marshal a wide range of neurobiological evidence to support this dual-process architecture of moral cognition in the brain. Importantly, some of the evidence goes beyond mere correlations found in brain-imaging experiments, by drawing on lesion studies and the manipulation of slow, deliberate moral thinking in study participants. Consider, for example, the moral judgments of people with deficits in their automatic emotional responses to ethically charged situations, such as individuals with psychopathy, damage to the vmPFC, and frontotemporal dementia (Koenigs et al. 2012; Koenigs et al. 2007; Mendez et al. 2005). As the dual-process model predicts, these patients tend to give more counterintuitive "utilitarian" responses to the sacrificial dilemmas (e.g., that it's morally acceptable to sacrifice the one in Push).

Greene also asserts, even more controversially, that automatic moral intuitions are often inflexible and unreliable (at least when applied to novel moral problems to which the intuitions were not attuned). This is part of an ambitious and provocative attempt to establish, roughly, the utilitarian moral theory that we always ought to maximize happiness, even if it requires sacrificing others in gruesome ways. We'll now turn to this debunking of deontological (or non-utilitarian) intuitions.

6.3.3 Are Some Intuitions Untrustworthy?

So far we have asked what drives moral judgment about sacrificial dilemmas, but that doesn't tell us whether such judgments are reliable. Much of the evidence does suggest that our moral intuitions that conflict with utilitarianism are driven by automatic emotional heuristics (Singer 2005). But is that a problem? Surely emotions can sometimes be a reliable guide, sometimes not (Berker 2009). Greene (2014) ultimately develops a more sophisticated critique of non-utilitarian judgments.

The idea is that such moral intuitions arise from areas of the brain associated with automatic emotional heuristics *that are being applied to novel situations to which they were not attuned*. Compare how motivated we are to gorge on sugary and fatty foods. Some 300,000 years ago, when starvation was a serious threat, it made good evolutionary sense for our brains to automatically present these foods as immensely valuable, but these powerful cravings can lead to obesity and other health complications in modern societies where calorie-dense foods are so readily available. Of course, the temptations can be overcome, but doing so can be exceedingly difficult. Automatic heuristics can fail in other contexts as well. "Save 15% of your paycheck for retirement" is sound financial advice for most adults, but not if you've just been diagnosed at the age of 35 with terminal brain cancer. Similarly, "Don't push people to their death" is a good moral rule, but it can lead us astray in extreme or unusual contexts, like that of war or strange moral dilemmas.

Why might we have this moral rule? Following Singer (2005), Greene suggests that our opposition to utilitarian resolutions of moral dilemmas is grounded in a gut-level aversion to prototypical violence (Greene 2013). An aversion to violence might be innate—instilled in our ancestors by evolution to reduce conflict and promote cooperation among members of small tribes. But a rigid aversion to violence might also be learned, through bad experiences with aggression or by witnessing it. We might be like rats who refuse to push a lever that electrocuted them in the past, despite recognizing that the lever no longer seems to have that effect (Cushman 2013; Crockett 2016; Greene 2017). Our familiar cast of dual-process brain structures do seem to underwrite such reinforcement learning in humans and other mammals (May et al. 2022).

Whether our automatic moral intuitions are innate or learned, Greene maintains that they are too inflexible. They are insufficiently sensitive to new information when applied to moral problems to which they were not attuned. Thus, we should distrust our automatic non-utilitarian intuitions when applied to modern, controversial moral problems. Return to the compass analogy. Following magnetic north isn't *always* an unreliable method of traveling north. It works well enough in many situations, like those areas of the globe where magnetic and true north match or when you're traveling such a short distance that the margin of error will be negligible. Similarly, Greene (2014) allows that many rules of thumb in ethics are fine to rely on, provided we've had some relevant "trial-and-error" experience with the issue. In most ordinary situations, it is wrong to lie, cheat, steal, and push people to their death. But trolley scenarios are unusual moral dilemmas, as are contemporary controversies in politics about abortion, euthanasia, novel brain interventions, punishment of addicts, and so on. This leads to the following form of argument (based on Greene 2014):

The Argument from "Unfamiliar" Moral Problems

1. Non-utilitarian judgments are generally driven by automatic (and emotional) heuristics.
2. Automatic heuristics are reliable only when they have been acquired through *sufficient trial-and-error experience*—either from the experiences of oneself (personal experience), others in the community (cultural transmission), or ancestors (genetic transmission).
3. We have not acquired sufficient trial-and-error experience with *novel (unfamiliar) moral problems*. These include moral issues that involve (i) recent cultural developments (e.g., the push dilemma, human cloning) or (ii) widespread disagreement (e.g., abortion, euthanasia).
4. So: Our non-utilitarian judgments are unreliable when applied to novel moral problems.

5. Many non-utilitarian judgments concern novel moral problems (presumably most dilemmas in which the needs of the many outweigh the needs of the few).
6. Therefore: Many of our non-utilitarian judgments are unreliable.

(Two notes: First, we're focusing on this formulation of Greene's argument—instead of his "Argument From Morally Irrelevant Differences"—since it relies more directly on the neuroscientific evidence, particularly in the first premise. Second, Greene aims to not only debunk our deontological or non-utilitarian judgments but also to establish the theory of utilitarianism. Additional premises would be needed to draw such a conclusion, but I'll leave that as an optional exercise for motivated readers.)

There are a number of ways to resist this creative argument. Some neuroimaging research does call into question the first premise. It's not clear that responses to these moral dilemmas cleave neatly into utilitarian versus non-utilitarian judgments. Some "utilitarian" responses seem to be driven, not by a concern to promote the greater good, but rather by anti-social tendencies to be comfortable with the harm of others (Kahane et al. 2018). Psychopaths, after all, are more inclined to endorse sacrificing one to save five (Koenigs et al. 2012). Nevertheless, responses to the sacrificial moral dilemmas do seem to recruit the sorts of brain areas implicated in the dual modes of cognition—thinking fast (automatic intuitions) and thinking slow (controlled deliberation). In the context of moral judgment, the dlPFC may be more involved in calculating the outcomes of an action while the vmPFC may help apply learned moral rules (or assigning values to act types). That might be enough for Greene's conclusion, or near enough.

More problematic is the third premise. Ample evidence suggests that our automatic moral intuitions—like automatic responses in the Cognitive Reflection Test and the Stroop task—are quite flexible and responsive to changing circumstances. They are frequently the product of sophisticated unconscious learning and reasoning that occurs over time (Mikhail 2011; Railton 2017; May 2018a). For example, contrary to Greene (2013), a meta-analysis suggests that our intuitions about sacrificial dilemmas aren't sensitive to mere pushing but rather to how involved the actor is in bringing about the harm, including whether the harm was intended instead of merely foreseen (Feltz & May 2017). We don't respond negatively to pushing a large man to his death to save five others because our brains developed an inflexible aversion to pushing or violence. Rather, we unconsciously learn that the moral rules in our community place significance on intended harm.

Indeed, although trolley problems and euthanasia are relatively novel problems in human history, non-utilitarian distinctions that drive our responses to such moral issues are familiar and ubiquitous. In some areas of ethics and the law, we treat intent as central while in others we hold someone "strictly liable" for bad outcomes even if they aren't intended. Some evidence does suggest that the moral distinction between intended and merely foreseen harm can be learned unconsciously by children through inferring the general structure of rules in their community (Nichols 2021). So our concern to not use others as a mere means to the greater good might arise from ample trial-and-error learning, from our ancestors in the Pleistocene, more recent human societies, and individual children growing up in such societies.

In general, our automatic intuitions, both within and outside the domain of ethics, are not fixed but rather malleable responses to changes in one's environment and circumstances. Consider how this plausibly worked with the recent gay rights revolution in places like the United States (Kumar & Campbell 2022; Kumar et al. 2022). Both ideological rationales and gut feelings had long grounded widespread condemnation of homosexuality and same-sex marriage, so why did moral opinions shift?

One factor, among many others to be sure, is moral consistency reasoning. Unlike race, sexual orientation is a largely concealable trait that is distributed approximately equally across the population. As gay people began to "come out" and disclose their identity, it was often *after* they had already developed close loving relationships with people opposed to homosexuality—people in their families, churches, schools, and workplaces. Suddenly, a diverse range of racial, socioeconomic, and religious groups were confronted with an inconsistency in their attitudes: "I accept my friend, uncle, or pastor and their romantic relationships as morally admirable and worthy of love and respect, yet I'm not extending those attitudes to strangers who are also gay." Such consistency reasoning encourages treating like cases alike, and a dual-process model is apt. Intuitive feelings toward the gay people one loves are reconciled with the slower reflective judgment that there is no morally relevant difference between the gay people in one's community and those outside of it. Many people, though certainly not all, eventually shifted their moral opinions accordingly. This is just one fascinating example of how gut feelings and slow deliberation, working together, can be flexible enough to respond to changing circumstances, even concerning contemporary moral issues.

This example points to another concern. Greene ultimately aims not only to challenge non-utilitarian intuitions but also to support utilitarian reasoning. That further argument assumes that slow, deliberative reasoning is a better moral guide in novel contexts than automatic intuitions. Yet, absent gut feelings of love and mutual respect for gay friends and family, people often used slow deliberation to concoct dubious rationalizations for denying equal rights to same-sex couples. Reasoning is often motivated to defend existing values in this way (see Chapter 8). So it's doubtful that slow deliberation alone—unaided by gut feelings—is a more reliable guide to novel moral problems.

6.4 Conclusion

Our gut feelings in ethics and politics aren't necessarily inflexible and unreliable heuristics, liable to lead us astray. They are the result of unconscious learning and reasoning over time and in the moment. Although all thoughts and feelings can lead us astray, we shouldn't cast aspersions on these ones. We've seen that in pathological cases a lack of gut feelings leads to profound deficits in decision-making, not a stroke of good luck wherein patients are freed from the burdens of irrational intuition. Thus, as impressive as a magic trick it would be, we cannot easily pull utilitarianism out of the neuroscientific hat.

None of this implies that morality is a mere matter of blind emotion divorced from reason. Research on both neurotypical and abnormal moral judgment shows that the reason/emotion dichotomy is dubious, or at least much blurrier than commonsense would suggest. Our moral intuitions, even when driven by automatic emotional reactions, involve much unconscious inference. The emerging picture of the moral brain is that of a sophisticated reasoning machine. When these brain areas are dysfunctional, as in psychopathy, we see entangled deficits in both reason and emotion.

So are psychopaths incapable of understanding right from wrong? As with other mental disorders (see Chapters 4 and 5), it depends on the case. Psychopathy and anti-social personality disorder present on a spectrum, so a diagnosis isn't tantamount to being completely incapable of distinguishing right from wrong. Perhaps at the extremes, these deficits preclude a minimal grasp of ethics. Even if so, it's not as simple as "psychopaths lack empathy, so they are morally incompetent." We must evaluate each case individually.

What about Dugan specifically, who repeatedly and methodically ended the lives of innocent people without remorse? Kent Kiehl, a leading psychopathy researcher who testified for the defense, reports that Dugan scored 38.5 out of 40 on the standard diagnostic test, the Psychopathy Checklist, placing him in the 99th percentile (Hagerty 2010). So Dugan is an extreme case, in contrast to most others diagnosed with psychopathy, let alone anti-social personality disorder. Combined with other facts about Dugan, the case for his being unable to discern right from wrong is fairly strong. Dugan's defense lawyers might be right that he should get life imprisonment as opposed to the death penalty. Importantly, the conclusion is not that Dugan should walk the streets a free man. He should be locked up, in a kind of quarantine from the public (Fine & Kennett 2004).

Our understanding of how moral judgment arises in the human brain is certainly provisional and incomplete. Most studies focus on evaluations of harm, leaving other moral values understudied, such as loyalty and fairness. Nevertheless, harm, care, and related values are core pillars of morality—arguably the very pillars that have cracked or crumbled in psychopathy. Our provisional picture of the "moral brain" might even be developed enough to aid investigation of a related issue in neuroethics: whether and how we can *improve* our moral thoughts, feelings, and behavior.

7
Moral Enhancement

We saw in the previous chapter that moral judgment can be rather unconscious and automatic. Although these processes often involve complex inference, they aren't perfectly reliable. There always seems to be room for moral improvement, even by one's own lights. Many people explore paths of self-improvement to become more compassionate toward fellow humans and animals, more courageous in the face of temptations and injustice, more humble and open-minded about controversial issues. Better attitudes and behavior might also help us more ethically address great societal challenges, such as climate change, mental health crises, global pandemics, and cruelty in animal agriculture. Can neuroscience help enhance our moral capacities ethically?

This chapter builds a presumptive case in favor of moral bioenhancement, before testing it against objections. We'll evaluate five key ethical concerns with going beyond treatment to enhancing our brains. Such endeavors could, for example, bypass one's agency, promote a problematic desire to master oneself, or lead to the rich getting morally richer. Although such concerns are to be taken seriously, we'll see that they are typically overblown. Pills and other brain interventions will work best and most ethically when they merely aid more traditional forms of character building, such as moral education and talk therapy. These work through our rational learning mechanisms rather than bypassing them in some posthuman fashion. The result is a realistic conception of moral bioenhancements that are no more problematic than traditional modes of moral improvement. To make our discussion concrete, we begin by considering the neurobiological manipulation of intelligence and compassion.

7.1 Microdosing Morality

Treatments for brain disorders are proliferating, from anti-psychotic medications to deep brain stimulation for movement disorders and depression. But it's possible to go beyond treatment and enhance our brains, to embrace "cosmetic neurology" (Chatterjee 2006). Students and professionals are already trying to outcompete others by altering their brain chemistry, using prescription stimulants (like Adderall, an amphetamine), psychedelics, and electrical brain stimulation. Leading the pack of cognitive enhancers (or "nootropics") is arguably modafinil, a drug that appears to boost dopamine in the brain by blocking transporters that clear it from synapses. College students, writers, tech workers in Silicon Valley, military pilots, and even public servants have openly discussed taking modafinil to increase their alertness, focus, drive, and working memory. It seems to provide all the benefits of a stimulant without the jitteriness, racing heart, and other common side effects.

Our concern in this chapter will be *moral* enhancement specifically, not cognitive enhancement generally. The previous chapter suggests that the two are linked. Given that our moral attitudes are heavily influenced by reasoning, cognitive enhancement should also improve our moral beliefs and behavior. However, "cognitive" is often restricted to conscious reasoning, which is only the tip of the inferential iceberg. We'll discuss various means to enhance one's moral character, to be a better person, through neurobiological interventions.

Oddly enough, many have sought moral enhancement through psychedelics, such as LSD (lysergic acid diethylamide), magic mushrooms (psilocybin), and ecstasy (methylenedioxymethamphetamine, or MDMA). These substances have been lamented as dangerous recreational drugs since the 1960s. Rigorous research on their mental benefits has only recently begun, as stigmas start to wane, but users of psychedelics often experience *ego-dissolution*, a feeling of being one with other people and nature (Nour et al. 2016; Pollan 2018; Forstmann et al. 2020). Self-interested concerns seem less significant from this perspective, perhaps similar to how one often feels while walking in the woods or taking in a grand vista. Such radical love, altruism, and compassion are pillars of many moral and religious traditions.

The effects of psychedelics can be powerful in their usual recreational doses, but some have sought more attenuated, more manageable effects with small amounts, a technique known as "microdosing." Ayelet Waldman, a writer and former public defender, attempted to improve her life using this technique with LSD. Waldman sought to not only treat her mood disorders but also to improve her relationships with others, to become a better person (Earp & Savulescu 2020). In her book *A Really Good Day* (2017), Waldman documents her experiences microdosing over the course of a month. Predictably, there were numerous and inconsistent effects. Although she sometimes felt a greater sense of well-being and joy on the days she microdosed, she also sometimes felt more irritable and had more trouble sleeping. Nevertheless, Waldman reported being generally able to approach marital conflicts more productively and to feel less guilt and shame when conflicts arose. Her children, who were informed of her experiment only after it was complete, reported that she was noticeably happier the prior month and less angry. It remains unclear whether directly manipulating one's brain chemistry in this way, in either small or more liberal doses, can make most of us better people, but the randomized controlled trials and personal experiments are only just beginning.

In addition to microdosing, Waldman recounts taking MDMA with her husband to help enhance their relationship. Some therapists have been using MDMA, ketamine, and psilocybin for decades to guide partners through relationship conflicts and to deepen their bonds. Waldman reports that after taking the drug

> we were transported emotionally back to our relationship's early and most exciting days, to the period of our most intense infatuation, but with all the compassion and depth of familiarity of a decade of companionship.

These feelings persisted for months, and Waldman and her husband take the drug every couple of years to rekindle their relationship. Far from the small, temporary effects of most drugs, a single session of MDMA was equivalent to years of couples therapy. If more people could experience greater relationship satisfaction and stability, that would be a major boon to society (Earp & Savulescu 2020).

Relationships and the families they often build are part of the social glue that holds our communities together. More generally, since self-centeredness is a regular enemy of virtue, psychedelics might have far-reaching moral benefits.

7.2 A Presumptive Case for Enhancement

Our topic of moral enhancement is nested within a broader debate about all biomedical interventions that allow one to perform beyond normal. Bionic limbs, for instance, might afford the ability to run faster, jump higher, or climb longer than any human in history—perhaps warranting labels such as "posthuman" or "transhuman."

Ethicists have ranged from being deeply dubious of bioenhancement to brimming with enthusiasm for it. Positions span a continuum of what we might call more "restrictive" versus more "permissive" (Giubilini & Sanyal 2015). *Restrictive* views regard enhancement as morally fraught either in principle or in practice (e.g., Kass 2003; Sandel 2004; Sparrow 2014). *Permissive* theorists believe that enhancement is in general morally acceptable, perhaps even an urgent necessity to avoid the collapse of civilization (e.g., Douglas 2008; Persson & Savulescu 2008; Buchanan 2011; DeGrazia 2014).

We'll eventually examine arguments for more restrictive positions on moral enhancement specifically. But we'll start with building a presumptive case in favor of a permissive position by considering *why* moral enhancement is worthwhile, *what* changes to our moral minds would need to be made, and *how* neurobiological modifications could yield such changes.

7.2.1 Why?

You might worry immediately that bioenhancement should be off the table because none of these moral ills are diseases or disorders in need of treatment. Healthcare providers often draw a sharp distinction between *treatment* for ailments and *enhancement* beyond normal capabilities. You wouldn't expect your physician to write you a prescription for a stimulant to enhance your performance on tests without a diagnosis of a mental affliction, such as attention-deficit/hyperactivity disorder (ADHD). Similarly, in competitive sports players are allowed to treat injuries but punished for taking steroids and other performance-enhancing drugs.

However, the treatment/enhancement distinction doesn't hold up well under the pressure of hard cases. Imagine two boys who are projected to have the same short stature of five feet, three inches (160 cm) but due to different causes (Daniels 2000). One of them has a brain tumor near the pituitary gland that causes a lower secretion of growth hormone; the other boy has short parents. Health insurance will typically cover growth hormone treatment for the first boy but not the other, which seems arbitrary.

Indeed, what counts as a deficit or enhancement is quite malleable. Left-handedness and homosexuality used to be considered defects in need of treatment. In the 1970s, the psychiatrist Robert Heath of Tulane University attempted to quell a man's homosexuality by stimulating the reward center of the patient's brain during intercourse with a sex worker. It's perhaps unsurprising that many theorists have roundly criticized the treatment/enhancement distinction as resting on subjective value judgments about what counts as normal versus an impairment (Wolpe 2002; Levy 2007: Ch. 3). Is grandiosity an ailment in need of treatment or an enhancement that helps one speak up in meetings and secure second dates? Don't hold your breath for a consistent, objective, non-arbitrary answer.

The treatment/enhancement distinction is particularly blurry when it comes to individual moral improvement. Consider the character Chidi Anagonye, from the philosophical comedy series *The Good Place*. Chidi is a professor of moral philosophy whose deep concern for doing what's right turns out, paradoxically, to be a moral conundrum. He regularly becomes so preoccupied with moral uncertainty that he and those around him suffer (which serves as a humorous example of the alienation problem in ethics). Imagine Chidi embarks on a journey of self-improvement with the aim of keeping his moral anxieties in check by means of psychotherapy, or psychedelics, or a transcranial direct current stimulation (tDCS) device fashioned together from parts readily available for purchase on the internet. Is he treating a disorder or enhancing himself to become "better than well"? It looks like a distinction without a difference.

Whether we call it treatment or enhancement, moral improvement generally seems desirable, even necessary. In the previous chapter, we saw that various moral attitudes are based on automatic emotional heuristics. Even if these are not unreliable across the board, they aren't perfect. Some studies suggest that one's moral judgments can be swayed by morally irrelevant factors, such as self-interest, mood, and the order in which information is presented (for review, see Doris 2015; Crockett & Rini 2015; May 2018a: Ch. 4). At any rate, the world would clearly be a better place if there were much less suffering, oppression, authoritarianism, alienation, and inequality. Even if the moral arc of the universe bends toward justice, many moral problems that have plagued humans for millennia remain in some form today. Women are often subjugated; ethnic, religious, and sexual minorities are oppressed; human trafficking and other forms of slavery persist; and gratuitous violence results from war, terrorism, and civil conflicts. Monumental harm can also arise from novel forms of immorality, such as biological warfare, anthropogenetic climate change, alienation and destabilization of communities, and the mass mistreatment of factory-farmed animals in exchange for modest gustatory gains.

We might not be equipped to handle these societal problems without direct, intentional manipulation of ourselves to be better. Conventional forms of moral improvement are limited. Explicit moral education can yield measurable improvement on a wide range of issues, from volunteering to animal ethics (Han et al. 2017; Schwitzgebel et al. 2020). But some research suggests that professional ethicists—who regularly study moral texts—don't always behave any better than the general public (Rust & Schwitzgebel 2014). Moreover, along with advances in technology and human intelligence come increased power to inflict catastrophic harm, from violent acts among terrorists to the intentional release of a deadly disease by an unhinged misanthrope (Persson & Savulescu 2008). In short, moral education can only go so far, and super-technologies could breed supervillains.

These great moral problems of the past, present, or future might seem overblown. Even so, moral progress is always a noble endeavor.

Why not be better if we can? That "if" is an important qualifier. Let's turn to whether such enhancement is even possible.

7.2.2 What?

Moral improvement by neurobiological means is possible only if it targets certain psychological states or processes. One might think that moral enhancement is just cognitive enhancement—improvements in domain-general capacities like attention, memory, and insight (Harris 2011: 106). Other ethicists focus on the reduction of problematic motivations, such as aggressive impulses and racial biases (Douglas 2008). But a richer model views moral behavior as generated by beliefs about appropriate ways to act *and* motivation to so act (May 2018a; DeGrazia 2014):

> Moral judgment + moral motivation → moral behavior

For illustration, consider the opportunity to discretely cheat on an important test. Failing the test would prevent you from getting into medical school, say, or keeping your job. If you remain honest, you will do so because you judge that it's the right thing to do and are sufficiently motivated to follow through. Those who cheat do so typically for one of two reasons. Either their motivation to do what's right is weaker than their self-interested desires, or they don't really think it's wrong to cheat. Some, like Thrasymachus in Plato's *Republic*, believe that cheating is acceptable if you can get away with it. Or at least that's how some people rationalize it in the moment (see Chapter 8).

This model of moral behavior is limited for at least two reasons. First, it's oversimplified at least because it leaves out self-control or willpower. Many well-meaning folks truly want to volunteer more often, turn the other cheek, let go of a grudge, or purchase more ethically produced (even if more expensive) products, but they can't bring themselves to do it. Nevertheless, self-control can be captured at least to some degree by strength of moral motivation. A violent impulse, for example, is easier to control if it is weakened, more difficult to control if it strengthened.

A second limitation is that our model is underspecified. Some behavior is motivated by a general desire to do whatever is right, a form of moral integrity (Batson 2016; May 2018a). But moral improvement would also require targeting more specific motivations and beliefs. Plausible candidates include greater compassion, sympathy, or empathy and the altruism these tend to produce (Persson & Savulescu 2008; Batson 2011; May 2011). Distinctively moral progress also plausibly requires more inclusivity and tolerance of other people and animals as well as greater equality and fairness among genders, minority groups, and social classes (Buchanan & Powell 2018; Kumar & Campbell 2022). Could we directly manipulate our brains to improve such characteristics?

7.2.3 How?

Traditional means of moral enhancement predominantly involve learning. We receive explicit instruction by teachers, parents, and community leaders, as well as indirect instruction through rewards and punishment, including social institutions like the criminal justice system. Throughout life, we are influenced by role models or moral exemplars (both real and fictional) and the arguments and ideas found in moral treatises and social critiques. Other traditional methods include therapy, meditation, humor, and retreats into nature to spur self-reflection. All of these techniques affect one's brain to be sure, but indirectly and typically through more familiar processes. Wearable devices that measure but don't manipulate brain waves are novel, but they too only change one's brain indirectly by providing feedback on one's neural activity.

Direct interventions on one's neurobiology would be decidedly *nontraditional*. These include brain stimulation, genetic engineering of psychological traits, and pharmaceutical drugs that manipulate neurotransmitters. Neural prostheses and brain-machine interfaces, such as Elon Musk's Neuralink, also count as nontraditional, though they are less likely to support *moral* enhancement, at least in the foreseeable future. Of course, the ingestion of psychoactive substances, such as peyote and ayahuasca, to aid moral learning and spiritual growth isn't particularly novel (Earp et al. 2018; Haidt 2012: 266). Nevertheless, virtue pills and other direct brain interventions are markedly different from typical forms of moral improvement.

Debates about human enhancement began to flourish around the 1990s with a focus on genetic engineering. Bioethicists primarily analyzed the ability parents might one day have to choose traits for their children that promote individual well-being, such as intelligence, disease resistance, and height. Ethical debates about genetic enhancement have only gained momentum with the advent of revolutionary technologies, such as CRISPR, which can effectively delete or replace specific DNA fragments with remarkable precision.

Our focus, however, will be on the enhancement of *moral* traits and through more direct neurobiological interventions. We will ask whether these interventions are morally suspect compared to more traditional forms of moral improvement. According to the parity principle from Chapter 3, direct brain interventions should not be considered morally suspect just because they are direct brain interventions, unlike indirect interventions on the brain, such as alterations of one's body or circumstances. Yet many traditional forms of self-improvement, being indirect changes on the brain, are perfectly morally acceptable, even laudable. The question is whether more direct neurobiological methods of moral improvement are problematic, for reasons other than the fact that they are direct brain interventions. But first we must determine whether such methods are available now or in the near future. Ethical problems with unlikely enhancements are innocuous, or they at least warrant little attention compared to other more pressing issues.

Neurobiological enhancements are not far-fetched science fiction. Brain-based interventions are already available, largely through off-label use of prescription drugs that have been around for decades. Students have used Ritalin, Adderall, and other stimulants to improve their focus and retention of science, why not also of ethics? A number of studies support the idea that psychoactive drugs and brain modulation devices can enhance moral traits (Table 7.1).

Consider recreational drugs. Researchers have shown that MDMA increases empathy and generosity, at least among a sample of men. By promoting "mystical experiences," psilocybin seems to boost mood,

Table 7.1 Potential Methods of Moral Bioenhancement

Intervention	Effect	References
MDMA (ecstasy)	increased empathy and generosity	Hysek et al. 2014
psilocybin	reduced ego; reduced authoritarianism	Studerus et al. 2011; Lyons & Carhart-Harris 2018
ayahuasca	increased tolerance, compassion, moral motivation	Harris & Gurel 2012: 212–213
beta-blockers (e.g., propranolol)	reduced racial bias	Terbeck et al. 2012
oxytocin	increased trust, cooperation, and generosity (with ingroup)	Van IJzendoorn & Bakermans-Kranenburg 2012; De Dreu 2012
SSRIs (e.g., citalopram)	increased cooperation and aversion to harm	Tse & Bond 2002; Crockett et al. 2010
deep brain stimulation (DBS) of hypothalamus	decreased impulsivity	Franzini et al. 2005
transcranial direct current stimulation (tDCS) of the prefrontal cortex	increased attention, learning, and memory; decreased aggression	Coffman et al. 2014; Choy et al. 2018
neurofeedback	Increased self-regulation	Sitaram et al. 2017

reduce egoism, and decrease authoritarianism. Users of ayahuasca, a psychedelic tea originating in South America, report being less judgmental, more tolerant of others, and more motivated to make a positive difference in the world.

Prescription medications also have moral effects. Some musicians take beta-blockers (e.g., propranolol) to reduce performance anxiety, but the effects also appear to help reduce implicit racial bias. Oxytocin, a hormone secreted by the pituitary gland, is crucial for bonding and naturally released during breast feeding, sexual intercourse, and other forms of physical connection. Administration of this hormone through a nasal spray appears to increase trust, cooperation, and generosity, at least among members of the same social group (although it's unclear whether this delivery method is truly effective). Some studies suggest that increased serotonin through the ingestion of selective serotonin reuptake inhibitors (SSRIs; such as citalopram) increases cooperation and aversion to harm.

Noninvasive activation and inhibition of neurons also produces morally relevant effects. Deep brain stimulation (DBS) of the hypothalamus has been shown to reduce impulsivity, at least among individuals with intellectual impairments. Participants who receive tDCS of the prefrontal cortex have exhibited decreased aggression as well as improvements in attention, learning, and memory, which might improve moral learning. People can also learn to manipulate their own neural activity by receiving feedback about it in real time and being rewarded for maintaining desirable brain waves. Some of these "neurofeedback" training regimens seem to improve self-regulation in both psychiatric patients and healthy individuals.

So a number of current drugs and devices have the potential to provide moral benefits (for further discussion, see Earp et al. 2014; Crockett & Rini 2015; Dubljevic & Racine 2017). Some of these might be placebo effects, but they are no less real for that; the benefits would just lie partly in how users interpret the treatment. Well-established protocols could allow consumers to use pharmaceuticals, supplements, or perhaps brain stimulation devices to aid certain moral training regimens. The putative moral enhancers are already available. Although deep brain stimulation is too costly and invasive for the task, consumers can cheaply build transcranial direct current stimulators, and drugs are relatively inexpensive and easily attainable.

Even if not science fiction, these examples are largely speculative, for three reasons. First, there are too *few studies*, let alone meta-analyses. More studies like these might not even yield practical applications to moral enhancement. Second, they often demonstrate *small effects* at best (Dubljevic & Racine 2017)—certainly no more powerful than the brain boosts afforded by a single workout or a hike in the hills (see, e.g., Basso & Suzuki 2017; Jones et al. 2021).

Some drugs even produce an inverted dose-response curve, wherein moderate doses can improve performance but higher doses produce no change or impaired performance (Glannon 2011: 117). Perhaps direct brain interventions are just too blunt, ill-suited to target specific moral faults without negative moral side effects (Harris 2011). Oxytocin appears to parochially increase compassion and loyalty toward one's own clan while decreasing tolerance of outsiders (De Dreu 2012). Finally, *external validity* is also questionable. The effects are sometimes restricted to subgroups (e.g., only men), and the interventions modify responses on rather artificial tasks (e.g., the ultimatum game), which prevents generalizing to the complex moral decisions people make in everyday life.

To chart a neurobiological path toward enhancement, we would need many more studies. However, we'll see that the path is chartable, provided neuroenhancements are used alongside more traditional forms of moral improvement. The previous chapter suggests that the best methods would not merely manipulate incidental emotions but tap into mechanisms of learning and reasoning.

Is this a morally dubious path for humanity to take? The foregoing considerations provide a presumptive or *prima facie* case for a negative answer. Barring powerful objections, we should probably consider moral bioenhancement ethical, given that moral improvement is welcome, perhaps necessary, and that individuals should generally have the liberty to choose their own life plans. So we start with a presumption in favor of citizens having the individual liberty to morally enhance—and perhaps of parents to enhance their children.

7.3 Ethical Concerns

Are there substantial reasons to think that enhancing our moral characters though neurobiological means is unethical? We'll critically evaluate five prominent objections: either neuroenhancements would be inauthentic, enslaving, perfectionistic, unfair, or unsafe. We'll start with the weakest arguments and move progressively toward more compelling concerns.

7.3.1 Authenticity

Biological methods of enhancement might seem ethically problematic in principle because they are in some sense unnatural, undignified, or inauthentic. The foremost proponent of this argument is the physician-bioethicist Leon Kass (whom we encountered in Chapter 3). Sometimes Kass (2003) objects to biomedical enhancements by appealing to "our" reactions of disgust toward them. He appeals to the "wisdom of repugnance" when evaluating the ethics of biotechnologies that have the power to manipulate or transform human nature. In these moods, Kass is offering an argument from intuition that, truth be told, has been a prominent form of philosophical argument.

One might demand further reasons beyond gut feelings. However, we have seen that gut feelings can be reliable guides in ethics, indeed in all forms of human judgment and decision-making (Chapter 6). Moreover, it can be unreasonable to expect a full articulation of the reasons behind one's intuitive reactions if they have been absorbed unconsciously, acquired through the trial-and-error experience of one's distant ancestors through evolution, one's community through cultural transmission, or even one's own experience over time. However, arguments from intuition are dialectically useful only if one's audience shares the intuition, and some evidence suggests that many people don't share the reaction of repugnance toward biotechnologies (see May 2016a, 2016b; Fitz et al. 2014).

Moreover, in philosophical analysis, we should try to uncover and interrogate the reasons behind our intuitive reactions, which Kass does attempt to do. One way Kass articulates the concern is that biological methods of self-improvement are undignified, inauthentic, or detached from meaningful forms of human activity. Unlike the ingestion of smart pills to gain an edge over a coworker, the ingestion of caffeine to improve wakefulness is dignified, according to Kass, because it is typically ingested in "forms and social contexts" that provide "meaning in human terms" (2003: 22). We don't ingest pure caffeine simply to increase wakefulness; we drink it in the form of coffee or tea as part of a morning routine or a book club. Whereas, according to Kass, with "biotechnical interventions that skip the realm of intelligible meaning, we cannot really own the transformations nor experience them as genuinely ours" (24). Brain interventions again are charged with risking inauthenticity, whether in the context of enhancement or treatment (recall Chapter 3).

Yet, like brain treatments, enhancements aren't doomed to flout authenticity or intelligible meaning. Many a truck driver has purchased pure caffeine pills and ingested them ethically as a means to remain alert on the road; millions of consumers use pure melatonin to aid sleep and CBD oil to relax and manage pain. Although drugs can be abused (more on this below), they are far from a gateway to a dystopian, let alone posthuman, future. Peyote, tobacco, fermented beverages, ayahuasca, and other psychoactive compounds in nature have long served humans in their cultural and contemplative endeavors. Some have used these substances more responsibly than others, but on the whole, mind-altering drugs have likely proliferated throughout human cultures because they promote meaningful and authentic improvements in creativity, bonding, collaboration, and group solidarity (Pollan 2018; Slingerland 2021).

Kass would likely regard these human practices as meaningful, unlike the use of nootropics, psychedelics, or brain stimulation as a sole means to self-improvement. But then the objection tackles a straw man. Proponents of bioenhancement have envisioned its use alongside traditional forms of moral improvement, playing an *adjunctive* role (Earp et al. 2018), just as antidepressant medications are used alongside talk therapy, exercise, and a healthy diet. Studies do consistently show that, for many psychiatric conditions, pharmaceutical treatments and talk therapy work best together (Cuijpers et al. 2014). When playing an adjunctive role, neuroenhancements can operate in perfectly meaningful contexts that promote authentic changes. Some clinicians already practice psychedelic assisted therapy, which helps patients integrate their mind-altering experiences with traditional tools of psychotherapy. Now, if the concern is that these contexts, while meaningful, bypass one's free will, then that is a distinct objection, to which we now turn.

7.3.2 Freedom

A related concern about moral bioenhancement is that it threatens valuable forms of freedom. Traditional means of self-improvement seem more compatible with viewing oneself as an agent, not a mere object to be manipulated. Through reflection or moral education, Kass writes, "we can see how confronting fearful things might eventually enable us to cope with our fears" or "how curbing our appetites produces self-command" (2003: 22). Kass's concern seems to be that biological means of self-improvement require a kind of reductionist attitude toward oneself, wherein one's agency is bypassed: "a drug that brightened our mood would alter us without our understanding how and why it did so" (22).

In a similar vein, John Harris (2011) argues that our "freedom to fall" remains only if moral bioenhancement is merely cognitive enhancement that improves our general capacities to reason, focus, recall, and the like. Then our moral knowledge can be improved while retaining the ability to freely choose to do wrong. If instead our moral motivations and emotions are directly manipulated, then the changes might bypass one's assessment of the reasons for acting (see also Habermas 2003; Sparrow 2014; Schaefer 2015). The absence of moral understanding might make direct brain manipulation similar to forming one's moral opinions simply based on what someone else tells you to believe (the problem of moral testimony). Shouldn't you decide for yourself on the basis of reasons?

Critics have responded that, although freedom has value, its value only goes so far. We should happily sacrifice considerable freedom to prevent abominations like human trafficking (DeGrazia 2014: 367). But moral bioenhancement wouldn't just occur in extreme cases, where restrictions on individual liberty are typically warranted to prevent significant harm, especially to vulnerable individuals. What about a man who aims to curb his misogyny? In any case, one might worry that direct brain manipulations threaten a more subtle form of mental freedom, a core aspect of which is "conscious control over one's mind" (Bublitz 2016: 95). Biomedically dampening one's implicit racial biases or amplifying one's compassion for others would largely fly under the radar of consciousness.

However, a neurobiological understanding of human agency suggests that moral bioenhancement is not inherently threatening to freedom, even if we were to directly manipulate our motivations and emotions. A theme of this book is that most people fail to accurately understand why they do what they do, yet this does not reveal their agency to be a sham. We've seen that it's a mistake to identify your freedom, autonomy, or self with conscious awareness (Chapter 2). It's equally problematic to conceptualize proper freedom as choice that is in opposition to emotion (*contra* Harris 2011; Bublitz 2016). On the contrary, human agency is driven largely by automatic and unconscious processes that blur the distinction between cognition and emotion (Chapter 6). To reject this form of agency as irrational, inauthentic, or unfree is to reject traditional forms of moral learning as well, which chiefly involve teaching children rules and habits that they only later, if ever, come to fully understand consciously.

To illustrate how this might work with moral bioenhancement, let's get concrete. Consider two hypothetical examples that combine traditional with neurobiological enhancements:

> *Altruism and compassion with psychedelics*: Alonzo is a decent person, but he comes to realize he is too often self-centered, which makes him stingy with his time, money, and affection. He wants to be more compassionate, generous, and other-regarding. He has tried multiple therapists, even read some philosophy, but old habits die hard. Alonzo needs to retrain his brain. So, while continuing therapy and self-reflection, he goes on a guided psilocybin retreat in The Netherlands to start anew with a rebooting of his brain and hopefully some fresh insight. Afterward, he begins microdosing LSD, following a set protocol, and he finds it remarkably easier to break his old habits and start forming new ones. Often his mood is brighter, and he finds himself more genuinely interested in the concerns of others. Their problems no longer seem like such burdens to spurn. Six months later he stops microdosing, after finding himself volunteering, donating more of his wealth to effective charities, and building stronger connections with his friends and family. Paradoxically, he finds all of these developments powerfully rewarding for himself, which reinforces these new habits of thought and action, even after he ceases microdosing. Nevertheless, two years later, after losing his father to Alzheimer's and his job to a global financial crisis, Alonzo finds himself turning inward and slipping back

into some more self-centered habits. So he attends another psychedelic retreat, which helps him course correct.

Inclusivity with oxytocin: Ever since she was a little girl, Ingrid had considered herself an animal lover. In high school, she learned about the horrors of factory farms and became a vegetarian for a month. It was too difficult to keep up. Thoughts about the mistreatment of farmed animals receded from consciousness. She began to wonder whether omnivorism is natural and necessary. Still, every time she thought carefully about the issue, it was clear she should give up eating most meat, since 99% of what she'd eat would come from factory farms. Ingrid wanted help—something that no amount of therapy, meditation, or ethics books alone would provide. What if she could strengthen her emotional bonds with farmed animals and solidify a vivid desire to "tend and defend" them? Being a mother and busy law student, she can't up and move to the countryside. She decides to temporarily foster a pig and while doing so takes small doses of oxytocin. Afterward, she adopts a vegetarian diet once again, and this time it sticks, even though she makes exceptions for special occasions. Once she has a dozen vegetarian recipes down, her new diet is surprisingly easy to maintain, even infectious. As many of her friends become inspired by Ingrid's ethical—not to mention healthier—diet, they too begin reducing their own meat consumption.

These are just two examples of how neurobiological interventions could aid moral improvement in the not-too-distant future, perhaps even the present. Other examples might involve using oxytocin to curb infidelity, beta-blockers to unlearn racial biases, and so on. In every case, the neurobiological interventions could harness emotions and unconscious processes to *facilitate rather than determine* one's reasoning and understanding (Earp et al. 2018). Moreover, the characteristics they enhance wouldn't just yield greater compliance with existing norms (Harris 2011; Buchanan & Powell 2018) but genuine improvement in the status quo as well. No threats to freedom; just autonomous individuals conducting their experiments in living.

Now, these are examples of personal journeys in moral enhancement. Some ethicists have suggested that societies might have a moral imperative to enhance citizens en masse, similar to fluoridating the water supply in the name of public health (Persson & Savulescu 2008). Such proposals threaten a different kind of freedom—to form one's beliefs and opinions without interference by governments or corporations (Bublitz 2016). They reanimate the dark history of eugenics, with its forced sterilizations and parochial conception of a good life (recall Chapter 3). In light of neurodiversity (Chapter 4), it's particularly worrisome for governments and other organizations to impose a particular vision of what it is to be a good person. As Frances Kamm puts it, "we are constantly surprised at the great range of good traits in people, and even more the incredible range of combinations of traits that turn out to produce 'flavors' in people that are, to our surprise, good" (2005: 13; see also Schaefer 2015).

Coercion and illiberalism are serious political concerns and should be avoided. In some countries it's possible "for a *bogus* science of moral enhancement to serve as a fig leaf for the pursuit of power and the interests of those already convinced of their own merit" (Sparrow 2014: 30). Such scenarios should be avoided, but the problem seems to be the authoritarianism, not the project of enhancement. Is moral bioenhancement likely to be authoritarian, even in liberal democracies?

Not necessarily. By self-medicating as it were, individuals could voluntarily seek out enhancements that would promote their own conception of the good life. Moreover, if the state were to play a role, it could simply encourage bioenhancement through research funding and perhaps insurance coverage. Governments needn't support any particular moral ideal either, for a new "liberal eugenics" would thoroughly embrace a pluralistic conception of the good life (Agar 1998). Some ethicists worry that even subtle nudges by those in power are manipulative and paternalistic. But they needn't be if designed to exploit rational learning mechanisms (Kumar 2016), which promote understanding and long-lasting improvements to one's character, as in the hypothetical cases above. State influence has the potential to be as benign as encouraging exercise, healthy diets, or mental health services. Of course, there is a debate to be had about whether the state should have any hand in moral education, but the issues there are not specific to biomedical enhancement.

The deeper problem with compulsory enhancement is practical, not moral. Such proposals are utterly infeasible—not because the neurotechnologies are worthless, but because people won't accept the mandates. If there is widespread opposition to compulsory vaccinations that alter one's body to prevent deadly diseases, we can expect even greater opposition to interventions that alter one's mind to improve virtue! At any rate, if moral neuroenhancement is to leave autonomy intact, it would have to occur voluntarily among individuals who supplement classical tools with modern technologies.

7.3.3 Character

A distinct concern with moral bioenhancement is not that it undermines human agency but that it expresses *too much* control. By directly manipulating core features of ourselves—our brains, our genes—one might inevitably engage in a project of self-improvement that expresses a problematic drive to treat oneself as an object to be controlled and perfected. Michael Sandel (2004) argues that this "drive to mastery" endangers our healthy "openness to the unbidden" or to what we can't control. Accepting limits to what we can control cultivates the virtue of humility rather than hubris. Of course, all moral improvement expresses a desire to master a certain skill—to become more kind, generous, sympathetic, respectful, loyal, impartial, or courageous. Traditional means to these ends, however, might be less likely to run amok, to involve an unhealthy obsession with achieving perfection.

One might immediately object that many moral flaws shouldn't be accepted as given, such as racial biases or violent aggression (Douglas 2008; Kahane 2011). However, the project of moral enhancement is not meant to ameliorate only the darkest of human impulses. What about Alonzo's project of cultivating saintly levels of compassion, or Ingrid's endeavor to withdraw her participation in a system of animal cruelty? Sandel's concerns about hubris might be more applicable, precisely because the aim is perfection—not just to rectify deep character flaws—which could lead to a vicious hubris. But what exactly is this vice and its corresponding virtue?

An openness to the unbidden might be thought of as a kind of grit or *resilience*. The idea isn't that we ought to accept character flaws, but rather that our attempts to stamp them out shouldn't come at the cost of this character *strength* (Chatterjee 2006). The hubris here might be thought of as a kind of weakness or fragility in the face of life's challenges and the great limits on one's ability to make the world conform to one's desires (compare the "moral flabbiness" concern in Buchanan 2011). Put this way, the character concern resonates with strands of Buddhism and Stoicism that counsel us to let go of what we can't control. Instead of seeing the world as something to be perfectly controlled, you ought to cultivate more (even if not total) acceptance of undesirable outcomes, at least one's you can do little to change. Of course, in the case of moral bioenhancement, we're imagining that you *can* change your character. Sandel's claim, however, is that the overall project of unconstrained enhancement will lead to the atrophy of resilience, which is needed in *other* aspects of our lives.

One problem with this argument is that resilience often comes precisely by changing oneself. As the great Roman emperor and Stoic philosopher, Marcus Aurelius wrote in his *Meditations*:

> You have power over your mind—not outside events. Realize this, and you will find strength.

Openness to the unbidden looks like the kind of fortitude that allows one to accept what one cannot control by adopting an attitude that is more compatible with one's circumstances. Instead of crying over spilled milk, one sees it as an opportunity to finally clean that crumb-filled countertop. Yet moral improvement, whether by traditional means or bioenhancement, could promote just such changes in attitude. Popular counseling techniques, like cognitive behavioral therapy, train one to replace problematic thought patterns, such as catastrophizing, with more productive attitudes (Lukianoff & Haidt 2015). As we've seen, bioenhancements are precisely meant to facilitate such changes in one's thoughts and emotions and thus stand to enhance resilience, not threaten it. Neurobiological tools are decidedly modern but using them to improve one's habits of thought and action would be recognizable to Aristotle and other virtue ethicists.

7.3.4 Fairness

The objections so far have charged enhancement itself with being inherently corrupting: it's inauthentic, coercive, or erodes character. Another rather different concern, discussed by neuroethicists and the general public, lies in some degree of optimism about enhancement being beneficial (Greely et al. 2008; Fitz et al. 2014). The worry is that the advantages would be unfairly distributed or produce greater inequality in society, as the rich get morally richer and the poor get morally poorer (McKibben 2003; Archer 2016). People of modest means already compete against wealthy individuals on an uneven playing field in education, work, politics, even dating. Shouldn't we mitigate, not aggravate, social inequalities?

Concerns about inequality arise on a global scale as well. Wealthier countries might devote more resources to the development of cognitive and moral enhancements that could instead aid research into the effective treatment of ailments that affect the poorest and least advantaged people around the world. As Michael Selgelid puts it, we already face an alarming 10/90 divide as it is: "Only 10% of medical research resources focus on 90% of the global burden of disease, and 90% of medical research resources focus on 10% of the global burden of disease" (2014: 11). Encouraging biomedical enhancement might support or exacerbate such disparities.

Interestingly, ethicists representing quite different perspectives have found such objections wanting. After all, modern societies already tolerate a great amount of inequality in order to promote individual liberty (Kass 2003: 24; Sandel 2004: 2; Greely et al. 2008). The children of wealthy parents already benefit not just from fancier homes but from better schooling, tutoring, and opportunities for advancement. Of course, two wrongs don't make a right. Perhaps we shouldn't embark on the project of enhancement if it would exacerbate already unacceptable levels of inequality.

A more powerful response to concerns about inequality denies the claim that it would inevitably result. The first step requires recognizing that, although we do sometimes compete with others in society, life isn't entirely or inherently competitive. Allen Buchanan puts the point vividly in relation to his own occupation: "I'm very happy that there are lots of philosophers who are more creative and insightful than I am" (2011: 114). Even better if one's colleagues, coworkers, and CEOs were more compassionate, inclusive, and fair. Although these traits can make one more competitive on the job market or in climbing the corporate ladder, they benefit others in most contexts.

The second step in the reply points out that the acquisition of beneficial traits, including enhancements, isn't always a "zero-sum" game. Often technological advances ultimately benefit everyone, not just the wealthy or elite members of society. Sure, wealthier individuals are early adopters of computers, mobile phones, and the internet, but now the benefits of those technologies have spread to people throughout the world. As Buchanan (2011) explains, the now widespread availability of cellular phones alone is remarkably beneficial. Cheap mobile phones have equipped marginalized communities in America to record police brutality, women in rural India to receive microloans, and oppressed citizens to organize anti-government protests during the Arab Spring. Moral enhancements could work similarly. Prescription and recreational drugs—the forms of moral bioenhancement most likely to be effective—are relatively inexpensive and attainable. Even if the rich outpace the poor in moral improvement, this result could benefit everyone. It might even lead elites to have more compassion for the masses and promote policies aimed at reducing inequality.

In sum, concerns about equality and fairness are to be taken seriously. But they don't appear to decisively sink biomedical enhancement, especially moral enhancement, provided there are likely to be many win-win scenarios.

7.3.5 Safety

We now come to the final concern about moral bioenhancement. All interventions come with side effects, many of which are not discovered until millions of patients have taken them for prolonged periods of time. Unexpected collateral effects are sometimes treated as weak objections to enhancement (Douglas 2008), but the risks are worth taking seriously. Concerns about the safety and effectiveness of medical treatments (recall Chapter 3) are only amplified when it comes to brain interventions for the purposes of enhancement. Our knowledge of how the brain works is so profoundly impoverished—and may not improve much in the medium term—that the risk of unintended harms is especially high (Wolpe 2002). Millions of people could end up causing long-term damage to the organ that not only houses their personality, memory, and intelligence but also regulates nearly all essential bodily functions. Experimenting with different forms of therapy, exercise, or diet is one thing; brain manipulation seems a riskier endeavor.

The treatment/enhancement distinction might help illuminate these risks. Earlier we saw that the distinction is blurry at best, but that's compatible with conceiving of treatment and enhancement as lying on a spectrum (Selgelid 2014). A relevant feature of paradigm treatments is that they target ailments, which can make for a simpler risk-benefit analysis of the side effects that inevitably occur with medical interventions, from pharmaceuticals to surgery. Patients and their physicians trade the risk of adverse side effects for a chance at eliminating or mitigating severe symptoms. With enhancement, there are generally less severe "symptoms" to balance against harmful side effects, which might speak against most, even if not all, neuroenhancement efforts.

Now, our analysis has deemed voluntary enhancement most ethical, so isn't it up to each competent individual to freely choose whether to take on the risks? Perhaps in an ideal world. But realistically, there will likely be great societal pressure to enhance. Partly that's because some aspects of life *are* competitive, which tends to produce an "arms race" toward being better than others or to merely keep up (McKibben 2003). As deeply social creatures, we are attentive to trends, especially among celebrities and others in society marked with status or prestige (Henrich 2015). The more that successful people pop virtue pills or experiment with brain stimulation, the more others will follow suit.

Of course, social pressure is a problem only if moral bioenhancment is independently problematic. Long-term overreliance on any intervention is concerning, especially amid insufficient investigation of side effects. Indeed, this might be the greatest problem with the versions of enhancement most likely to arise in the near term: excessive long-term use of drugs and do-it-yourself brain stimulation devices (Dubljevic & Racine 2017). Part of the problem is that these are external interventions on internal bodily states and chemicals, which runs up against *homeostasis*—the body's ability to maintain functional stability in an everchanging environment. Homeostasis is involved in the development of drug tolerance (Chapter 5), but it's also responsible for some negative side effects. For example, the long-term ingestion of anabolic steroids among athletes leads to various health problems, including shrunken testicles in men. As the steroids introduce excessive quantities of testosterone in the body, the brain seeks to maintain balance by ramping down internal production in the testes, causing them to shrink. The effect is similar to how muscles will atrophy over time if unused, whether because one lies in bed all day or moves around through the assistance of bionic limbs. However, long-term overuse is neither inevitable with, nor specific to, moral enhancement.

Overreliance on enhancers is avoidable for several reasons. First, most putative moral enhancers are not habit-forming, unlike many recreational drugs (recall Chapter 5). Deep brain stimulation can target dopamine-producing structures in the reward center, such as the nucleus accumbens, but those areas lie deep within the brain and thus cannot be stimulated without invasive surgery. Other devices, such as tDCS and transcranial magnetic stimulation, are noninvasive but less precise and limited primarily to stimulating the brain's surface (the cerebral cortex). Psilocybin, oxytocin, and many other drugs don't manipulate dopamine. Some drugs do, like modafinil, but without the euphoria that often encourages abuse. Of course, any consistently rewarding behavior can be reinforced and become an obsession. Like exercise addicts, some people might become so obsessed with moral improvement that their own health and well-being languishes, similar to patients with scrupulosity who develop unhealthy compulsions driven by an obsession with following moral rules (Chapter 4. Sec. 4.3.1). But such cases would be rare.

Second, drugs and brain stimulation can be used temporarily to aid one's agential capacities of learning and reasoning, which promote the development of habits or traits without long-term dependence on the intervention. Consider what I'll call the *melatonin model*. Melatonin, beloved by many globe-trotters, is a hormone produced by the pineal gland in the brain that primarily controls the body's circadian rhythms. I've used melatonin myself, particularly when enduring up to a 17-hour time difference after traveling between the United States and Australia. Proper use of melatonin for jet lag is temporary: you take a single pill a few hours before bedtime in the new time zone, perhaps repeating this an extra day or two if necessary. A single dose can be enough to retrain your brain into a new circadian rhythm. No abuse, dependency, or shrunken pineal gland. One could apply the melatonin model to moral bioenhancement as well. Indeed, it's precisely the model adopted by Alonzo and Ingrid in the above vignettes. Both used drugs *temporarily* to *facilitate* changes in brain function.

Overreliance isn't specific to neuroenhancement either. Such problems arise for purely therapeutic interventions advocated by opponents of enhancement (a *tu quoque* or "you too" rejoinder). One can become overreliant on caffeine, counseling, or a friend's lent ear, for that matter. Should you never drink coffee or attend therapy because you might become dependent? No, for that presumes a false dichotomy. A third option is to responsibly utilize these tools either temporarily or in moderation as sources of support that teach new skills. One can kick away the ladder after using it to climb to new heights (as Wittgenstein might put it).

Ultimately, the risk of side effects is largely an issue of *prudence* rather than ethics. It is wise for individuals to enhance their brains safely and responsibly, but they generally have the autonomy to choose how costs are weighed against benefits, for both the treatment of ailments and the enhancement of character. The direct manipulation of brain chemistry for moral improvement, even if unwise for some people, can be done ethically.

7.4 Conclusion

Let's now return to the case of Ayelet Waldman, who ingested psychedelics in an attempt to be a more positive and agreeable person. Although the relationships with her family and friends were not in disrepair, she sought to enhance them through a neurobiological means of self-improvement. Is her project likely to be undignified, inauthentic, unfair, unsafe, or otherwise erode her character?

We began with a presumptive case for moral bioenhancement, deeming it morally acceptable unless we have good reasons to reject it. There are no doubt some important concerns with moving beyond treatment to enhancement generally, including moral enhancement specifically. There are some risks, particularly to coercion, resilience, inequality, and safety. But many of these risks are small—the kind we accept in other areas of self-improvement. As Buchanan puts it, *concerns aren't arguments* (2011: 144). At least the concerns we've examined don't appear to be *decisive* considerations against biomedical enhancement, especially moral enhancement with its potential to benefit others in a win-win fashion. Waldman carried out her enhancement project voluntarily, responsibly, and temporarily in an effort to acquire new insights that contribute to changes that would survive the conclusion of her experiment. By resembling the melatonin model, her project seems to pass ethical muster.

We are thus left with a form of permissivism regarding such endeavors. We should be wary of overuse, abuse, overhype, and premature adoption of novel neurotechnologies, but that is true of any biomedical intervention (*tu quoque*). Even if direct brain stimulation devices prove useful for consumers—a dubious prediction in my estimation—their wise use should be welcomed by ethicists. Out with anxious alarmism, in with cautious optimism.

The moral gains, of course, might turn out to be meager. Perhaps just some big city writers and suburbanites improve their marriages or become more ethical consumers. That's minor moral improvement in the grand scheme of things. But it's not as though progress would move at a faster clip with *fewer* items in the moral toolbox. Moreover, pessimism tends to underestimate the power of incremental moral progress (Kumar & Campbell 2022). For example, modest neuroenhancements could combine with other factors to produce gradual improvements in social justice by reducing discrimination, in social inequality by decreasing egoism, and in both animal welfare and global warming by reducing meat consumption. Of course, colossal societal problems like climate change require rapid strides forward, not incremental progress. But large-scale social change can gain momentum quite rapidly, as with the drastic decline in anti-gay attitudes in the United States (discussed in Chapter 6).

Rapid change is most likely to occur when individual efforts combine not only with traditional forms of moral improvement but also with legal and other structural changes to produce a cascade of social influence. Recall Ingrid, for example, whose dietary changes influenced others not through sanction but positive peer influence. Successful experiments in living are more likely to be copied by others and lead to a snowball of social change (Henrich 2015; May & Kumar 2023). Then, as consumer demand for plant-based alternatives shifts, it sends both economic and political signals that can lead to new products and legislation that increase animal welfare while decreasing greenhouse gases.

The social influence here is not mere mimicry. We are inspired by the behavior of others because it serves as evidence about how to behave, similar to how we rely on reviews of products and restaurants as reasons for what to buy and where to dine (Cialdini 2006: Ch. 4). In this way, others' behavior can link up with our own reasoning to produce moral progress (Kumar & May 2023). We are by nature deeply social creatures with reasoning machines between our ears. Of course, this moral equipment can lead to moral regress or stagnation too, as the bad behavior of others helps us rationalize doing it ourselves. In the next chapter, we consider just such motivated reasoning and how it leads to bad behavior, even within neuroscience itself.

PART V
JUSTICE

8
Motivated Reasoning

The previous two chapters suggest that our moral decisions are primarily grounded in both conscious and unconscious reasoning, and thus improving our moral characters requires forms of reasoning. However, human reasoning, including conscious deliberation, is often covertly shaped by one's existing values. How much of our reasoning is biased?

Neuroscience ably reveals motivated reasoning in split-brain patients but also neurotypical individuals, including scientists themselves. Whether it's neuroscience or physics, all inquiries are subject to bias. Chapter 3 touched on this topic in the context of medical hubris and gentle medicine; now we dig more deeply into these issues and the psychological mechanisms underlying them. Confabulation, rationalization, and other forms of motivated reasoning can make anyone biased in their collection or assessment of evidence. We deceive ourselves into thinking that our reasoning is pure while others are biased, but none of us is Lady Justice, whose blindfold represents the ideal of objectivity. Nonetheless, we'll see that there is reason to be cautiously optimistic about human reasoning and its ability to produce scientific knowledge through a marketplace of competing ideas and evidence.

8.1 Split-Brain Self-Deception

The human brain has two distinct hemispheres that communicate with one another through the *corpus callosum*. When this neural highway is severed, often to treat seizures from epilepsy, the two hemispheres no longer communicate effectively with one another. In the absence of crucial information from one side of the brain, patients often concoct a story to make sense of their behavior.

Such "confabulation" is easily discernable in split-brain patients, partly because the left and right sides of one's visual field are linked to the opposite hemisphere. Moreover, interpreting and communicating one's experiences linguistically is, for most people, primarily housed in the left side of the brain. With the corpus collosum severed, the information from the right hemisphere can't be transferred to the left hemisphere to be interpreted and articulated. So, when an image is shown to the right hemisphere, by presenting it to only the left side of the visual field, the patient's brain registers the image but is not fully aware of it and can't describe it.

To illustrate, consider two examples of confabulating split-brain patients, whom we'll call "Carol" and "Carl."

- **Carol** had a series of images shown to her left ("interpreter") hemisphere, one of which was quite out of the ordinary: a picture of a naked woman. When the nude appeared, Carol identified it as such and giggled. When it was presented to her right hemisphere, however, she again chuckled but confabulated an explanation for why: "I don't know . . . nothing . . . oh—that funny machine." (Gazzaniga 1967: 29)
- **Carl** was tasked with a matching game. Out of a row of images, which two best relate to a pair of pictures recently presented to him? The trick was that only one picture was presented to each visual field, and thus each image was registered by only one side of his brain. The "interpreter" hemisphere saw a chicken claw while the other half saw a house covered in snow. Of the eight images in a row before him, the best matches were the snow shovel and chicken head, which Carl correctly selected (see Figure 8.1). But why did he select the snow shovel, when his interpreter hemisphere can't really see the snowy home, which was presented to the other hemisphere? Instead of professing ignorance, Carl concocted a reason just to make sense of his intuitive selections, saying "you have to clean out the chicken shed with a shovel." (Gazzaniga 1983: 534)

The confabulations such patients construct not only help explain their behavior but also to do so in socially acceptable terms. Patients seem to be motivated to make sense of their behavior in ways that others will accept.

MOTIVATED REASONING 207

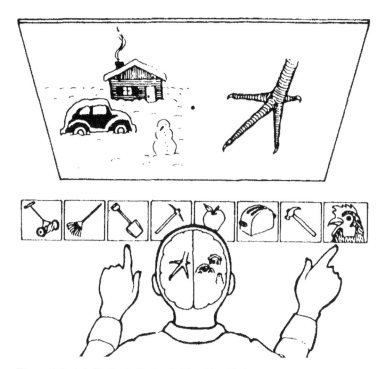

Figure 8.1 A Split-Brain Patient's Matching Task
The patient fixes his gaze on the center dot while pictures are flashed briefly on the screen, so that each hemisphere of his brain sees a different image. The task is to find the best match for each image among a row of other pictures. Despite lacking communication between the two hemispheres, the patient concocts an explanation for why he chose the matches he did.
Source: Gazzaniga (1983). Reprinted with permission of the publisher.

Similar forms of confabulation can be found in other neurological patients, such as those who deny having symptoms (anosognosia). Even when a brain injury yields paralysis on one side of the body, for example, patients sometimes insist that they can move the paralyzed limbs but just aren't in the mood to do so (Ramachandran 1996). Again, a story is concocted to justify their behavior—or lack thereof. Because some part of the patient's mind seems to recognize the truth, these cases are often described as ones involving self-deception.

However, self-deception and confabulation are not exclusive to psychopathology. These clinical cases reveal what occurs less conspicuously in everyone. We all tell stories to ourselves to make sense of our experiences and to rationalize our behavior. When José Delgado stimulated a portion of his study participants' brains that made their heads turn, he found that they tended to spontaneously provide explanations for their movements, such as "I am looking for my slippers" or "I heard a noise" (1969: 44). *Homo sapiens,* true to our name, can't accept that we act for no reason, so we regularly concoct stories to rationalize a host of choices and opinions. Indeed, our reasoning is generally motivated by our particular values and preferences. Prosecutors and defendants interpret the very same evidence in ways that favor their own case. Lawmakers of opposing political parties see the same facts as fitting with their own policy proposals. We not only rationalize unexpected behaviors but also interpret the world in ways that fit with our existing goals and values.

Is human reasoning perpetually biased? In this chapter, we'll see that it is, but not always in objectionable ways. The stories we tell ourselves and others to make sense of the world aren't always inaccurate, misleading, or irrational. Even reasoning in neuroscience is shaped by one's goals and values, such as desires to acquire grant funding, promote pet theories, and secure jobs for one's lab members. Such goals can lead researchers to oversell their findings, ignore methodological problems, and rationalize questionable research practices. Nevertheless, a marketplace of competing data and ideas tends to produce knowledge. Understanding how motivated reasoning works in science ultimately helps us draw on empirical evidence more carefully in neuroethics and everyday life.

8.2 Reasoning Motivated by Values

The confabulation neurologists observe in split-brain patients is alive and well in all of us. One theme of this book is that the human brain is a reasoning machine, even when it comes to moral cognition. Nevertheless, reasoning can be nudged toward certain conclusions by our desires and preferences.

8.2.1 Motivated Reasoning

It's familiar enough how ordinary reasoning can be influenced by one's desires, whether consciously or not. A teenager's desire to fit in with his peers who smoke can lead him to doubt the severity of the health risks or inflate the benefits so that they seem to outweigh the costs. A smoker might deny such addled reasoning, but other examples involve more self-awareness. The actor Matthew McConaughey (2020) describes struggling with his resolution to take on more challenging roles. At one point he was offered $5 million to star in yet another romantic comedy. After turning it down, the offer increased to $8 million, then $10 million, and eventually $14.5 million. McConaughey decided to reread the script:

> And you know what? It was a better script. It was funnier, more dramatic, just an overall higher quality script than the first one I read with the $5 million offer. It was the same script, with the exact same words in it, but it was far superior to the previous ones.

Despite ultimately declining the offer, the actor's judgments and perceptions were being pulled in a new direction by more immediate monetary drives.

Such motivated thinking manifests in many cognitive processes. Confirmation bias, for example, is our tendency to search for and interpret new evidence as supporting conclusions that one already accepts (Kahneman 2011: 81). Not all beliefs are formed via inference, of course. Sometimes we just take our perceptions at face value and simply believe what we see. A banana in the distance might just look yellow. How could that seemingly objective observation be shaped by your desires? Even here, though, some scientists argue that observations can be shaped by one's goals and values—so-called cognitive penetration of perception (but see Firestone & Scholl 2016). The distant banana might in fact be more green than yellow but look simply yellow because you want or expect it to be ripe. If that's right, then even the purportedly objective data on which science is based seems infected with subjectivity! Let's set that heated dispute aside and just focus on clear cases of inference, which clearly can be influenced by one's own motivations. Even if we don't always *see* what we want to see, we can certainly *justify* what we want to justify. And much of our reasoning is open to being so motivated.

Indeed, cognitive biases often work through reasons. Instead of merely opting for the conclusion one prefers, human beings curiously come up with reasons, even if dubious ones, in order to justify their decisions to others and, importantly, to themselves. Coming up with reasons for a specific conclusion is just what we colloquially call "rationalization," which is often used in a pejorative sense but has a wider application as well (see Davidson 1963). Sometimes we make a choice or form a belief automatically or intuitively and only afterward—post hoc—come up with a justification for why, and one that doesn't necessarily correspond with the reasons that actually drove one to the conclusion in the first place. Imagine being asked whether, hypothetically, it's morally acceptable for someone to clean their toilet with the national flag, to eat their pet that had been run over by a car, or to engage in consensual protected intercourse with an adult sibling. Most participants in studies automatically condemn such "harmless taboo violations" without being able to articulate appropriate justifications (Haidt et al. 1993; Stanley et al. 2019). Indeed, as we've seen, we often rapidly and automatically judge actions as right or wrong without always being aware of exactly why (Chapter 6). Reasoning, at least conscious reasoning, is often there interpreting, not generating, our intuitive responses.

However, reasoning and rationalization can also occur *before* a decision—ante hoc—in order to justify it in the first place (May 2018a: Ch. 7). The most familiar ante hoc rationalization is a paradigm of motivated reasoning, which has been studied extensively (Kunda 1990; Ditto et al. 2009). You want to believe that your favorite sports team will win, so you first rationalize that the star player's injury is but a flesh wound. Or you want a beer with lunch, and because you first justify it as deserved, given how busy the morning has been, you imbibe.

Construed broadly, however, *motivated reasoning* is just reasoning shaped by one's goals, desires, or preferences. This needn't be irrational at least because one's inferences can be driven by the desire for truth, accuracy, and consistency (Kunda 1990; Campbell & Kumar 2012). So motivated reasoning is neither virtuous nor vicious in itself, even though the term is often used pejoratively to denote forms of reasoning guided by motives other than truth.

Whether motivated by truth or other values, reasoning can occur before or after the relevant conclusion is drawn or decision made (ante hoc or post hoc). For example, a detective might begin with a hunch as to the thief's identity, but her attempts now to investigate the truth can be motivated purely by a desire to seek the truth. Similarly, Beck may go into therapy already thinking he's a loser, but his present attempts to scrutinize that core belief are motivated by a desire for self-knowledge, not wishful thinking.

Importantly, to accept the existence, even prevalence, of motivated reasoning is not to accept the postmodernist doctrine that truth is always relative and objectivity impossible. The point, rather, is a commonsense one: while truth and objectivity are possible, humans are fallible, and conflicts of interest can get in the way. Such biases can certainly conflict with the goal of acquiring knowledge, given its fundamental commitment to truth and justification. But this epistemic commitment alone can't neutralize motivated reasoning or rationalization, given that they work by generating justifications, even if spurious ones. Moreover, given the level of self-deception that frequently co-occurs with rationalization, the influence of one's goals or values often goes unnoticed.

Motivated reasoning is often associated with wishful thinking or "claiming that something is the case because one wishes it were the case" (Brown 2019: 227). But the two phenomena are distinct for at least two reasons. First, again, "motivated reasoning" needn't be a pejorative term, as when one's reasoning is influenced by a desire to be accurate. Second, "wishful thinking" often connotes the forming of a belief that would promote one's narrow self-interest, but motivated reasoning is not restricted to a certain class of desires. Partisan citizens who interpret all the president's actions in a positive light, even those detrimental to their own economic interests, exhibit motivated reasoning even if not wishful thinking. Similarly, the deliberations of a conscientious judge might be motivated by a powerful desire for justice, but that is not wishful thinking. In practice, many cases of motivated reasoning are appropriately described as wishful thinking. Nevertheless, the former provides a broader and more unified understanding of

Table 8.1 A Taxonomy of Motivated Reasoning

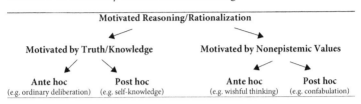

Reasoning, whether conscious or unconscious, can be influenced by different desires before (ante hoc) or after (post hoc) the conclusion is drawn or a decision is made. These two parameters (the motive and timing) explain a wide range of well-known psychological phenomena, from ordinary deliberation to confabulation.

when values (in the form of motivations) guide reasoning, whether in problematic or acceptable ways (see Table 8.1).

8.2.2 Biased Reasoning

The rationalizations in motivated reasoning are sometimes conscious. A key function of conscious deliberation in human beings is to convince others or ourselves of our intuitive verdicts rather than to uncover the truth (Mercier & Sperber 2017). Often this amounts to post hoc rather than ante hoc rationalization, however. Importantly, motivated reasoning can be unconscious and nonetheless ante hoc, powerfully influencing the intuitive verdicts themselves. When rationalizations are ante hoc and unconscious, they are particularly apt materials for motivated reasoning that produces problematic wishful thinking.

A large body of research suggests that reasoning motivated by values is ubiquitous. A meta-analysis of "moral licensing," for example, suggests that people will implicitly justify morally questionable, but personally advantageous, behavior to themselves when they have recently engaged in virtuous acts or affirm their virtuous traits (Blanken et al. 2015). In one study, participants were more likely to cheat if they had recently supported environmentally friendly products (Mazar & Zhong 2010). This is just one form of motivated moral reasoning, wherein people will unconsciously rely on whatever moral principles help justify a desired verdict (Ditto et al. 2009). A similar phenomenon is "motivated forgetting," in which we rationalize morally dubious acts or a better self-image by failing to recall past infractions or relevant moral rules (Stanley & De Brigard 2019).

The literature suggests that in many circumstances people aren't willing to rationalize fully breaking the rules, but they are happy to "bend" them. One series of studies examined under what conditions people will be dishonest when motivated to earn extra cash in an experiment (e.g., Mazar et al. 2008). Participants were told they would receive money for each math problem solved within a limited amount of time. When payment was based merely on self-reported success, most participants dishonestly reported solving more problems than they did, but just a few more. Most people can rationalize to themselves cheating a little but not a lot (Ariely 2012), due to their conflicting commitments to morality and self-interest (May 2018a: Ch. 7). As a final example, there is even some evidence that belief in free will is often accepted in order to justify punishing others (Clark et al. 2014).

Clearly, motivated reasoning is not restricted to certain domains and is particularly suited to rationalizing choices that are personally beneficial but otherwise questionable. Some evidence speaks to how political views can shape reasoning about science. One study asked a large sample of Americans about their opinions about climate change and assessed their competence in math and science (Kahan et al. 2012). While the more scientifically savvy liberals in the sample perceived climate change as more threatening to humanity, the more savvy conservative respondents perceived *less* risk. Apparently, a greater familiarity with math and science only made participants better able to rationalize their preferred stance on this now politicized issue. A recent meta-analysis suggests that this tendency to evaluate information more positively simply because it favors one's own political views ("partisan bias") is equally present among both liberals and conservatives (Ditto et al. 2019). Is it possible that scientific reasoning is also influenced by scientists' own values?

8.3 Bias in (Neuro)Science

8.3.1 Values in Science

Motivated reasoning is such a core part of the human condition that it naturally occurs in both everyday life and the scientific enterprise (Koehler 1993; Nosek et al. 2012; Stegenga 2018: 108). Reasoning motivated by values can even influence scientific investigations. For example, researchers motivated to detect a positive effect of a new drug may inadvertently use experimental designs more likely to produce the desired outcome and later rationalize their protocol as unbiased to peer reviewers. Similarly, if a researcher wants badly to publish in a prestigious journal, they might rationalize engaging in questionable research practices that will produce publishable results.

Since one's values generally give rise to corresponding motivations, they can influence various decisions made during scientific investigation. For example, a researcher's values and goals can sway choices about how to test hypotheses, to describe the results, and to assess the evidence (Elliott 2017), and corresponding labels are often given, such as "design bias" and "analysis bias" (Stegenga 2018: Ch. 10; Fanelli et al. 2017). Even the decision to report a particular finding (or a null result) can be influenced by a researcher's desire to construct a manuscript narrative that is more likely to survive peer review—a form of *publication bias* (Franco et al. 2014). Such decisions are arrived at through reasoning—sometimes deliberate, sometimes unconscious—which makes a framework of motivated reasoning apt.

Many philosophers of science have argued that values in science are inevitable and aren't inherently problematic (e.g., Longino 1990; Kitcher 2001). For example, as Elizabeth Anderson (2004) documents, prior to the 1990s many researchers studying divorce consistently looked only for negative effects on children, which presumed "traditional family values." To even look for positive or neutral effects of divorce on children, it took researchers with a different set of values that arose from a more feminist approach to the issue. Similarly, we saw in Chapter 5 that the brain disease model of addiction is often explicitly justified by a desire to reduce stigma, improve treatment, and reform overly punitive drug policies. These are noble goals. So it's not necessarily problematic for values to influence science, especially when they open new avenues of neglected inquiry. The problem is when values become self-fulfilling prophecies or "operate to drive inquiry to a predetermined conclusion" (Anderson 2004: 11). This concern in philosophy of science has been called "the problem of wishful thinking," which is a form of motivated reasoning.

Wishful thinking can be problematic in science. Less noble goals, such as self-interest, can lead to poor reasoning and research practices. Since around the year 2010, a number of unsettling events have yielded something of a crisis in science. Chief among these events is the realization that many studies cannot be replicated. For example, when a large group of scientists attempted to carefully replicate 100 psychological studies, only about 39% succeeded (Open Science Collaboration 2015). The problem is not just with social science either. A recent attempt to replicate 53 published findings in cancer research was only able to confirm 11% (Begley & Ellis 2012), while another effort reports a similarly low success rate of 20–25% (Prinz et al. 2011). How did we get here, and how do we grapple with it as consumers and producers of science?

8.3.2 Scientific Misconduct

One factor is fraud and other forms of outright misconduct. In a wide range of disciplines—from psychology to biology and oncology—papers have been retracted due to fabricated data. The researcher with the highest number of retracted papers, according to RetractionWatch.com is Yoshitaka Fujii. An astounding 183 of his scientific papers have been retracted, most of them published between 1990 and 2010 in anesthesiology, ophthalmology, and related fields. The papers primarily report clinical trials on the effectiveness of drugs and procedures to reduce nausea after surgical operations. Fujii's findings seemed too good to be true, which prompted the anesthetist John Carlisle in 2012 to investigate them (Stroebe et al. 2012; Marcus & Oransky 2015).

Such cases of fraud are plausibly driven by desires for personal gain. In order to acquire funding, a research position, or just recognition among one's peers, a researcher rationalizes misconduct as acceptable. Indeed, such motivated reasoning sometimes leads scientists, including prominent neuroscientists, to rationalize sexual harassment of their students (Engber 2018).

8.3.3 Questionable Research Practices

Scientific misconduct is rare, but the greater source of the replication crisis is likely that scientists sometimes engage in practices that they either know or should know will bias their results. Various "questionable research practices" make one's studies more likely to produce a statistically significant result (see, e.g., Nosek et al. 2012; Peterson 2019). Many scientists have powerful personal, professional, and ideological motivations to engage in such practices in order to rack up more publications, especially in more prestigious journals, which prefer exciting findings that substantially advance the cutting edge of research. One recent study collected anonymous responses from over 2,000 psychological scientists about their own engagement in 10 questionable research practices (John et al. 2012). The vast majority of respondents (91%) admitted to engaging in at least one of them. Of the practices, three stand out as most common, given that about half of respondents (45–65%) reported engaging in them:

- selectively reporting studies that "worked" (excluding null results, for example)
- deciding whether to collect additional data after checking to see whether the results were significant (a form of "p-hacking")
- failing to report all of a study's measures

Although the survey attempted to incentivize honesty, some respondents probably remained reluctant to reveal such misdeeds even anonymously.

Another questionable practice on the rise is the reporting of and reliance on "marginally significant" results. A p-value of less than 0.05 is the conventional threshold for statistical significance (see the appendix to Chapter 1), yet some researchers report slightly higher p-values as significant or "marginally significant" to ultimately support a hypothesis. Over the past few decades, this questionable practice has increased substantially in psychology (Pritschet et al. 2016). The choice to rely on marginal significance can be motivated by the desire to publish or to advance a desired conclusion. One potential example of both motivations is the widely cited—and apparently only—empirical attempt to demonstrate that blind auditions in orchestras increase the number of women who win auditions by reducing discrimination or implicit bias (Goldin & Rouse 2000). However, the media and the authors themselves tout the desired conclusion based largely on marginally significant effects with large standard errors (for discussion, see Pallesen 2019).

Another practice influenced by personal goals is the failure to disclose aspects of one's methods or data that could impact conclusions. An example can be found in one of the most famous studies in psychology, the "Stanford Prison Experiment" led by Philip Zimbardo in 1971. As the story goes, Zimbardo randomly assigned healthy male students at Stanford to play the role of either guards or prisoners over the course of two weeks in a basement on campus. Zimbardo shut the study down after only a week because the situation had apparently devolved into guards mistreating prisoners so badly that some begged to be released. However, it appears Zimbardo misrepresented the study's design and observations (Blum 2018). According to new interviews and old uncovered transcripts of discussions with participants and others present, it was revealed that Zimbardo essentially encouraged the mistreatment, that the prisoners were not quite free to leave for any reason, and that the pleas to be released were likely faked just so the students could get back to their lives (in one case to go study for an important exam).

Some problematic practices are more prevalent in or specific to neuroscience. False positives and false negatives, which won't ultimately replicate, are more likely when studies contain low numbers of participants or trials, making some statistical inferences weaker. And many areas of neuroscience tend to employ notoriously small sample sizes, typically around 20 participants in neuroimaging (Szucs & Ioannidis 2020). Some studies involve a single crucial observation that is difficult to repeat in unusual circumstances or with inaccessible populations. Studies of rare brain disorders, for example, are sometimes published in top journals like *Nature* and shape the field with only a sample of two patients (e.g., Anderson et al. 1999). With small samples and rare circumstances that are difficult to repeat, findings are more likely to be influenced by biases (Ionnidis 2005).

Yet neuroscience research is even less likely to be confirmed or replicated by other labs because it's so expensive. In neuroimaging, for example, each study participant usually spends about an hour in the MRI scanner, which typically costs at least US$500. Even if researchers are interested in replicating existing research, funding bodies rarely support such endeavors. Like high-impact journals, they want to see reports of exciting novel findings.

Much of neuroscience also involves highly complex technologies and statistical inferences that are still being understood and improved. For example, one team of researchers sought to demonstrate a common statistical problem in brain imaging that increases the chances of false positive results. They made their point vividly—and humorously—by presenting data from a functional magnetic resonance imaging (fMRI) scan of a dead fish, which showed elevated neural activity when the researchers instructed the Atlantic salmon to take on the perspective of others (Bennett et al. 2010). This clearly false positive result was made possible by failing to employ an important statistical correction when performing many tests simultaneously ("multiple comparisons"), which had gone unheeded by far too many investigators. Neuroscientists rapidly attempted to implement various statistical corrections in their fMRI analysis software packages, which was used in thousands of published papers. But a group of researchers eventually discovered that one prominent correction method in the software packages continued to allow for an inflation in false positives (Eklund et al. 2016; see also Poldrack 2018). It's thus important to remember not only that neuroscience remains in its infancy, but that it also often employs extremely complex technologies to study the most complicated and least understood organ on the planet.

Of course, questionable research practices are not specific to neuroscience or even the social sciences. One recent study asked over

800 scientists working in ecology and evolutionary biology, for instance, about how often they and their colleagues engage in questionable practices (Fraser et al. 2018). The researchers also directly compared their data to surveys of psychologists and found markedly similar results, leading to the conclusion that questionable research practices are "broadly as common in ecology and evolution research as they are in psychology" (p. 9). For example, about two thirds (64%) of respondents said they had cherry-picked which results they reported in articles by omitting null findings that were not statistically significant. And over half (51%) admitted to claiming that unexpected findings were predicted in advance. Another study mined articles in the PubMed database to estimate the likelihood of *p-hacking*, defined as acts where "researchers collect or select data or statistical analyses until nonsignificant results become significant" (Head et al. 2015: 1). Studies in the database included many disciplines in the natural sciences—including biology, chemistry, medicine, and geoscience—yet the authors conclude that "p-hacking is widespread in the scientific literature" (11). Of course, these concerns are only exacerbated by conflicts of interest, such as pharmaceutical companies who fund clinical trials of drugs (see Chapter 3).

Indeed, science has long been influenced by financial conflicts of interest, politics, and other biases. However, the recent replication crisis and high-profile cases of misconduct have renewed concerns about the generation of biased data and conclusions. We'll see that a researcher's preferences or values can contribute to the rationalization of experimental designs or interpretations of data that will bring the researcher personal gain or support a favored ideology.

8.4 What Motivates Scientists?

Why do scientists, like everyone else, sometimes cut corners or uncritically employ methods that lead to poor evidence? A key factor is motivated reasoning, particularly since research practices regarded as merely "questionable" provide enough of a fudge factor—enough wiggle room—to justify rule-bending to oneself or one's research group. With motivated reasoning as our framework for understanding the influence of values on science, we should consider what motivates scientists.

8.4.1 Ultimate Goals in Science

We have already encountered several common motives that can influence an investigator's reasoning, including financial gain, career advancement, ideology, and even truth. However, at any given time multiple motivations can arise that serve quite different end goals.

It is thus imperative to distinguish two kinds of goals, motivations, or desires. On the one hand, *instrumental* (or extrinsic) desires are those one has as a means to achieve another goal, such as the desire to take a pill to relieve a headache. *Ultimate* (or intrinsic) desires, on the other hand, are those one has for their own sake, such as the desire to relieve a headache. It is tempting to treat all desires as instrumental except for the desire to gain pleasure or to avoid pain (as the theory of psychological egoism would have us believe). But there is ample empirical evidence that humans ultimately desire more than their own self-interest, including helping others and doing what's right (Fiske & Rai 2014; Batson 2016; May 2018a: Ch. 6). Power, fame, prestige, and knowledge are also plausibly valued intrinsically.

Scientists have many ultimate goals, whether held consciously or unconsciously, but six distinct categories stand out (Table 8.2). Scientific reasoning is often guided by the desire to produce *knowledge* for its own sake, which is commonly identified as the ideal. However, scientists can also be motivated to produce novel and interesting results as a means to other ultimate goals, such as recognition and social status. The desire for such social *credit* can lead to questionable or otherwise poor research practices, which can frustrate the ultimate aim of acquiring knowledge (Nosek et al. 2012; Tullett 2015). Poor practices can also be rationalized as a means to achieve the ultimate goal of promoting or upholding one's favored *ideology*. Since one regards the ideology as correct, truth (or acceptance of it) is typically the ultimate goal. However, landing on the truth by luck via the path of wishful thinking does not amount to knowledge; sound evidence

Table 8.2 Some Sources of Motivated Reasoning in Science

Ultimate goal	Examples
Knowledge (production or acquisition of it)	accurate theories, genuine experimental effects, explanatory unification
Ideology (promoting the acceptance of it)	research supports egalitarianism, theism, denigration of conservatism
Credit (acquiring it)	reputation improvement and maintenance, career advancement, academic promotion and honors
Profit (acquiring it)	speaker fees, honoraria, book sales, higher salary
Altruism (promoting the interests of others)	helping one's students and postdocs get publications and jobs
Spite (harming one's rivals)	retaliating against other researchers by preventing their work from being published or publicly disparaging it

is required. Thus, rather than a truth motive, I prefer to speak of a "knowledge motive," which sharply distinguishes it from the ideology motive (contrast Bright 2017).

Some of these motives are ultimately self-interested (e.g., profit and credit), but others are not. The desire to produce knowledge is certainly not egoistic, but neither is the motivation to support an ideology or even to settle a grudge with rivals (*spite*), provided we appropriately understand these as goals desired for their own sakes, not as a means to personal gain. Researchers, like all humans, can also be motivated by *altruism*, where the ultimate goal is the promotion of another person's interests (Batson 2011; May 2011). Altruism is generally laudable, but it can lead to nepotism and bias the objective evaluation of work by one's students, friends, and mentors. That's why most scientific publication involves anonymous peer review, though publication is but one aspect of scientific advancement, and practitioners know that anonymity is often breached.

Whether self-serving or not, our framework of motivated reasoning suggests that any of these six ultimate goals can sway scientific investigation toward furthering them. The means to these ends can involve the production of quality data, as when one aims to produce knowledge or even to support one's favored ideology, given that disciplinary norms do value quality data and underexplored questions. However, the scientific process also values certain hot topics, as well as novel, counterintuitive findings, so a means to acquire credit, profit, and even altruism can involve fabricating data, questionable research practices, and the sabotaging of rivals.

Of course, science is conducted not only by individuals but also by large communities. Sometimes it's appropriate to ascribe motives to such groups of researchers, as when a particular laboratory is motivated to achieve collective credit or to promote their favored theory. However, the values within a community do not always reflect the motivations of each individual within it, particularly when it comes to dominant assumptions, ideologies, and stereotypes. Often the prevailing framework in a research community will match the motivations of the individuals within it. For example, many scientists have been unconsciously motivated to uphold (or at least not flout) stereotypes about divorce as inherently damaging to a family (Anderson 2004), about testosterone as a masculine hormone (Fine 2010), and about illegal drugs ravaging the brain (Hart 2013). But individual motivations and dominant community values can diverge. Suppose, for instance, that environmentalism is the most widely accepted ethic within ecology. Some individual ecologists might produce work that supports (or avoids conflicting with) conservationist policies, not for the ultimate goal of promoting conservation but as a necessary means to achieve profit or credit within the community's accepted framework.

Thus, we can ultimately understand the effects of community-level values in terms of the motivations of individual scientists. But, again, to understand the values that influence scientific practice, it is essential to distinguish between the ultimate and instrumental goals of individuals. The question now is which ultimate motivations are most prevalent among scientists.

8.4.2 What Motivates Most Scientists?

It is often difficult to know for sure what ultimately motivates people, let alone most scientists. A natural place to start is to ask them. Since some of the ultimate goals are self-serving (profit and credit), some scientists won't be fully truthful when self-reporting their motivations. Nevertheless, interviews, anonymous surveys, and case studies provide some relevant evidence.

In 2009, collaborating with the American Association for the Advancement of Science, the Pew Research Center (2009) surveyed over 2,500 scientists about political issues and the nature of the scientific enterprise. Respondents were primarily in the natural sciences (namely, biological/medical, chemistry, geosciences, physics/astronomy), with only 19% in the "other" category. Most worked in academia (63%) with the rest in government, industry, nonprofits, or other sectors. Most of the scientists reported opting for their careers in order to "solve intellectually challenging problems," "work for the public good," or "make an important discovery." Remarkably, though, a third acknowledged that a "financially rewarding career" was very or somewhat important, and the number jumps to about half (51%) for the scientists working in industry. Given the stigma attached to doing science for the money, these self-reported attitudes are likely an underestimation of the reality, particularly among early career researchers who are often paid little for the hours they work and the education level they have attained. These data suggest what is fairly commonsense. Scientists are highly motivated to solve challenging problems and produce knowledge that makes a difference in the world. But they also want to benefit personally from it.

Perhaps the greatest personal gains are not profit but social credit, such as recognition or career advancement. Indeed, competition is fierce across all the sciences. In a focus group setting, over 50 researchers from the biomedical, clinical, biological, and behavioral sciences reported no positive effects of competition among practitioners in their fields (Anderson et al. 2007). Instead, even though the scientists were not explicitly asked questions about competition, their responses regularly turned to competition and how it often leads to secrecy, sabotage, soured relationships, scientific misconduct, and interference with peer review. Multiple participants mentioned the "practice of taking photographs of poster presentations in order then to publish the results first" (451). Some participants reported that since "ideas get stolen constantly" sometimes fellow scientists will omit certain details of their research protocols in presentations or publications. Many researchers may go into science primarily with a desire to produce knowledge, but its competitive structure can inculcate desires for recognition and career advancement.

Vivid examples of the competition for credit and status can be found in cases of fraud, although they go well beyond mere bias in science. Consider, for instance, what motivated Dietrich Stapel, the infamous Dutch social psychologist. An extensive report by his employer, the University of Tilburg, found that for at least a decade Stapel manipulated and fabricated data in experiments that were eventually published in over 30 peer-reviewed articles. Stapel studied the social influences on human behavior, but there is no theme in his work that supports a particular moral or political ideology, such as socialism or conservatism. There doesn't even appear to be a particular theory of the human mind that Stapel's work supports. He wasn't known for an overarching framework, such as prospect theory, or even a famous mechanism, such as confirmation bias, moral licensing, or the fundamental attribution error. Stapel also didn't seem to accrue much financial gain from, say, high-profile speaking engagements or a self-help book centered on a key finding, such as "power posing." His own rationalization is that he was on a "quest for aesthetics, for beauty" in the data he reported, but a *New York Times* interviewer reports that Stapel "didn't deny that his deceit was driven by ambition" (Bhattacharjee 2013)—that is, credit or social status.

More common than fraud is the exaggeration or misrepresentation of research, which can be particularly easy to do in neuroscience given its infancy and complexity. For example, one group of researchers claimed to uncover the secret political attitudes of swing voters by scanning the brains of just 20 participants in the lab (Iacoboni et al. 2007). The scans were conducted during the 2008 presidential race in the United States, and the authors of the study argued that participants who rated Hilary Clinton unfavorably were conflicted about this judgment because they exhibited greater activity in the anterior cingulate cortex. Of course, like other brain areas, the cingulate has more than one psychological function (see the problem of reverse inference in Chapter 9). So we can't draw such specific conclusions about participants' attitudes, let alone most swing voters (Poldrack 2018). Yet the researchers skipped peer review and published a report of their findings directly in *The New York Times*. Such sensationalistic, overreaching claims are plausibly motivated by the desire to achieve recognition (the credit motive).

Of course, similar stories of questionable research practices also crop up elsewhere in the sciences (Stroebe et al. 2012). And the behavior is largely explicable in terms of the desire for personal gain. Profits in science, particularly academia, are not large, but the rewards of social credit are substantial. Concern with competition and social status is a natural feature of human life, grounded in our having evolved to live in groups saturated with social hierarchies and norms (Churchland 2011; Henrich 2015; Kumar & Campbell 2022). One of the most powerful drives among deeply social creatures like us is to acquire and maintain status, pride, or respect among peers. If to achieve such social status and approval we will engage in violence, p-hacking is a breeze. This powerful motive is common among human beings generally, not just scientists.

Overall, the framework of motivated reasoning reveals how values can influence all areas of science. Even research in the natural sciences is susceptible to various values, including moral, political, and other ideological motivations that otherwise seem endemic to social science. Moreover, ideological motives are generally minor compared to other motivations present in both domains, particularly credit but also profit. Of course, in some cases research has been influenced by ideology. Progressive values appear to have influenced psychological studies of conservatism and prejudice (Duarte et al. 2015), and staunch ideological opposition to government regulation has influenced climate science (Oreskes & Conway 2010). However, particular instances don't make for general trends across the sciences. We've seen that the basic motivations throughout science are the same, including desires for credit, profit, ideology, and knowledge. Incentives are also similar (e.g., publish or perish, acquire grant funding), as are the methods (experiments, interviews, meta-analyses, theory building, case studies, etc.). Accordingly, questionable research practices arise equally in all scientific domains, including all areas of neuroscience.

8.4.3 Optimism

Is scientific investigation hopelessly flawed? Not at all. Motivated reasoning sometimes engenders wishful thinking, but it isn't always a flaw. Even post hoc rationalization and confabulation can serve a valuable purpose in trying to make sense of one's automatic and unconscious attitudes (Gazzaniga 1967; Bortolotti 2010; Summers 2017; Cushman 2020). Psychotherapy, for example, might inaccurately identify the source of one's marital problems as narcissism, but the diagnosis might not be far off and can promote greater self-understanding in other facets of one's life.

Even if motivated reasoning were always inappropriate for the individual, it can often lead to knowledge in science at the group level. Individual biases can be tempered by mechanisms of *self-correction*, including anonymous peer review, conflict of interest disclosures, and replication efforts. Much like Adam Smith's invisible hand of the market, the system can produce a common good from self-interested individuals (see Solomon 2001, though she rejects the analogy). Mechanisms of self-correction don't function nearly as well as one would hope (Estes 2012; Nosek et al. 2012; Stroebe et al. 2012), but studies of collective deliberation have shown that individual biases can produce knowledge when people who disagree about a controversial topic hash it out (Mercier & Sperber 2017). In this way, recent game-theoretic models suggest that the motives of individual scientists, even if self-centered, can produce a greater good through a competitive marketplace of ideas (e.g., Zollman 2018; Bright 2017). The adversarial nature of scientific research can thus be beneficial to knowledge production.

No doubt science remains one of the best tools we have in our knowledge-producing toolkit, and we have several reasons to be optimistic about its fundamental soundness. First, the scope of bias is limited. Few scientists are frauds, and the system is to some degree self-correcting, even if not as much as one would hope. Although some findings can't be replicated, others have been reproduced and are corroborated by other empirical findings, meta-analyses, and explanatory frameworks. Second, while bad motives take reasoning in the wrong direction, good motives can steer it on the right track, and accuracy and rigor are both prized in science. Third, the problem of motivated reasoning is not specific to scientific inquiry (*tu quoque*). We can all agree that humans produce great amounts of knowledge, and yet our reasoning is often motivated. If we can produce knowledge outside of science, we can do so within it.

Moreover, scientific norms and practices are already improving and will continue to progress. Large-scale replication efforts are becoming more common, as are preregistration of studies in which researchers publicly declare their planned hypotheses and analyses in advance. Many researchers are posting their raw data to promote transparency and to make replication efforts easier to carry out. And scientists are engaging in earnest discussions about how to improve publishing models so as to limit the incentives to publish underpowered studies with small sample sizes. Social norms and behaviors in science can and do improve.

8.5 Conclusion

Having one's reasoning motivated by goals is a fundamental part of human life, including the working lives of scientists, not just the curious confabulations of neurological patients. We're deceiving ourselves if we think that we're immune to motivated reasoning.

The takeaway is *not* that split-brain patients or scientists are deliberate liars. Fraudsters are, but they are few and far between. Forms of motivated reasoning are more frequent but driven primarily by unconscious forces. Nevertheless, recall that we aren't only our conscious minds, and we can be responsible for choices made in ignorance of all the factors that influence them (Chapter 2). So the perpetrators of questionable research practices aren't entirely blameless. Like the CEO of a corporation, one is responsible to some degree for letting poor practices flourish on one's watch.

Even though motivated reasoning is pervasive, it doesn't preclude the acquisition of knowledge. Nevertheless, we should approach evidence with vigilance, especially when our topic is the brain, one of the most mysterious organs on the planet. In the next chapter, with the power of motivated reasoning on our minds, we examine whether neuroscience is developed enough to rely on in high-stakes situations, or, instead, whether it frustrates the aims of justice in the courtroom and violates the rights of individual consumers.

9
Brain Reading

If scientific reasoning can be so biased, shouldn't we be particularly worried about attempts to peer into our minds through brain reading? Courts are beginning to draw on neuroscience to inform criminal and civil liability. And corporations are using brain-based methods for detecting consumer preferences, to get the masses hooked (or even more hooked) on their products. Concerns about justice, privacy, and the health of society might make one deeply suspicious of using neuroscience in such contexts, especially when life, death, and injustice are on the line in courts of law.

Keeping with our cautious optimism, we'll see that it's unclear whether such alarmism is warranted. Concerns about neuromarketing are often based on overinflated claims about the power of brain imaging to uncover our deepest desires. Yet some neuroscientific technologies do provide useful evidence in the law, at least as useful as sources of evidence we already permit (an argument from parity). The benefits are modest, but this also limits the damage brain reading can do. Moreover, the meager benefits can be amplified when combined with other tools we already possess in our legal toolbelts.

9.1 Exoneration by EEG

In August 1978, Terry Harrington was convicted of the murder of a parking lot security guard in Iowa. Though he had an alibi and maintained his innocence, the 17-year-old was primarily convicted on the testimonies of other teenage accomplices and almost no physical evidence. Harrington was sentenced to life in prison without the possibility of parole. In the years following, he continuously tried to appeal his case but was rejected by the courts until two decades after his conviction (*Harrington v. State of Iowa* 1997). The appeal was based on new evidence: multiple witness recantations, newly discovered police reports containing evidence of another suspect, and "brain fingerprinting" evidence.

Brain fingerprinting uses electroencephalography (EEG) to record electrical activity on the surface of a person's brain through a cap that contains many small electrodes placed on the scalp. Dr. Larry Farwell, a psychophysiologist, developed the proprietary technique and claims that it reveals when someone is familiar with facts about a crime. The EEG cap monitors a particular pattern of brain activity—the well-known P300 brain wave—which reportedly occurs when an individual *recognizes* a piece of information. The P300 wave occurs so fast that it's automatic and involuntary, so it apparently can't be controlled or faked like the physiological arousal measured by traditional polygraphs or "lie detectors" (Langleben 2008). Harrington was exposed to sensitive information about the crime as well as information he certainly knew, which functioned as a control condition. Analysis of Harrington's brain activity suggested that he didn't recognize the details of the murder, but he did recognize information consistent with his alibi. Harrington's lawyers presented this evidence in court to support his innocence (Farwell & Makeig 2005).

The new evidence, including the EEG results, led the court to overturn Harrington's conviction and grant him a retrial. In 2003, he was given reprieve by the governor of Iowa, which thereby released Harrington after having served 25 years in prison, without needing a retrial. Though Harrington's exoneration wasn't solely based on the brain fingerprinting technology, its admission as a sufficiently reliable piece of evidence set a precedent for future use by other courts.

Brain reading promises a direct line into the minds of others, unmediated by their lies or lack of self-knowledge. Sometimes the best way to find out what someone is thinking is just by asking them. However, we've seen that much of our mental lives is unconscious (Chapter 2), that we form automatic intuitions without always knowing their complex source (Chapter 6), and we often concoct stories to rationalize our behavior (Chapter 8). So, when a person has reason to lie, is self-deceived, or is simply unable to communicate, we can't rely on their self-report of what's going on in their mind.

Neurobiological detection of mental states could circumvent these barriers and help jurors, interrogators, physicians, and marketers understand what people truly think and feel, and perhaps how they will behave in the future.

Several ethical issues arise with the use of novel neurotechnologies, especially in the courtroom. Justice, harm, and privacy are the primary concerns. Will premature adoption of neurotechnologies unjustly convict an innocent person or confuse the jury into acquitting a criminal? Will peering into people's minds obliterate the shred of confidentiality that most of us are clinging to in the modern world? In this chapter, we'll focus on the use of brain-based technologies in the courtroom and afterward briefly discuss their use on consumers.

9.2 Unjust Verdicts

Neuroscientific evidence is increasingly used in legal proceedings. Even if still used sparingly, it seems "neurobiological evidence is now a mainstay of our criminal justice system" (Farahany 2016: 508; see also Davis 2017). Such evidence can inform a wide range of judgments about the mental states and capacities of individuals in the courtroom. These include guilty knowledge, malicious intent, legal insanity, competence to stand trial, amenability to rehabilitation, the capacity for self-control, liability to reoffend if released on parole or probation, severity of psychological injuries for civil disputes, and even bias among jurors (Sinnott-Armstrong et al. 2008; Glenn & Raine 2014; Hirstein et al. 2018; Aharoni et al. 2022).

The primary ethical issue in all of these cases is injustice and harm from reliance on poor evidence or premature adoption (Wolpe et al. 2005; Levy 2007: 144; Satel & Lilienfeld 2013: 95). Recall the case of Brian Dugan from Chapter 6, the inmate diagnosed with psychopathy who committed numerous murders and sexual assaults. During his trial for the murder of 10-year-old Jeanine Nicarico, Dugan's defense lawyers used functional magnetic resonance imaging (fMRI) to try to spare him from the death penalty. The defense admitted that Dugan knew right from wrong and thus was legally sane; their claim instead was that Dugan's brain abnormality impaired his self-control. This was one of the first times fMRI was used as evidence to prove a brain abnormality caused diminished control (in 2009 for the 1983 crime). If the neurobiological evidence is weak, overreliance on it in this case could unjustly reduce punishment for some truly heinous crimes. In other cases, such as Harrington's, junk science risks setting a criminal free, which would be unjust and risks harm to society if the individual is liable to reoffend after release. Similar concerns about harm and injustice arise for judgments about parole, sentencing, damages awarded to plaintiffs, and so on. There are many ways poor evidence can impede justice.

Should we be pessimistic about the prospects of brain reading? Many commentators worry that neuroimaging in particular does not provide sufficiently strong evidence to outweigh the dangers it brings for misinterpretation or misuse (e.g., Morse 2006b; Levy 2007: Ch. 4; Sinnott-Armstrong et al. 2008; Poldrack et al. 2018). Others defend a more optimistic take, emphasizing that neurobiological data provide additional evidence of brain dysfunction and psychological capacities (e.g., Glannon 2011: 79–80; Glenn & Raine 2014; Gaudet et al. 2014; Aharoni et al. 2022).

A useful approach to resolving this dispute lies within common legal standards. When determining whether to allow proposed evidence, most courts in the United States follow the Federal Rules of Evidence. Rule 403 articulates a reasonable guide:

> Evidence may be excluded if its **probative value** is substantially outweighed by the **danger** of unfair prejudice, confusion of the issues, or misleading the jury, or by considerations of undue delay, waste of time, or needless presentation of cumulative evidence.

The rule essentially instructs courts to balance (a) the *strength* of the evidence against (b) its *dangers*. We've already seen in the previous chapter that neurobiological evidence, like all scientific evidence, can be poor in quality and subject to bias. But is there a special problem here? We'll consider neuroscience's probative value and potential dangers before weighing them against one another.

9.3 Too Unreliable?

Neuroimaging and related technologies are incredibly complex with inherent trade-offs. The technology that helped exonerate Harrington is older than fMRI and doesn't rely on tracking relatively slow blood flow. Instead, EEG measures electrical activity with a high "temporal resolution," meaning it can track quick changes in brain waves, down to milliseconds. However, EEG can't pinpoint with great precision *where* these changes in electrical activity occur (low spatial resolution), partly because the electrodes aren't well-suited to detecting changes below the brain's surface. In contrast, fMRI scanners can detect changes in blood flow anywhere in the head, though only in the range of seconds, not milliseconds.

On top of these trade-offs, it bears emphasis that any brain-reading technique involves many, many links in an inferential chain (see the appendix to Chapter 1). The more links, the more opportunity for weakness, error, or motivated reasoning. The strength of neurobiological evidence is also limited by its subject matter, namely diverse nervous systems that follow complicated paths to generate thoughts and behavior. Courts often seek to uncover a *particular* person's mental states or psychological capacities, yet the research is largely based on *average* brain structure and function, which presents the *group-to-individual problem* (Poldrack et al. 2018). These concerns are important enough, but let's consider in detail some further constraints on the probative value of brain reading.

9.3.1 Nominal Normality

One issue is that it's difficult to define neurologically "normal" with precision. Brain scans might be used to show that an offender like Dugan has abnormal brain activity, but judgments of abnormality are shaky, given that there is wide variation in human brain structure and function. We saw in previous chapters that human agency, rationality, and mental health present along a continuum, and there is increasing evidence of cognitive diversity across cultures (Henrich 2020). So talk of what's "normal" or "abnormal" in the brain is often nominal at best

(Daniels 2000; Washington 2016). The problem is exacerbated in many criminal and psychiatric contexts. When the behavior and psychological traits of defendants or patients are already expected to deviate from the average, any purported brain abnormalities might be particularly uninformative.

We can, of course, identify mean (average) brain activity. But means provide an illusion of uniformity when the standard deviations are high (see Figure 9.1), which is common in neurobiological measures. As Walter Sinnott-Armstrong, Adina Roskies, and their co-authors put it: "Most neuroscientific studies using fMRI report group averages, but individual functional profiles can vary so much that it is not unusual for most individuals to differ from the group average" (2008: 362). So, demonstrating that someone like Dugan has "abnormal" brain structure or function might tell us little, except that he is just like everyone else in deviating from the average (Satel & Lilienfeld 2013: 110).

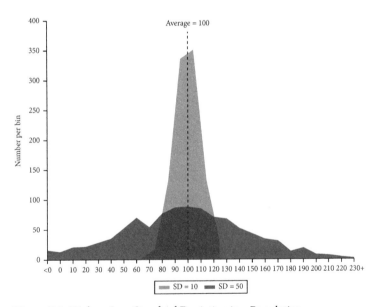

Figure 9.1 High vs. Low Standard Deviation in a Population

Samples from two populations with the same mean (100) on some hypothetical measure, but different standard deviations (SD).

Source: Wikimedia/JRBrown.

Problems of normality also plague attempts to discern truth from lies, a common aim of brain reading. Companies—with clever names like "No Lie MRI"—and researchers have been trying to detect deception from brain activity alone (for review, see Langleben 2008). Neuroscientists have identified several areas of the brain that tend to be more active when participants are engaging in intentional deception, compared to telling the truth. Further research using functional neuroimaging claims to identify deception in particular individuals with up to 78% accuracy. However, such studies all require cooperative participants who are engaging in deception under highly artificial contexts (Levy 2007: 138–140). Slight movements and heavy breathing can render neuroimaging data utterly worthless, even when a subject is constrained by the MRI head coil. Poor external validity thus prevents generalizing to many real-world situations, where uncooperative defendants or patients can render the process unreliable.

Now, we shouldn't impose an impossibly high standard here. Satel and Lilienfeld lament that no study has shown that a specific brain region is "consistently activated in all people when they fib, and consistently silent when they do not" (2013: 89). The implicit standard here trades one extreme for another. The recognition of a cognitive continuity among human brains allows neurobiological evidence to reveal where someone falls on that spectrum. Even if judgments of "normality" aren't informative, we can perhaps discern to what *degree* one has, say, moral knowledge or self-control.

9.3.2 Low Base Rates

Another concern about the probative value of neurobiological evidence is that some uses are particularly prone to yielding *false positives*. That is, tests might suggest that a defendant has a brain abnormality or neurological condition when she doesn't (Wolpe et al. 2005; Sinnott-Armstrong et al. 2008).

The problem lies in the rarity of many neurological conditions, their low "base rates." The concept, often deployed in medicine, is straightforward: the *base rate* is simply the prevalence of some property among a group of individuals. A physician, for instance, might be interested in detecting a disease, such as Huntington's, in some patients through testing blood samples. But tests are always imperfect: they can yield false positives or false negatives. Suppose that the blood test only produces false positives, and at a rate of 5%. Is this a reliable test? It depends on how prevalent the disease is in the population tested. Imagine the prevalence varies by country. In High Country 40% of people have the disease, while in Low Country the base rate is only 2% (see Figure 9.2). If health professionals randomly test a person from each population, what is the probability that the patient has Huntington's, given a positive test result?

You might think the answer is 95% for each population, but it depends greatly on the base rate. In High Country, 400 people out of every 1,000 has the disease. The blood test will accurately catch these 400 people, because it doesn't yield any false negatives. Of the remaining 600 people, however, 5% will be false positives (about 30 people). So 430 people would receive a positive test while only 400 have the disease, making the probability 93% (400/430) that a person in the High Country has Huntington's given a positive test. Not bad. Prior to the test, each person in this country could only ascertain that she has a 40% chance of having the disease, whereas a positive test result updates the probability to 93%.

Now consider Low Country, where the disease is rare. Only 20 out of every 1,000 people has Huntington's there. The test will accurately report these 20 positive results, because again it doesn't yield

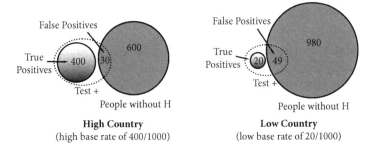

Figure 9.2 High vs. Low Base Rates in a Population

Two populations with different base rates of some property H (e.g., Huntington's disease).

false negatives. However, 980 people don't have the disease, and the test will report 49 (5%) as positive, yielding a total of 69 people with a positive test result. What's the probability, then, that any individual has Huntington's in the Low Country, given a positive test result? The answer is only 29%! After all, only 20 of the 69 positive test results are accurate. Prior to the test, each person in the Low Country could only ascertain that they have a 2% chance of having the disease, and a positive test result increases the probability to only 29%. The very same test isn't so useful in a different context.

The lesson for neurobiological evidence should be clear. Serious brain abnormalities are rare (a low base rate), which can yield a high rate of false alarms, even with rather precise tools for detecting the abnormalities. Matters are exponentially worse if the diagnostic methods for identifying the abnormalities are imprecise. We must exercise caution when evaluating legal evidence regarding rare neurological conditions, yet that is exceedingly difficult for humans to do. We can be quite good at statistical reasoning in some contexts, but we're particularly prone to neglect base rates (Kahneman 2011).

Nevertheless, our hypothetical examples focus exclusively on the one test for a disease, when in reality there is often other evidence to add into the mix. For example, some rare brain abnormalities are large tumors that show up with great precision on a structural brain scan. Recall Weinstein's arachnoid cyst, which was nearly the size of an orange (Chapter 2). Other brain differences that purport to reveal reduced psychological functions are much more subtle, such as those in psychopathy. However, we don't have to use brain imaging alone to provide evidence of psychological dysfunction. The Psychopathy Checklist, for example, assesses a person's behavior and criminal record to yield a diagnostic score. So, even if brain imaging provides only a 29% probability that a defendant has a brain disorder, other pieces of evidence can bump that probability up much, much higher.

9.3.3 The Thought-Action Gap

Another cluster of concerns about probative value emphasizes the gulf between brain activity and action. The law is often concerned with intent and other elements of mens rea, but largely only when causally related to criminal actions and one's ability to control them. Yet many brain abnormalities, assuming we can accurately identify them, only indicate abnormal thoughts and feelings, not specific behaviors for which one can be held legally liable. Several factors contribute to this gap.

First, brain imaging only provides correlations between the brain and behavior. Consider Dugan whose brain scans indicated abnormal brain structure and function consistent with psychopathy. These abnormalities are correlated with psychopathic traits and behavior, but we cannot conclude from correlations alone that these brain abnormalities *caused* his decisions to repeatedly abuse and murder young girls. It could be that his deviant behavior led to the abnormalities, similar to how repeatedly carting passengers around London's web of streets increases gray matter volume in the hippocampus of taxi drivers (Maguire et al. 2006). In Dugan's case, the expert witness, Kent Kiehl, was careful to stress that the neuroimaging evidence only showed that Dugan's brain was different, not that the abnormality caused his actions. Yet defense lawyers, like Weinstein's, often need to show that a defendant's brain abnormalities contribute causally to the criminal behavior, not vice versa.

Second, even if we're able to identify the direction of causation, the brain abnormalities might merely cause deviant *desires* that don't necessarily cause the resulting action. Consider the case of Kevin who had deviant sexual desires consistent with Klüver–Bucy syndrome (Chapter 1). Although Kevin's brain surgery was likely responsible for the deviant desires, he didn't always act on them. Indeed, the judge in his case ultimately accorded Kevin some responsibility for downloading child pornography because Kevin did so only at home, refraining from such activities while on his work computer. In other words, deviant desires don't necessarily preclude self-control. Many neurotypical people experience deviant thoughts or desires but don't act on them. So the mere existence of such mental states does not necessarily tell us much about criminal liability.

9.3.4 Reverse Inference

Instead of focusing on brain abnormalities, we could use neurobiological evidence to uncover relatively normal mental states or capacities, such as deception, intent, juror bias, and moral or legal knowledge. In these cases, there will be less concern about the gap between thought and action, though issues of normality and base rates remain (Wolpe et al. 2005). However, another issue impedes our ability to discern specific mental states and functions from brain activity: the dreaded problem of "reverse inference" (Poldrack 2006).

Ultimately, we want to know how brain activity gives rise to psychological states and functions. Even in this book we've examined, for example, what the reward pathway tells us about self-control in drug addiction (Chapter 5) and what activity in the amygdala and other brain areas tells us about the role of reason and emotion in moral judgment (Chapter 6). Yet identifying specific functions of brain areas can be problematic. Any one anatomical area typically has a diverse range of psychological functions. For example, the ventromedial prefrontal cortex processes fear but also reward-based learning, among many other things. Similarly, the temporoparietal junction (TPJ) is involved in ascertaining what others are thinking and feeling (so-called theory of mind or mind-reading). But this brain area also facilitates many other functions, including daydreaming and other forms of mind-wandering, given that it's part of the brain's "default mode network" (see the "inferior parietal lobule" identified in Buckner et al. 2008). How can we conclude from, say, heightened activity in the TPJ that participants making moral judgments of attempted harm are ascertaining the actor's intent? After all, this brain area isn't just associated with mind-reading but also mind-wandering.

Herein lies the crux of the problem of reverse inference, to be contrasted with unproblematic forward inference. Suppose that activation of the TPJ is well correlated with both mind-reading and mind-wandering. We can then safely infer (forward) that when someone is mind-reading (or mind-wandering) they have heightened TPJ activity. But we cannot necessarily infer (reverse) from heightened TPJ activity that a person is mind-reading rather than mind-wandering (see Figure 9.3). The problem arises because, despite some localization of function in the brain, it only goes so far. There is a one-to-many (not a one-to-one) mapping between brain activity and mental states or functions.

The problem arises for inferring mental states or capacities from any neurobiological method that only correlates brain activity with mental

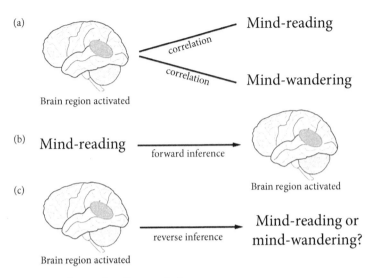

Figure 9.3 Forward vs. Reverse Inference
An illustration of the difference between forward and reverse inference in neuroimaging. (a) The scientific literature shows a *correlation* between activity in a brain region, such as the TPJ, and multiple psychological processes, such as mind-reading and mind-wandering. (b) *Forward inference* would be concluding that there is activity in the TPJ because the person is engaged in mind-reading. (c) *Reverse inference* would be concluding that the person is mind-reading based on observing heightened activity in the TPJ. This is problematic because the person could actually be mind-*wandering*, given that the region has multiple psychological functions.

states, including EEG. The P300 brain wave, for example, is associated with recognizing a stimulus, but also attention and memory. In a systematic review of nearly half a century of research, one authority on the subject writes: "A singular overarching explanation for this neuroelectric phenomenon has proven difficult, primarily because the P300 is observed in any task that requires stimulus discrimination—a fundamental psychological event that determines many aspects of cognition" (Polich 2007: 2137). We can safely infer in a "forward" manner that a P300 wave is occurring when a person recognizes a fact about a crime. However, we cannot necessarily infer in a "reverse" way that a defendant must recognize the fact given the presence of the P300 wave. Reverse inference arguments take this form:

1. If mental event M occurs, then this brain event B occurs.
2. Brain event B occurred.
3. So:
   Mental event M occurred.

Prior correlational studies support the first premise, but the conclusion doesn't follow. As Poldrack (2006) points out, this is a logical fallacy (namely, "affirming the consequent").

Is neuroscience doomed to such fallacious reasoning? Not necessarily, since reverse inference needn't be flawed if enriched with further conditions, premises, or evidence.

First, consider further study conditions. Reverse inference is stronger when drawing on studies in which the particular task that participants are engaging in makes one psychological function of the given brain area more likely than its other functions (Hutzler 2014). For example, if the experimental task is specifically designed to elicit memory recall, then it is likely that the individual is recalling a memory rather than imaging it for the first time.

Second, consider further premises. Even if the experimental task makes multiple psychological states plausible, such as memory recall and attention, the hypotheses being tested might make competing predictions about them (Machery 2014). For example, the hypothesis that Harrington knows incriminating facts of the crime might predict that he will both recall *and* pay more attention to them, compared to mundane statements that mean nothing to him. The hypothesis that Harrington doesn't know the incriminating facts of the crime might predict no P300 wave in response to such stimuli, since they should not have any significance to him. Observation of brain activity can therefore *better support* one hypothesis over another, even if the activity is associated with multiple psychological functions.

Finally, we needn't rely exclusively on merely correlational evidence. Reverse inferences can be combined with psychological tests, witness recantations, and other evidence to build an overall case for exoneration. Neuroscientists can also avoid the problems with reverse inference to some degree by "decoding" mental states from patterns of brain activity. Studies have already used this method to predict with 85% accuracy whether a participant in the scanner is imagining a face or a house (Haynes & Rees 2006). Such decoding works by using the tools of machine learning to identify patterns in brain activity. The method has its own limitations, but it demonstrates how neuroimaging needn't always rely on the dubious assumption that individual brain areas have only one relevant psychological function.

In sum, inferring mental states from brain activity can be based on unproblematic forms of reverse inference that are well supported by other converging evidence. Reverse inference is a serious problem, but it can be overcome with vigilance.

9.4 Too Dangerous?

Even if neurobiological evidence is generally reliable, its use in the courtroom and elsewhere is suspect if we can't properly apply it. Here the concern is that neurobiological evidence is liable to *mislead, confuse,* or *bias* the audience, whether composed of judges, juries, patients, or consumers. The new neuroscience, with its shiny brain images that paper over underlying complexities, might induce what Stephen Morse (2006b) cheekily dubs "brain overclaim syndrome." Experts might be able to discern subtleties in the data, but some commentators worry that a "great danger lies in the abuse of neuroimaging data for presentations to untrained audiences, such as courtroom juries" (Canli & Amin 2002: 425).

9.4.1 Neurobabble

An initial danger is that audiences overinflate the probative value of neuroscientific talk. Press coverage is rife with exaggerated claims about how neuroscience proves that certain experiences are real or that particular therapies like acupuncture truly alleviate pain. The assumption seems to be that "seeing" activity in the brain provides definitive, objective proof of the mental phenomenon (Racine et al. 2005). Some experiments suggest that, in general, neuroscientific descriptions and brain images do bias our evaluation of their evidential value.

In one series of studies, Deena Weisberg and her collaborators (2008) had participants read an explanation for why it's so easy for one to assume that most other people know what one already knows. Participants were randomly assigned to read either a good or bad psychological explanation of this "curse of knowledge" phenomenon, only some of which included superfluous neuroscientific claims such as "brain scans indicate" and "frontal lobe brain circuitry." The researchers found that participants appropriately rated the good explanations more satisfying than the bad ones, but they also rated the merely psychological explanations as less satisfying than the ones with extra neuroscientific lingo. Neuroscience experts, in contrast, did not rate the superfluous "neurobabble" as more satisfying.

One potential example of neurobabble's power is a program developed in the late 1990s by government officials in Georgia. While governor, Zell Miller proposed an initiative to give a tape of classical music to every child born in the state to boost their budding intelligence (Goode 1999). Miller proposed allocating $105,000 from the state's annual budget to provide each newborn Georgian with a CD of classical music. (In the end, not a dime of taxes went toward this effort, because record companies jumped in to provide the music for free.) The proposal was based on just one or two studies that found that briefly listening to Mozart slightly boosted the IQ of college students, not babies. However, this prominent example doesn't show that people are especially liable to misappropriate neuroscience specifically. In fact, the studies on the "Mozart effect" clearly didn't involve any brain-based data. (Brain changes are only implicated because the issue is increased intelligence in child development.) What this case reveals is that all evidence, including scientific evidence, can be misunderstood and overhyped.

Neuroscience does trade heavily in brain images, which might be particularly liable to mislead. One study reports that brain images alone can artificially inflate the credibility of scientific arguments (McCabe & Castel 2008). The researchers had participants read several texts making empirical arguments for conclusions like "meditation enhances creative thought" and "playing video games benefits attention." Participants were randomly assigned to read passages that included a brain image, other images (a bar graph or topographical map), or text only. Across several experiments, the arguments were rated more favorably when they included a brain image specifically.

These studies are a good start, but ironically they are too often thought to have proved definitively that people are easily bamboozled by neuroscience. There are several reasons to remain cautious. First, although the researchers have found an effect of neuroscientific explanations on participants' ratings, the differences were rather *small*. In the neurobabble study (Weisberg et al. 2008), nonexperts rated the bad psychological explanations on average as just *slightly* unsatisfying (around -1 on a scale from -3 to 3) and rated the bad neuroscientific explanations around the neutral point (0 on the scale), so not outright satisfying. Similarly, McCabe and Castel (2008) found that arguments with brain images "made sense" more than arguments alone but only by less than a quarter of a point on a 4-point scale. Of course, these effects are "statistically significant," but that only means (roughly) that the results aren't likely due to chance. Even if the results aren't a matter of chance, they tend to be small and don't demonstrate a flip in participants' attitudes (see May 2014b on the emotional manipulation of moral judgments).

Some studies do show stronger effects, especially when combined with other sources of evidence. One experiment found that more study participants will judge that a hypothetical defendant is not guilty by reason of insanity if the description of her psychosis is paired with a brain image and expert testimony (Gurley & Marcus 2008). However, a second concern is that we shouldn't put too much stock in a handful of studies. We should be especially cautious in light of the replication crisis and when the studies don't tend to use large sample sizes (Open Science Collaboration 2015; Machery & Doris 2017). Indeed, some later experiments using thousands of participants in a mock trial found no effect of brain images on perceived credibility of legal arguments or judgments of a defendant's culpability (Schweitzer & Saks 2011; Schweitzer et al. 2011b). More studies with larger samples, and eventually meta-analyses, are necessary before drawing firm conclusions, let alone prohibitions on the use of neuroscience in the courts and elsewhere.

Third, although some of the studies attempt to simulate real-world contexts, it's unclear whether we can generalize from these lab studies to the real circumstances in which life, death, and justice are on the line (Sinnott-Armstrong et al. 2008: 370). Juries and patients might be much less inclined to overrate the value of neuroscientific evidence in real judicial proceedings, where the stakes are much higher and the adversarial nature of the process allows presentation of both sides. One study does suggest that potential jurors are not unduly swayed by fMRI evidence when they read a cross-examination that questions its validity (McCabe et al. 2011).

Finally, and this is perhaps the most important issue, people are not necessarily "fooled" just because they find an explanation slightly more compelling when it includes extra bells and whistles that correspond to what is already in a text. Reading is arduous, especially when it features scientific and mathematical facts. Pictures are worth a thousand words, as they say, and our eyes are less likely to glaze over when facts are paired with figures. As many artists, activists, and orators know, images and provocative language help capture the audience's attention and to make relevant information more vivid and easier to comprehend (McGrath 2011; May 2018b). Sometimes non-evidential factors like images can *enable* one to better see or appreciate evidence, without the enabling condition illicitly serving as evidence itself (Burge 1988: 654–655). What might seem superfluous as a source of evidence is integral to comprehension or appreciation. That the light is on isn't an extra reason to believe there's a spider on the wall, but it sure enables you to notice it. Indeed, even if brain images shift one's judgments in a certain direction, they might not be misleading but rather increasing the accuracy of one's judgments, depending on whether the argument or explanation at hand should be regarded as sound or compelling (Sinnott-Armstrong et al. 2008: 370).

In the end, these studies don't demonstrate that brain images or neurobabble hoodwink nonexperts. What we have are a *handful* of experiments that *tentatively* suggest that people in *artificial* contexts will *sometimes* find psychological arguments and explanations *slightly* more satisfying when the texts are enriched with brain images or neuroscientific lingo. So do we have reason to think that neuroscientific evidence is particularly liable to mislead? Like all scientific evidence, it can be spun. We've seen that scientists themselves can massage evidence to support their own goals (Chapter 8), which can even affect medical interventions (Chapter 3). In Chapter 5, we saw that neurobiological evidence can be used to promote models of addiction that arguably hinder, or at least don't help, recovery and sensible drug policy. But there is little evidence that neuroscience is significantly more misleading than other forms of evidence that we allow in the courts. Discouraging the use of such evidence risks being too paternalistic, betraying a skepticism about the ability of judges, jurors, and other citizens to discern good from bad evidence.

9.4.2 Neuroredundancy

A remaining danger is that neurobiological evidence might just be a waste of time. Even if it provides some minimal probative value, the evidence might typically be an instance of "neuroredundancy" (recall Satel & Lilienfeld 2013: 22; see also Morse 2006a). To make sure a neuroimaging method is accurately revealing mental states and capacities, we must calibrate them against behavioral measures, such as self-report, eye-trackers, and tasks that otherwise reveal one's preferences or biases (like the implicit association test). Shouldn't we just cut out the middleman and use these behavioral tools? As Neil Levy says, it seems mind-reading is "best done, today and for the foreseeable future, from outside the mind" (2007: 149).

However, we should think of neurobiological markers less as middlemen and more as trainees that can go on to do their own work. To correlate brain activity with bias in jurors, we do have to rely on behavioral measures of bias, but once we have a neurobiological marker we can kick away the ladder, so to speak, and only look at the brain activity. Once calibrated, neuroimaging techniques can be used to directly uncover mental states and capacities even when the individual is motivated to deceive.

Sometimes neurobiological measures of psychological tendencies can even outperform behavioral tests. Consider the many areas of the law that are concerned with assessing the risk that a defendant or prisoner will reoffend, relapse, or respond to treatment. Measures of a defendant's brain activity might be more reliable than interviews, questionnaires, or criminal history. One landmark study measured the brain activity of over 90 inmates while they engaged in an impulse control task, then tracked whether the men reoffended a few years after being released from prison (Aharoni et al. 2013). The researchers found that the probability of rearrest was significantly higher for individuals who exhibited lower activity in the anterior cingulate cortex, which is involved in impulse control. Importantly, the lower brain activity was a better predictor of rearrest than age, psychopathy score, lifetime prevalence of drug abuse, or even performance on the impulsivity task. Such methods show the potential of neuroscience to not just aid judgments of culpability but also risk assessments that inform a wide range of decisions, from sentencing to parole.

Of course, studies like these are only preliminary and retain low probative value. Conducting a study of 90 individuals is one thing, but applying neuroprediction to a particular inmate outside of that data set is another (Poldrack et al. 2018). To avoid false positives (or negatives), the test would need to be highly precise, particularly if there are low base rates of the relevant brain responses. Nevertheless, neuroprediction demonstrates that brain activity can be useful above and beyond other assessments of risk. The traditional alternative is subjective assessment of risk by a clinician, which is regularly allowed into legal proceedings despite being far from reliable. In one study, clinical judgment was only slightly better than chance at predicting future violence in a psychiatric population (Lidz et al. 1993). Risk assessment, which is ubiquitous and here with us to stay, is just one example of how evidence can be improved by the addition of neurobiological data (Aharoni et al. 2022). Neuroscience isn't doomed to redundancy.

9.5 Balancing and Parity

Brain-based evidence has a number of specific limits and dangers. After examining the literature at the time of their writing, Sinnott-Armstrong and his co-authors conclude that brain images specifically should not be used as legal evidence: "Their moderate dangers 'substantially outweigh' their minimal probative value, so brain images fail the balancing test . . . and should not be admitted into trials" (2008: 371).

However, neurobiological evidence appears to pass the balancing test, at least because the purported dangers aren't moderate. The evidential value of neurobiological evidence certainly remains low. Even if problems like reverse inference can be overcome with sufficient care, a number of limitations cannot be easily dismissed, such as problems of normality and low base rates. And these limits on probative value apply to nearly all brain-based data, not just fMRI. So it might be overly optimistic to assert that the "shortcomings of proffered brain scan evidence and testimony do not lie in the scan technology itself, but in its application" (Gaudet et al. 2014: 44). Nevertheless, absent significant dangers, minimal probative value is enough to pass the balancing test.

With only minimal probative value, one might remain skeptical of introducing neuroscience into the courtroom or elsewhere. Perhaps we should err on the side of caution. But we should remember that no piece of evidence stands alone; it can be combined with other sources of evidence in a *cumulative* fashion (Glannon 2011: 73; Aharoni et al. 2022). Accumulation of empirical evidence for a conclusion is unlike a deductive argument that collapses if one of the premises is unsupported.

Compare memory-based testimony, which is now well-known to be far from reliable. Like perception (see the appendix to Chapter 1), the brain's method of memory formation and recall is more like an artist's constant reconstruction of an image from limited materials than taking a high-resolution photo that can be recalled the same way every time. Elizabeth Loftus (1997) and her collaborators have demonstrated in over 200 experiments conducted over the course of decades that people can develop false memories of events simply by receiving some misinformation. Participants in one study viewed a video of a car accident near a stop sign, but those who randomly received the suggestion that there was instead a *yield* sign tended to later recall seeing one. In another study, adult participants read stories of events from their childhood, ostensibly recounted by their relatives. One of the events, which claimed the participant was lost in a shopping mall at the age of five, was totally made up by the experimenters. Yet a quarter of the participants claimed to recall the fabricated event, even in later follow-up interviews.

False or distorted memories have arguably led to numerous false convictions, which can be devastating even if overturned, as illustrated by the tragic case of Steve Titus. In 1980, he was falsely convicted of rape in Seattle because the victim chose his image out of a photo lineup. The police only captured a picture of Titus because, like the perpetrator, he was a bearded white man driving a blue car on the night of the crime (National Registry of Exonerations, n.d.). Police eventually arrested Edward Lee King who confessed to the crime, but by that time Titus had lost his job, savings, and fiancé. Titus sued the Port of Seattle but died of a heart attack at age 35 before the civil trial could be resolved.

Despite the flaws in testimony from victims and eyewitnesses, this type of evidence is regularly allowed in trials. Why? Like many other forms of evidence, it's imperfect, but it can add some probative value to the overall argument. The lesson from false convictions is not that we shouldn't trust the memories of victims at all, but rather that we should accord them the meager weight they deserve. The error is in the process, in the miscarriages of justice that occur.

Many other forms of evidence also have limited probative value that can be dangerously exaggerated. In addition to clinical risk assessment (discussed above), we can include DNA analysis. In 2015, the U.S. Department of Justice and the Federal Bureau of Investigation (FBI) discovered serious flaws in its method of analyzing hair samples, which tended to overstate forensic matches and therefore facilitated false convictions. As *The Washington Post* reported, this is "one of the country's largest forensic scandals, highlighting the failure of the nation's courts for decades to keep bogus scientific information from juries" (Hsu 2015).

There are certainly reasons to be concerned about the misuse of neurobiological evidence. We've seen that medical interventions, even when scientifically tested, are often less effective and more harmful than most patients or physicians recognize (Chapter 3). Part of the explanation is that scientists are human too and thus susceptible to motivated reasoning (Chapter 8). So shouldn't we doubt the value of novel neurotechnologies in legal proceedings? Not necessarily. As with medical interventions and scientific knowledge generally, we should recognize the limitations without resulting to all out despair.

Established science isn't perfect, but it's some of the best evidence we have. It's at least as good as the evidence typically brought to bear in the law.

In other words, we have the materials for an *argument from parity*. Even when neurobiological evidence is weak and imperfect on its own, so too are many other forms of legal evidence. We should treat like cases alike, lest we operate with an inconsistent double standard. Of course, when two beliefs or policies are inconsistent, we can resolve the conflict in one of two ways. We could disallow testimony, DNA analysis, clinical risk assessment, and other forms of evidence with only minimal probative value. But then we're left with even less evidence on which to ground justice in an already flawed judicial system. So perhaps it's better to resolve the inconsistency in the other way, to allow neurobiological evidence despite its minimal probative value. When matters of justice hang in the balance, the more useful tools, the better.

Let's return to the case of Terry Harrington. Brain fingerprinting does have serious limitations. Few of Farwell's studies have been published in peer-reviewed journals, and its proprietary technique uses secret methods of analysis that cannot be independently verified or reproduced anyhow (Wolpe et al. 2005: 43; Levy 2007: 136). For these reasons alone, brain fingerprinting is arguably suspect. That said, the court might not have made a grave mistake in allowing the EEG evidence. If it played any role in the proceedings, Harrington was not exonerated by EEG alone but also by witness recantations and new evidence about alternative suspects.

In the end, the proprietary nature of brain fingerprinting isn't inherent to EEG, brain imaging, or other neurobiological evidence. There are certainly limitations inherent to most neuroscience research, such as nominal normality and reverse inference, but these are relatively minor and surmountable. It also matters that the stakes are high with false imprisonment and other serious wrongs hanging in the balance. Adding more tools to the judicial toolbox can help enhance or corroborate other sources of evidence. So we should generally welcome the introduction of neuroscience into the courtroom.

Indeed, we should also expect brain reading to have useful applications in medicine. Brain scanning, for example, can help determine whether a patient is in a minimally conscious state. Brain imaging is also positioned to aid in the early detection of psychiatric illness, such as suicidal thoughts (Just et al. 2017). When combined with other reliable tools, brain-reading technologies might improve health in addition to justice.

9.6 Neuromarketing

So far we've been optimistic about the use of brain reading. What about its use on consumers?

One concern is that consumers will be swindled by junk neuromarketing, similar to how jurors might be swayed by brain images. Entrepreneurs are already capitalizing on neurohype, claiming that their brain supplements or smartphone apps can harness neuroplasticity to dramatically improve your intelligence and memory. Celebrity doctors are hawking expensive brain scans to diagnose and treat psychiatric disorders. Some commentators lament that these are unethical brain *scams* (Satel & Lilienfeld 2013: 27). Efforts to swindle with science are certainly problematic, especially among vulnerable populations, such as psychiatric patients (Murphy et al. 2008). But these problems aren't specific to neuroscience. Snake oil salesmen are an inevitable feature of the marketplace. So let's set this issue aside and focus instead on how consumer neuroscience might obliterate privacy, or what semblance we have left of it in the digital world.

9.6.1 Privacy Problems

Corporations are always eager to learn more about consumer preferences before investing in new products or marketing campaigns. Surveys and focus groups provide only limited information, because introspection is fallible, as are the confabulations we come up with to explain our stated preferences (recall Chapter 8). Members of a focus group might say they prefer one advertisement over another, but it might not lead more people to buy the product. Even when we know our preferences through introspection, the desire to appear normal can prevent us from being truthful (which psychologists call "social desirability bias"). For example, most people won't say they are attracted to sexual intercourse among step-siblings, yet "big data" suggest that it's one of the most popular genres on pornographic websites (Stephens-Davidowitz 2017).

Brain reading, in contrast, promises direct access to consumers' thoughts and desires. Efforts to uncover our consumer or political preferences are already well underway (Ariely & Berns 2010). Leading marketing firms, such as Nielsen, have consumer neuroscience divisions that aim to help clients fine-tune advertisements by reading the brains of sample consumers using EEG or fMRI. Large companies, such as St. Joseph Aspirin, have already taken advantage of such services.

The long-term goals of neuromarketing are not limited to bionic focus groups. Facebook has worked with researchers at UC San Francisco to develop a brain-computer interface that allows users to write a text message by simply attempting to speak. After years of work, the team was able to successfully build a neural prosthesis that was surgically implanted into a stroke patient's brain who had lost the ability to articulate speech (Moses et al. 2021). Connected to a computer, the device allowed the patient to reply to simple text prompts in kind, such as "I am very good" in response to "How are you?" Well-funded start-ups like Neuralink are also in the mix, building brain-computer interfaces that help paralyzed individuals regain the ability to move their limbs using only their minds.

Of course, these tech companies aren't intending to become medical device developers. Their press and website content explicitly state that their ultimate goal is to market brain-computer interfaces to the general public. Some direct-to-consumer devices are already available or in production, typically matching the price of a new gaming console. Consumers can purchase wearable devices that employ EEG technology to provide biofeedback about the user's sleep patterns, for instance.

If brain-reading technologies are fully unleashed on consumers, their thoughts and desires might be impossible to conceal. Privacy concerns are particularly pressing as powerful corporations develop brain-computer interfaces that decode neural activity. Multinational tech companies and big box stores would not only know your search and purchase history, they could also gain direct access to your once private thoughts and desires. Some ethicists have called for government regulation of the "exploding trove of neurodata" that companies are acquiring (Kreitmair 2019: 159). Others have called for explicit recognition of a right to "cognitive liberty" that prohibits government surveillance of citizens' thoughts without their explicit consent (Wolpe et al. 2005).

These privacy concerns should be taken seriously, not only for the potential violation of a putative right to cognitive liberty. Encroaching on mental privacy could also harm citizens through abuse of the information by hackers and government, including law enforcement who can demand access to corporate data in the name of investigating and preventing crime. The FBI has demanded that Apple unlock suspects' iPhones, for example, and police departments are already using warrants to acquire the location data that Google stores on its users. Finally, society suffers if consumers become even more hooked on social media and other products that appear to increase depression and anxiety while fomenting political polarization (Twenge et al. 2020; Rini 2017; Nguyen 2020). The stakes are high.

9.6.2 Avoiding Alarmism

How alarmed should we be about neuromarketing? Privacy and related concerns rest on the assumption that brain reading holds unprecedented power and will be widely adopted by corporations and consumers alike. Yet this chapter casts serious doubt on that assumption.

We are remarkably far from powerful, precise brain reading. Neuroscientists can use brain activity alone to discern with reasonable accuracy whether a person is thinking about or imagining one kind of thing rather than another. Yet without brain imaging I can predict with 50% accuracy whether you're thinking about a face or a house. All I have to do is flip a coin—and restrict the task to a choice between only two options. Lesley Stahl, the host of *60 Minutes*, once asked neuroscientist Marcel Just whether a machine will one day be able to read complex thoughts like "I hate so-and-so" or "I love the ballet because . . ."

The distinguished professor replied, "Definitely... and not in 20 years. I think in three, five years" (CBS News 2008). Recent neuroimaging studies conducted by Just's lab have been able to decode one of 240 specific thoughts, such as "The judge met the mayor" or "The window was dusty" (Wang et al. 2017). But Stahl's question was about whether and when neuroscientists will be able to identify one among the *myriad* complex thoughts or desires an individual might have. Over a decade later, we remain astronomically far from that mark, let alone being able to roll it out into consumer applications.

It's entirely predictable why. First, the brain itself imposes constraints, such as high standard deviations in the data. Human brains are so complex and so diverse that making inferences about a single consumer's thoughts is nearly impossible to do without exorbitant sums of time and money. Technology does tend to improve exponentially, but some of the limitations of neuroimaging and other techniques are inherent to how the brain works. Functional neuroimaging *might* be cheap in a century, but blood won't flow to recently activated neurons any faster than two to six seconds. That's a built-in biological limitation. Second, brain-reading technologies themselves are limited. They typically have low signal-to-noise ratios and rely on long chains of statistical inference that allow many opportunities for weakness or error.

One might insist that privacy is threatened whether or not the technology is reliable. We might even be more concerned about the acquisition and use of brain data if it's often inaccurate! However, being driven primarily by the profit motive, corporations are ultimately responsive to poor marketing data or wasteful projects that hurt the bottom line. Indeed, soon after its breakthrough with UCSF, Facebook's Reality Labs announced that it is refocusing its efforts away from head-mounted brain-computer interfaces to wearable technologies that track neural activity in the user's wrist. Such devices would use electromyography (EMG) to merely decode movements such as swiping, typing, and clicking—not thoughts or desires. Similarly, as *Forbes* reported, Nielsen shut down most of its consumer neuroscience offices (Dooley 2020). The move was ostensibly due to the coronavirus pandemic of 2020, but the pandemic put economic constraints on virtually all aspects of business, and corporations don't cut their strongest assets. The decimation of Nielsen's consumer neuroscience operations suggests that the cost isn't worth the benefits and that existing methods of marketing are proving to be sufficient. It seems reality is catching up with the hype surrounding brain reading.

The comparison to existing methods of mind-reading is key. Your preferences can already be gleaned from overt behavior, such as your purchases, internet search history, and relationships to others and their "digital footprints." The retail giant Target reportedly uses purchases and other consumer behavior to predict when a shopper is pregnant, in order to send them coupons for diapers, formula, and other baby products (Duhigg 2012). As Levy puts it, "the kinds of powers that neuroscience promises in the near future pale in comparison to the mind reading and control techniques already in existence, in power and in precision" (2007: 154–155).

Indeed, brain reading is probably inferior in the medium to long term. Information about a person's behavior is often more valuable than their mere thoughts (thus sidestepping the thought-action gap). Consumers and criminals alike have myriad thoughts and desires that come and go, but corporations and courts want to know which ones lead to *action*. Even one's appearance can betray one's values and preferences, as facial recognition technology can identify a person's political orientation with 72% accuracy, just based on a single photo from their social media or dating profile (Kosinski 2021). Researchers have also been able to use machine learning to predict some severe psychiatric disorders based on one's writings and speech (McFarlane & Illes 2020). So, although it might seem that neurobiological data will provide "unprecedented insight into the mental health states of technology users" (Kreitmair 2019: 158), the insight is already precedent in one's overt behavior.

We shouldn't let neurohype serve as a distraction or diversion from more formidable threats to privacy. It would be odd for consumers to express fears about their cognitive liberty while continuing to give away treasure troves of even more telling behavioral data in the form of digital footprints on the internet and location data on their phones. Neuroscientific tools will surely improve over time, but so will the analyses of big data used to analyze consumer behavior, which will further optimize marketing campaigns and targeted ads. These methods will arguably always outcompete neurobiological data in terms of affordability, availability, and accuracy.

9.7 Conclusion

There are many potential applications of brain reading, and many of them present ethical concerns about privacy, safety, and justice. But recall that mere concerns aren't decisive arguments (Buchanan 2011: 144). Many of the concerns have been overblown. For example, some jurors might be hoodwinked by neuroscientific evidence, but these concerns have been inflated by a few early studies reporting small effects that could not be replicated. Moreover, we must compare any potential dangers to the benefits of enriching legal systems that are already awash in meager evidence, such as eyewitness testimony. By parity of reasoning, we should allow neuroscientific evidence, despite its similarly limited probative value.

In contrast, we should avoid alarmism about the use of brain reading in the marketplace. Concerns about privacy and safety are legitimate to a degree, but again comparisons are key. Consumer behavior is already monitored and deciphered with precision in the digital age, while our understanding of the brain remains dismal. Massive, well-funded companies are already discovering that brain reading can easily turn into a money pit. While commentators fret about brain reading, consumers continue to have their minds more readily and efficiently read by their digital footprints. If mental privacy is a serious concern, it's not because of neuromarketing.

Why is it that neurobiological data are useful in the courts but not in the marketplace? Can't brain-based information be combined with behavioral data to improve existing techniques to read consumer preferences? There are two main reasons for the asymmetry. First, neuromarketing doesn't scale well in terms of time and money. Effective brain-reading technologies are inordinately expensive and require massive computing power. The return on investment would need to be much higher than the brain can deliver, now or in the foreseeable future. Second, companies already have relatively cheap access to a large set of information about consumer behavior, and there is nothing analogous for the courts to lean on. In other words, the law is informationally impoverished and doesn't need to use expensive neurotechnology on most defendants, let alone most consumers. Corporations, in contrast, already have much more information at their disposal that allows them to read minds at scale. Neuroredundancy becomes a formidable problem in the marketplace because meager probative value isn't worth the cost.

In the next and final chapter, we'll take a step back and do even more comparisons like this across the distinct but interrelated topics of this book. Sometimes neuroscience is illuminating or threatening; other times it isn't. It should be clear that it's pointless to paint with a broad brush. All of our neuroethical analyses require nuance.

PART VI
CONCLUSION

10
Nuanced Neuroethics

We've seen that neuroethics is complicated by novel technologies, mysteries of the brain, and human foibles. Each chapter has tackled rather distinct topics, but together they suggest a unified approach to neuroethics. In this concluding chapter, we draw out some general lessons and return to the grim case of Kevin's brain surgery. A nuanced approach emerges that is *neither alarmist nor incredulous* and reconceives human agency as *less conscious and reliable*, but *more diverse and flexible*, than we ordinarily think. An overarching lesson for medicine, law, cognitive science, and public policy is one of *cognitive continuity*: disordered and neurotypical minds are more alike than they are unalike. By avoiding alarmism and embracing nuance, neuroscience and philosophy can work together to improve the human condition through a better understanding of it.

10.1 Back to Kevin's Brain Surgery

Recall the case of Kevin (from Chapter 1) who had portions of his temporal lobe and amygdala removed to treat debilitating seizures. I promised that we would provide an answer to whether he is morally culpable for possessing child pornography. This case can be seen as tying together many threads from the previous chapters, which demonstrates how blurry the division is between the ethics of neuroscience and the neuroscience of ethics.

Recall that Kevin's illicit behavior followed the removal of a brain tumor that led to Klüver–Bucy syndrome. It matters little whether Kevin had a brain disease or mental disorder as such (Chapters 4–5), but the neurological details inform whether his agency was likely impaired and whether his behavior was likely to improve after treatment (Chapter 9). His moral responsibility rests on the capacity to know right from wrong and to control his behavior in light of that knowledge. Portions of the temporal lobe and amygdala appear to be central to moral cognition but recall that there is no one moral module in the brain (Chapter 6). Rather there is a set of spatially distributed networks that subserve moral knowledge, which fits well with Kevin's statement that he continued to know it was wrong to download illegal pornography. It's also unlikely that his self-control was completely impaired, for that too is not entirely housed in the temporal cortex or amygdala. And Kevin was indeed able to refrain from downloading pornography on his work computer. Like most bad behavior, Kevin's deviant desires probably led him to rationalize his actions as ultimately harmless, a victimless crime (Chapter 8). It's not his fault that he had those deviant desires, but that's true of any person's desires (Chapter 2). What matters is how he responded to them.

So, is Kevin morally responsible for his crime? Our nuanced approach to neuroethics suggests that he is, at least to some degree. Some amount of blame and punishment are warranted since Kevin had substantial control and moral knowledge. He did change drastically as a person after the brain surgeries, becoming moody and hypersexual in ways his wife found to be unprecedented in their relationship. But we've seen that people undergo transformative experiences throughout the normal course of life, such as puberty and parenthood (Chapter 3). So there is nothing special about deep personality changes resulting from medical interventions in the brain. Nevertheless, insofar as Kevin's character and values took a dark turn, moral improvement might be appropriately aided by further brain interventions, from brain stimulation to psychedelics (Chapter 7). Perhaps some reduced punishment is appropriate since Kevin's self-control was probably diminished by particularly powerful desires that he was unaccustomed to controlling. But that's not a hard-won victory funded by his brain abnormality. Fluctuations in free will occur often in everyday life among the neurotypical (Chapter 2).

Like this analysis of Kevin's case, our tour through neuroethics has been balanced. Despite acknowledging neuroscience as an important and exciting frontier in the quest for human health and knowledge, we have not traded in alarmism and speculative prognostications. From the foregoing chapters, we can now extract five principles that make up a nuanced approach to neuroethics:

1. **Humility**: Avoid alarmism and neurohype.
2. **Scrutiny**: Approach evidence with vigilance.
3. **Complexity**: Recognize the complexity of human agency.
4. **Continuity**: Emphasize continuity over categories.
5. **Harmony**: Blend philosophy and neuroscience.

Let's consider each in turn.

10.2 Avoid Alarmism and Neurohype

Neuroethicists commonly stake out one of two extreme positions. Either they defend an alarmist fear of the new frontier or a hubristic futurism that too eagerly seeks a radical transformation of human nature and society. The truth is somewhere in between. Consider some examples from the previous chapters.

We saw that some commentators have proclaimed that humans lack any semblance of free will and that the criminal justice system must be radically reformed. Others have been more prone to disregard the science as making no difference whatsoever. Careful attention to both disciplines suggests a more moderate position. The neuroscience does show that we're less free than we tend to think because our actions can be influenced by factors that limit our control, choice, or coherence. But *less free doesn't mean unfree*. Indeed, we've seen that a large class of people are (sometimes) appropriate targets of praise and blame, even those with mental disorders and addictions. Like the concept of solidity (as opposed to witches), free will can turn out to be a bit different from what we initially expected.

However, this shouldn't be very surprising. We regularly mitigate blame as we learn of others' constraints, whether external or psychological. Our resentment toward an ineffectual boss, an irritable spouse, or an inattentive friend softens after learning about their extenuating circumstances, such as divorce, anxiety, stress at work, chronic pain, an unusually hectic schedule, a cancer diagnosis, or responsibility to care for an infant or ailing parent. And, unfortunately, such trials and tribulations are common in ordinary life. Importantly, we do not necessarily let one another off the hook entirely, for such circumstances do not regularly cause us to lose total control or act incoherently. Nevertheless, our ordinary practices are already sensitive to the fact that, although humans possess remarkable powers to control their actions in light of reasons, we are not gods. We are limited creatures, rarely working in ideal circumstances, and thus our imperfect freedom is fluid: it varies across time and space.

We also needn't be alarmed by brain manipulation treatments, just because they affect one's personality. Transformative experiences are a normal part of life. Even better if they can be undertaken voluntary, in contrast to puberty, bereavement, and other life-altering experiences that happen without our consent. Nevertheless, we should avoid neurohype by being clear-eyed about the risk-benefit ratios of brain interventions, particularly given an impoverished knowledge of the brain that will remain for much longer than futurists realize.

Scientists and philosophers have also drawn on neuroscience to demonstrate that many of our moral beliefs are based on unreliable biases and emotions. Some have even argued that many of us don't know right from wrong or that a controversial theory in ethics (utilitarianism) is true. Some critics have attacked such skeptical arguments by insisting that the science shows no such thing and is irrelevant. Again, a moderate stance is most defensible. Brain science does suggest that moral judgment is largely unconscious and automatic, but that doesn't mean it's inflexible or irrational. The brain is a sophisticated reasoning machine that can learn complicated patterns and rules unconsciously. Slow deliberation isn't always a better guide, for it can concoct rationalizations of our biases.

We should also soberly recognize the technological and ethical limits of neuroscience without banishing it as too dangerous or corrupting. Moral bioenhancement, for example, needn't be dystopian. There are legitimate concerns about safety, unfairness, and the corruption of character, but we must remember Buchanan's dictum: *mere concerns aren't decisive arguments* (Buchanan 2011: 144). Our moral attitudes are largely formed over time through experience, learning, and reasoning, much of it unconscious. So the most effective forms of moral improvement through brain enhancement—whether from microdosing psychedelic drugs or noninvasive brain stimulation—will work through our implicit learning mechanisms, much like traditional techniques, such as education, discipline, nutrition, sleep, and exercise. Indeed, direct brain manipulation will likely be useless in the long term unless combined with such traditional methods, just as cochlear implants only provide some functional hearing when paired with auditory training programs after surgery. In the end, bioenhancement isn't a panacea but rather like caffeine and drugs, which can be used responsibly to aid learning, creativity, and social engagement.

There is certainly room for moral enhancement, at least because problematic forms of motivated reasoning are pervasive. Scientists themselves are no exception to this rule, which should make us cautious about misuses of neuroscience (or any science) that thwart justice, privacy, or the health of society. But alarmism is unwarranted. An impoverished knowledge of the brain means that other methods for mind-reading the masses are more worrisome. At the same time, neuroscience can serve as corroborating evidence in courtrooms that lack big data on defendants.

10.3 Approach Evidence With Vigilance

Extreme positions in neuroethics are even more likely if we are overly credulous toward neuroscience. If novel discoveries, methods, and technologies are taken at face value, it makes sense to ring the alarm bells about ethical dangers, such as unreliable legal evidence, invasion of privacy, manipulation of patients' personalities, and unfair moral enhancement. The other extreme is to celebrate the neuroscience as providing simple resolutions to centuries-old problems of free will, blameworthiness, and moral knowledge. But matters are never so simple on such complex topics as ethics and the brain.

A key antidote to alarmism and overhype is vigilance. Not all science is created equal, and doing *good* science is hard. Scientists are people too, which means they are fallible. Take care to avoid overhyping the science that is characteristic of "brain overclaim syndrome" (Morse 2006b). Instead, embrace humility about its powers, including the prospects of brain interventions. Neuroscience has the power to improve human health and knowledge, but we should continue to prioritize traditional routes to brain health, such as exercise, education, sleep, and diet (Presidential Commission 2015: 46).

The powers of motivated reasoning should make us especially careful when reporting on or evaluating neuroscience. The tools and results of brain science are particularly attention grabbing, which motivates journalists, researchers, and policymakers to downplay subtleties that would dampen enthusiasm or complicate the plot of an otherwise simple and compelling story. Our values and preconceived notions can also leave assumptions unexamined and reinforce stereotypes. Research on sex/gender differences in the brain, for example, can rationalize traditional gender roles as "hardwired" (Hoffman & Bluhm 2016). More generally, we need to check our own assumptions about what is neurologically normal or defective.

At the same time, nuance also requires us to avoid painting with a broad brush. Examples of unethical experiments, sloppy science, and harmful medical interventions shouldn't overshadow the many times when science advances our knowledge and health. Systematic empirical investigation of the world is one of the best tools we have for advancing human knowledge. Broad skepticism about science is no more warranted than uncritical acceptance.

10.4 Recognize the Complexity of Human Agency

The prior two lessons together prescribe a measured approach to ethical issues in neuroscience that is *neither alarmist nor incredulous*. We can also glean important insights about the human condition. Overall, the arguments in this book suggest a nuanced conception of human agency as *less conscious and reliable* but *more diverse and flexible* than is often supposed (see Table 10.1).

Much of one's mental life is unconscious and automatic, but an emerging consensus in neuroscience is that the brain is a flexible learning machine. Brains are "hard-wired" to some degree, but they are ultimately designed to rewire themselves to adapt to their circumstances (see neuroplasticity discussed in the appendix to

Table 10.1 Lessons for Human Agency

Less conscious	Chapters 2, 6, 8
Less reliable	Chapters 6–9
More diverse	Chapters 3–5
More flexible	Chapters 3–7

Chapter 1). Much of this rewiring is relatively unconscious, but rationality is not constantly dependent on conscious awareness. In fact, much irrationality, such as confabulation and post hoc rationalization, is conscious. The unconscious mind certainly has its biases and limitations too, but it is also adept at learning over time, so much so that we often find ourselves with intuitive knowledge that we can't consciously articulate. We have a sense of which outfit would be too dressy for a particular occasion, which text reply will be most tactful, whether lying in a certain circumstance would be wrong, and so on. Such knowledge is neither innate nor inflexible but rather intuitive and inferential (and not exactly emotional, even if twinges of "affect" help guide the process).

We are most directly acquainted with our own conscious thoughts, but human identity and agency are more complex and fluid than we can witness in any one moment in time. Like the CEO of a corporation, our conscious minds set agendas, monitor progress, and integrate information across the entire agency. Importantly, though, you are the agency, not just your conscious mind. In addition to consciously weighing pros and cons, you unconsciously monitor cocktail parties for salient information, implicitly mimic others to promote cooperation, automatically apply principles to moral dilemmas, and so much more. All of this agency is carried out through exercises of conscious willpower but also through developing habits and structuring your environment to facilitate goals. The dual-process architecture of our minds allows us to flexibly shift between unconscious and conscious processing, automatic intuition and deliberation, thinking fast and slow.

Recognizing the complexity of human agency has helped support a nuanced approach to issues in neuroethics. Mental disorders, including substance use disorder, can certainly impair a patient's rationality or ability to control her behavior, but that is different only in degree from ordinary life. Addicts and other individuals struggling with psychic problems deserve compassion, but they also deserve empowerment to exercise the agency that is required for better mental health. Brain manipulation treatments can lead to drastic changes in a patient's personality, but that's normal in human life, filled as it is with transformative experiences. Human agency doesn't just take the form of a neurotypical thinker sitting on a rock with head perched on fist.

10.5 Emphasize Continuity Over Categories

The final lesson is perhaps the most radical. Throughout this book, it has proved useful to resist dubious dichotomies, such as free/unfree, blameworthy/exempt, competent/incompetent, treatment/enhancement, rational/emotional, and ill/well (and even textbook/monograph). Our nuanced neuroethics ultimately prizes continuity over categorical thinking. More generally, we have recognized a *continuity* in human agency and mental health, such that *we are more neurologically alike than unalike.*

How did we get to this conclusion? It has taken a *dual adjustment* to our conceptions of the neurologically typical and atypical. Consider first how we often think of neurotypical individuals as being deliberate, rational, and mentally well. Yet philosophical reflection and neuroscience suggest that differences among individual brains and circumstances vary so wildly that the minds of "neurotypical" people are rather variable and heterogeneous, both within and across cultures. We've seen that the typical mind arises from largely automatic and unconscious processes, including motivated reasoning. Even the self is so dynamic that it undergoes radical transformations throughout life. Normal agency, including among scientists, isn't always quite as uniform and idyllic as it might seem at first blush.

Now consider how we've adjusted our conception of the neurologically atypical. Many individuals with mental disorders, addictions, and brain abnormalities are thought of as lacking agency, rationality, self-control, and thus responsibility. But many addicts and psychiatric patients are capable of self-control and are competent enough to make choices about their lives, including whether to undergo brain interventions. Patients regularly exhibit agency as well as irrationality, which helps explain why the distinction between treatment and enhancement is blurry at best. Some brain diseases and abnormalities can certainly rob individuals of their agency or rationality, but these are the exception rather than the rule.

This dual adjustment reveals that people in general are more neurologically alike than unalike. At first there seemed to be a marked difference in the amount of agency and rationality in the two camps, like an imbalanced scale. But we've seen that there is *less* agency, rationality, and mental health among the neurotypical and *more* of these among the disordered. So, rather than emphasize categories, such as the neurotypical and neurodivergent, we should imagine human agency (including rationality and mental health) as lying along a continuum with anchor points at each end (see Figure 10.1). Recognizing the great continuum of agency helps resist the chauvinistic, albeit tempting, thought that neurotypical individuals represent a rigid norm and that deviations are differences in kind, as opposed to merely degree. (The continuum might likewise help us appreciate cognitive similarities between humans and other animals.)

It doesn't even make sense to place categories of individuals in one place along the continuum. Not only do symptoms vary greatly among individuals with a neurological condition, human agency in the neurologically typical and atypical is *fluid*. Like neurotypical people, individuals with autism, Alzheimer's, major depression, and

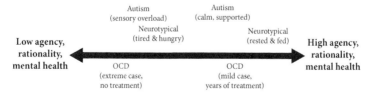

Figure 10.1 The Great Cognitive Continuum

Examples of how both neurologically typical and atypical individuals experience fluctuations in agency, depending on the severity of their condition, circumstances, and environmental triggers.

other conditions have good days and bad days, as well as fluctuations throughout the day depending on circumstances and triggers. Temple Grandin (1995/2006) frequently refers to "tantrums" that she and other autistic individuals have when they experience changes in routine, sensory overload, etc. Similarly, a series of grueling meetings, subtle slights, and a traffic jam can cause a neurotypical person to fly off the handle. Stressors, anxieties, and cognitive distortions vary across individuals and time, but they all can tax our nervous systems and ultimately our agency.

We should thus treat like cases alike, but how should we treat them? A continuity between the neurotypical and atypical might seem to threaten agency for everyone. Many people consider disorders like addiction to impair one's agency, even free will (Clarke-Doane & Tabb 2022). Does that mean no one really has control over their behavior? Not necessarily. We've seen that freedom and responsibility come in degrees (Chapter 2), and partly for that reason it's regularly appropriate to mitigate blame for neurotypical individuals (Chapter 4). So, yes, we should treat like cases alike, but that just means that we should evaluate agency on a case-by-case basis, not based on whether someone is or isn't diagnosed with a neurological or psychiatric condition. And, when we do hold someone accountable despite their having mental maladies, we should keep in mind Pickard's principle: *distinguish responsibility (and agency) from blame* (Pickard 2011). Just because someone is responsible for a bad outcome doesn't mean it's appropriate to hurl blame and indignation.

A similar approach to mental health is warranted. We could say, as many advocates of neurodiversity in autism do: "See, the mentally 'ill' aren't ill at all; it's just another perfectly legitimate way of being." Autism, for example, can be construed as not only a different mode of thought but also one that is in no way inferior to neurotypical agency. Rather than focus on the struggles of autistic people to navigate social situations, self-advocates often highlight the advantages their condition confers, such as pattern recognition, mathematical acuity, and empathic connections with nonhuman animals. To demonstrate how autism is often implicitly construed as inferior, some autistic self-advocates have asked us to imagine treating neurotypical individuals as having a deficit. A humorous example is the satirical website for the

Institute for the Study of the Neurologically Typical. Here's an excerpt of how the subject of study is characterized:

> *Neurotypical syndrome* is a neurobiological disorder characterized by preoccupation with social concerns, delusions of superiority, and obsession with conformity. . . . Neurotypical individuals often assume that their experience of the world is either the only one, or the only correct one. (Quoted in Brownlow 2010: 250)

This fictional institute shines a light on how autism is typically treated by clinicians and family members as a defect, as something to be corrected. Advocates within the neurodiversity movement have forcefully pushed back, saying that autism is a mere difference, not a deficit.

A different attitude that cognitive continuity makes available is that we're all mentally ill to some degree or other. Perhaps we should follow the Stoic teaching that "everybody is mad" (Ahonen 2019: 7); we are all works in progress somewhere along the spectrum of imperfection. Now, this might be a distinction without a difference since we're operating with a continuous spectrum of agency and mental health. Is the glass half empty or half full? We all move about on the great continuum. Often it will be helpful to recognize everyone's similar faults or struggles. Humans seem to build more solidarity and acceptance by acknowledging their shared vices more than their shared virtues, by erring on the side of humility over arrogance.

From which end of the continuum should we calculate one's distance? It might depend on the individual and the particular time in their life. Grandin (1995/2006: 50) has said, "If I could snap my fingers and be nonautistic, I would not. Autism is part of what I am." Yet she notes that other people with autism, such as Donna Williams, say, "Autism is not me. Autism is just an information processing problem that controls who I am." Grandin believes that they are both right because "we are on different parts of the autism spectrum." Grandin values her "ability to think visually" and has found her "place along the great continuum."

Either way, emphasizing continuity over categories promotes social integration and the reduction of mental health stigma. People often treat mental illness as rare and categorical—something *others* suffer from. Some societies, in contrast, treat mental health and disorder as forming more of a continuum (see Goldstein & Godemont 2003). For example, in Zanzibar, an island off the coast of Tanzania, people with schizophrenia who experience hallucinations are regarded as being taken over by spirits, which happens to everyone from time to time, though to a lesser degree among the neurotypical (McGruder 2002). Rather than being stigmatized or "othered," individuals with schizophrenia are integrated into the community and appear to enjoy better overall health. A similar approach is available for all psychiatric conditions if we embrace cognitive continuity.

10.6 Blend Philosophy and Neuroscience

Neuroethics is still nascent, with many moral problems and insights on the horizon. We need both neuroscience and philosophy (among other disciplines) working together to improve mental health and human knowledge with moral integrity.

Neuroscience and philosophy might seem odd bedfellows. One is a hard science; the other is a core discipline of the humanities marked by armchair reflection. Yet not long ago philosophy and neurobiology were not so distinct. René Descartes made advancements in neurophysiology and even famously (though erroneously) proposed that the pineal gland is the point at which the brain interacts with the ethereal world of the soul. Since that time, neuroscience and philosophy formed distinct disciplines, which has produced some rifts between them. Some philosophers believe that neuroscience is too fledgling and dispassionate to illuminate the human condition, while some neuroscientists balk at speculative intrusions into brain science.

Neuroethics calls for an end to any such divisions. The discussions throughout this book suggest some specific antidotes to chauvinism from either side.

For the neuroskeptics, consider that neurobiological evidence is more important than ever. There are advantages and drawbacks to any one scientific field or methodology. In the wake of the replication crisis in science, we need more good data, not less of it. Methodological problems that plague individual researchers, labs, and disciplines can be overcome, but only by drawing on the best evidence from all corners of research in both the humanities and sciences. It's not that neuroscience is immune to the same problems or that it alone will save the day. Rather, neuroscience plays an important role as *corroborating* evidence. Some critics are particularly dubious of brain imaging, but keep in mind that *there's more to neuroscience than fMRI*. Other studies—on brain abnormalities, neurostimulation, psychopharmacology—aren't merely correlational or rife with problematic reverse inference.

Some theorists doubt that neuroscience can help answer perennial questions in moral theory, because the evidence is weak or the results can be too easily misinterpreted. But that alone concedes that there are pressing ethical questions about the misuse of neuroscientific evidence and technologies. And we've seen that even a modest understanding can provide some useful evidence for theorizing in moral philosophy when combined with research in other domains, such as psychology, anthropology, psychiatry, and legal theory. Neuroscience is often overhyped, but it needn't be. Sober accounts of the science still raise important new issues (such as moral enhancement and brain reading) or inform age-old philosophical problems (such as free will and moral knowledge).

For those skeptical of the value of philosophy, consider how it has aided neuroethics.

The philosophical literature is a treasure trove of distinctions that clarify concepts (e.g., epiphenomenalism vs. determinism vs. physicalism), hypothetical scenarios that can serve as stimuli (like trolley dilemmas), and unconventional ideas that can shape theory and practice (such as transformative experiences and medical nihilism). Since the late 1990s, philosophers have also increasingly collaborated with scientists to help uncover the mind's mysteries (e.g., the concept of free will, the importance of moral character to one's identity, and the brain processes underlying moral cognition). Philosophical analysis—especially careful argument—often brings clarity to complex ethical issues, not necessarily uncertainty and hairsplitting. Moral philosophy, although sometimes abstruse, has a rich history (and present!) that can push theorizing in new directions without being inherently far-fetched or alarmist.

The line between ethicist and scientist is becoming increasingly blurred, yet each ultimately provides indispensable checks and balances against one another. Developments in neurobiology inform our understanding of the human condition and raise moral problems that philosophers then help to critically evaluate. We might think that scientists working in a particular area are best positioned to police it, but researchers in any one domain are (unconsciously) motivated to emphasize its successes and downplay its faults. That too is a good thing; armchair critics can be overly dismissive of important research. Rather than privilege any one discipline or method, our best bet is a collaborative endeavor brimming with mutual respect and vigilance.

Bibliography

Abumrad, J., & Krulwich, R. (2013). *Blame*. Episode of *Radiolab*. New York Public Radio.

Ackermann, R., & DeRubeis, R. J. (1991). Is depressive realism real? *Clinical Psychology Review* 11(5): 565–584.

Agar, N. (1998). Liberal eugenics. *Public Affairs Quarterly* 12(2): 137–155.

Aharoni, E., Abdulla, S., Allen, C. H., & Nadelhoffer, T. (2022). Ethical implications of neurobiologically informed risk assessment for criminal justice decisions. In De Brigard & Sinnott-Armstrong (Eds.), pp. 161–193.

Aharoni, E., Sinnott-Armstrong, W., & Kiehl, K. A. (2012). Can psychopathic offenders discern moral wrongs? A new look at the moral/conventional distinction. *Journal of Abnormal Psychology* 121(2): 484–497.

Aharoni, E., Vincent, G. M., Harenski, C. L., Calhoun, V. D., Sinnott-Armstrong, W., Gazzaniga, M. S., & Kiehl, K. A. (2013). Neuroprediction of future rearrest. *Proceedings of the National Academy of Sciences* 110(15): 6223–6228.

Ahonen, M. (2019). Ancient philosophers on mental illness. *History of Psychiatry* 30(1): 3–18.

Alexander, B. K., Coambs, R. B., & Hadaway, P. F. (1978). The effect of housing and gender on morphine self-administration in rats. *Psychopharmacology* 58(2): 175–179.

Alloy, L. B., & Abramson, L. Y. (1979). Judgment of contingency in depressed and nondepressed students: sadder but wiser? *Journal of Experimental Psychology: General* 108(4): 441.

Alzheimer's Association. (2019). Alzheimer's disease facts and figures. *Alzheimer's & Dementia* 15(3): 321–387.

American Psychiatric Association (2013). *Diagnostic and statistical manual of mental disorders* (5th ed.).

Anderson, E. (2004). Uses of value judgments in science. *Hypatia* 19(1): 1–24.

Anderson, M., Ronning, E., Vries, R., Martinson, B. (2007). The perverse effects of competition on scientists' work and relationships. *Science and Engineering Ethics* 13(4): 437–461.

Anderson, S. W., Bechara, A., Damasio, H., Tranel, D., & Damasio, A. R. (1999). Impairment of social and moral behavior related to early damage in human prefrontal cortex. *Nature Neuroscience* 2(11): 1032–1037.

Appelbaum, P. S. (2007). Assessment of patients' competence to consent to treatment. *New England Journal of Medicine* 357(18): 1834–1840.

Archer, A. (2016). Moral enhancement and those left behind. *Bioethics* 30(7): 500–510.

Ariely, D. (2012). *The honest truth about dishonesty*. Harper Collins.

Ariely, D., & Berns, G. S. (2010). Neuromarketing: the hope and hype of neuroimaging in business. *Nature Reviews Neuroscience* 11(4): 284–292.

Arpaly, N. (2002). *Unprincipled virtue: an inquiry into moral agency*. Oxford University Press.

Arpaly, N. (2005). How it is not "just like diabetes": mental disorders and the moral psychologist. *Philosophical Issues* 15(1): 282–298.

Arpaly, N. (2022). Quality of will and (some) unusual behavior. In King & May (2022), pp. 14–32.

Arvan, M. (2020). *Neurofunctional prudence and morality: a philosophical theory*. Routledge.

Bargh, J. A., & Chartrand, T. L. (1999). The unbearable automaticity of being. *American Psychologist* 54(7): 462–479.

Barnes, E. (2016). *The minority body: a theory of disability*. Oxford University Press.

Baron, R. A. 1997. The sweet smell of . . . helping: effects of pleasant ambient fragrance on prosocial behavior in shopping malls. *Personality and Social Psychology Bulletin* 23(5): 498–503.

Barrett, H. C., Bolyanatz, A., Crittendend, A. N., Fessler, D. M. T., Fitzpatrick, S., Gurven, M., et al. (2016). Small-scale societies exhibit fundamental variation in the role of intentions in moral judgment. *Proceedings of the National Academy of Sciences*, 113(17): 4688–4693.

Basso, J. C., & Suzuki, W. A. (2017). The effects of acute exercise on mood, cognition, neurophysiology, and neurochemical pathways: a review. *Brain Plasticity* 2(2): 127–152.

Batson, C. D. (2011). *Altruism in humans*. Oxford University Press.

Batson, C. D. (2016). *What's wrong with morality?* Oxford University Press.

Baylis, F. (2013). "I am who I am": on the perceived threats to personal identity from deep brain stimulation. *Neuroethics* 6(3): 513–526.

Beauchamp, T. L., & Childress, J. F. (2019). *Principles of biomedical ethics* (8th ed.). Oxford University Press.

Begley, C. G., & Ellis, L. M. (2012). Raise standards for preclinical cancer research. *Nature* 483: 531–533.

Berker, S. (2009). The normative insignificance of neuroscience. *Philosophy & Public Affairs* 37(4): 293–329.

Bennett, C., Baird, A. A., Miller, M. B., & Wolford, G. L. (2010). Neural correlates of interspecies perspective taking in the post-mortem Atlantic salmon: an argument for proper multiple comparisons correction. *Journal of Serendipitous and Unexpected Results* 1: 1–5. First presented at the Human Brain Mapping conference in 2009.

Berridge, K. C. (2017). Is addiction a brain disease? *Neuroethics* 10(1): 29–33.

Berridge, K. C., & Robinson, T. E. (2016). Liking, wanting, and the incentive-sensitization theory of addiction. *American Psychologist* 71: 670–679.

Bertrand, M., & Mullainathan, S. (2004). Are Emily and Greg more employable than Lakisha and Jamal? A field experiment on labor market discrimination. *The American Economic Review* 94(4): 991–1013.

Berryessa, C. M. (2018). The effects of psychiatric and "biological" labels on lay sentencing and punishment decisions. *Journal of Experimental Criminology* 14: 241–256.

Bhattacharjee, Y. (2013). The mind of a con man. *The New York Times Magazine*. https://www.nytimes.com/2013/04/28/magazine/diederik-stapels-audacious-academic-fraud.html.

Bjorklund, P. (2004). "There but for the grace of God": moral responsibility and mental illness. *Nursing Philosophy* 5: 188–200.

Blair, R. J. R. (2007). The amygdala and ventromedial prefrontal cortex in morality and psychopathy. *Trends in Cognitive Sciences* 11(9): 387–392.

Blackmore, S. (2005). *Consciousness: a very short introduction*. Oxford University Press.

Blanco, C., Secades-Villa, R., Garcia-Rodriguez, O., Labrador-Mendez, M., Wang, S., & Schwartz, R. P. (2013). Probability and predictors of remission from life-time prescription drug use disorders: results from the National Epidemiologic Survey on alcohol and related conditions. *Journal of Psychiatric Research* 47(1): 42–49.

Blanken, I., van de Ven, N., & Zeelenberg, M. (2015). A meta-analytic review of moral licensing. *Personality and Social Psychology Bulletin* 41(4): 540–558.

Bluhm, R., Cabrera, L., & McKenzie, R. (2020). What we (should) talk about when we talk about deep brain stimulation and personal identity. *Neuroethics* 13(3): 289–301.

Blum, B. (2018). The lifespan of a lie: the most famous psychology study of all time was a sham. Why can't we escape the Stanford Prison Experiment? *Medium*. https://medium.com/s/trustissues/the-lifespan-of-a-lie-d8692 12b1f62.

Bortolotti, L. (2010). *Delusions and other irrational beliefs*. Oxford University Press.

Bortolotti, L. (2015). The epistemic innocence of motivated delusions. *Consciousness and Cognition* 33(C): 490–499.

Bourget, D., & Chalmers, D. (2013). What do philosophers believe? *Philosophical Studies* 170(3): 465–500.

Brewer, J. A., & Potenza, M. N. (2008). The neurobiology and genetics of impulse control disorders: relationships to drug addictions. *Biochemical Pharmacology* 75(1): 63–75.

Bright, L. K. (2017). On fraud. *Philosophical Studies* 174(2): 291–310.
Broome, M. R., Bortolotti, L., & Mameli, M. (2010). Moral responsibility and mental illness: a case study. *Cambridge Quarterly of Healthcare Ethics* 19(2): 179–187.
Broughton, R., Billings, R., Cartwright, R., Doucette, D., et al. (1994). Homicidal somnambulism: a case report. *Sleep* 17(3): 253–264.
Brown, M. J. (2019). Is science really value free and objective? From objectivity to scientific integrity. In K. McCain & K. Kampourakis (Eds.), *What is scientific knowledge? An introduction to contemporary epistemology of science*. Routledge, pp. 226–242.
Brownlow, C. (2010). Re-presenting autism: the construction of "NT syndrome." *Journal of Medical Humanities* 31(3): 243–255.
Brownstein, M. (2018). *The implicit mind: Cognitive architecture, the self, and ethics*. Oxford University Press.
Bublitz, C. (2016). Moral enhancement and mental freedom. *Journal of Applied Philosophy* 33(1): 88–106.
Buchanan, A. (2011). *Better than human*. Oxford University Press.
Buchanan, A., & Powell, R. (2018). *The evolution of moral progress: A biocultural theory*. Oxford University Press.
Buckner, R. L., Andrews-Hanna, J. R., & Schacter, D. L. (2008). The brain's default network: anatomy, function, and relevance to disease. *Annals of the New York Academy of Sciences* 1124(1): 1–38.
Burge, T. (1988). Individualism and self-knowledge. *The Journal of Philosophy* 85(11): 649–663.
Burkett, J. P., & Young, L. J. (2012). The behavioral, anatomical and pharmacological parallels between social attachment, love and addiction. *Psychopharmacology* 224(1): 1–26.
Campbell, R., & Kumar, V. (2012). Moral reasoning on the ground. *Ethics* 122(2): 273–312.
Canli, T., & Amin, Z. (2002). Neuroimaging of emotion and personality: scientific evidence and ethical considerations. *Brain and Cognition* 50(3): 414–431.
Caramazza, A., & Shelton, J. R. (1998). Domain-specific knowledge systems in the brain: the animate-inanimate distinction. *Journal of Cognitive Neuroscience* 10(1): 1–34.
Caruso, G. D. (2012). *Free will and consciousness: a determinist account of the illusion of free will*. Lexington Books.
Caruso, J. P., & Sheehan, J. P. (2017). Psychosurgery, ethics, and media: a history of Walter Freeman and the lobotomy. *Neurosurgical Focus* 43(3): E6.
CBS News. (2008). How technology may soon "read" your mind. *60 Minutes*. https://www.cbsnews.com/news/how-technology-may-soon-read-your-mind/

CDC. (2021). *Drug overdose deaths in the U.S. top 100,000 annually.* Centers for Disease Control, National Center for Health Statistics. https://www.cdc.gov/nchs/pressroom/nchs_press_releases/2021/20211117.htm.

Chadha, M., & Nichols, S. (2021). Experiential unity without a self: the case of synchronic synthesis. *Australasian Journal of Philosophy* 99(4): 631–647.

Charland, L. C. (2002). Cynthia's dilemma: consenting to heroin prescription. *American Journal of Bioethics* 2(2):37–47.

Chatterjee, A. (2006). The promise and predicament of cosmetic neurology. *Journal of Medical Ethics* 32(2): 110–113.

Choy, O., Raine, A., & Hamilton, R. H. (2018). Stimulation of the prefrontal cortex reduces intentions to commit aggression: a randomized, double-blind, placebo-controlled, stratified, parallel-group trial. *Journal of Neuroscience* 38(29): 6505–6512.

Christen, M., & Müller, S. (2018). The ethics of expanding applications of deep brain stimulation. In Johnson & Rommelfanger (Eds.), pp. 51–65.

Chudek, M., McNamara, R. A., Birch, S., Bloom, P., & Henrich, J. (2018). Do minds switch bodies? Dualist interpretations across ages and societies. *Religion, Brain & Behavior* 8(4): 354–368.

Churchland, P. S. (2006). Moral decision-making and the brain. In J. Illes (Ed.) *Neuroethics: defining the issues in theory, practice, and policy.* Oxford University Press, pp. 3–16.

Churchland, P. S. (2011). *Braintrust: what neuroscience tells us about morality.* Princeton University Press.

Cialdini, R. (2006). *Influence: the psychology of persuasion* (Rev. ed.). Harper Business.

Cipriani, A., Furukawa, T. A., Salanti, G., Chaimani, A., Atkinson, L. Z., Ogawa, Y., . . . & Geddes, J. R. (2018). Comparative efficacy and acceptability of 21 antidepressant drugs for the acute treatment of adults with major depressive disorder: a systematic review and network meta-analysis. *The Lancet* 16(4): 420–429.

Clark, A. (2016). *Surfing uncertainty.* Oxford University Press.

Clark, A., & Chalmers, D. J. (1998). The extended mind. *Analysis* 58(1): 7–19.

Clark, C. J., Luguri, J. B., Ditto, P. H., Knobe, J., Shariff, A. F., & Baumeister, R. F. (2014). Free to punish: a motivated account of free will belief. *Journal of Personality and Social Psychology* 106: 501–513.

Clarke, R. (1993). Toward a credible agent-causal account of free will. *Noûs* 27(2): 191–203.

Clarke-Doane, J., & Tabb, K. (2022). Addiction and agency. In King & May (Eds.).

Clapton, E. (2007). *Clapton: the autobiography.* Broadway Books.

Corbetta, M., & Shulman, G. (2002). Control of goal-directed and stimulus-driven attention in the brain. *Nature Reviews Neuroscience* 3(3): 201–215.

Coyne, J. (2012). Why you don't really have free will. *USA Today*. https://usatoday30.usatoday.com/news/opinion/forum/story/2012-01-01/free-will-science-religion/52317624/1.

Coffman, B. A., Clark, V. P., & Parasuraman, R. (2014). Battery powered thought: enhancement of attention, learning, and memory in healthy adults using transcranial direct current stimulation. *Neuroimage* 85: 895–908.

Crockett, M. J. (2016). How formal models can illuminate mechanisms of moral judgment and decision making. *Current Directions in Psychological Science* 25(2): 85–90.

Crockett, M. J., Clark, L., Hauser, M. D., & Robbins, T. W. (2010). Serotonin selectively influences moral judgment and behavior through effects on harm aversion. *Proceedings of the National Academy of Sciences* 107(40): 17433–17438.

Crockett, M. J., & Rini, R. A. (2015). Neuromodulators and the (in)stability of moral cognition. In J. Decety & T. Wheatley (Eds.), *The moral brain: a multidisciplinary perspective*. MIT Press, pp. 221–235.

Cuijpers, P., Sijbrandij, M., Koole, S. L., Andersson, G., Beekman, A. T., & Reynolds III, C. F. (2014). Adding psychotherapy to antidepressant medication in depression and anxiety disorders: a meta-analysis. *World Psychiatry* 13(1): 56–67.

Cushman, F. (2013). Action, outcome, and value: a dual-system framework for morality. *Personality and Social Psychology Review* 17(3): 273–292.

Cushman, F. A. (2020). Rationalization is rational. *Behavioral and Brain Sciences* 43(e28): 1–59.

Damasio, A. R. (1994). *Descartes' error: emotion, reason, and the human brain*. Avon Books.

Daniels, N. (2000). Normal functioning and the treatment-enhancement distinction. *Cambridge Quarterly of Healthcare Ethics* 9: 309–322.

D'Arms, J., & Jacobson, D. (2014). Sentimentalism and scientism. In J. D'Arms & D. Jacobson (Eds.), *Moral psychology and human agency*. Oxford University Press.

Dart, T. (2015). "American Sniper" jurors: defendant was using PTSD diagnosis as an excuse. *The Guardian*. http://www.theguardian.com/us-news/2015/feb/25/american-sniper-trial-jury-eddie-ray-routh-ptsd-excuse.

Davidson, D. (1963/2001). *Actions, reasons, and causes*. Reprinted in his *Essays on actions and events*. Oxford University Press.

Davis, K. (2017). *The brain defense: murder in Manhattan and the dawn of neuroscience in America's courtrooms*. Penguin Press.

Davis, R. A., Epstein, C. H., Klepitskaya, O., Sharp, C. S., Ojemann, S., Abosch, A., & Heru, A. M. (2017). Disambiguating the psychiatric sequelae of Parkinson's disease, deep brain stimulation, and life events: case report and literature review. *American Journal of Psychiatry* 174(1): 11–15.

De Brigard, F., & Sinnott-Armstrong, W. (Eds.) (2022). *Neuroscience and philosophy*. MIT Press.

Decety, J., & Cacioppo, S. (2012). The speed of morality: a high-density electrical neuroimaging study. *Journal of Neurophysiology* 108(11): 3068–3072.

Decety, J., & Lamm, C. (2007). The role of the right temporoparietal junction in social interaction: how low-level computational processes contribute to meta-cognition. *The Neuroscientist* 13(6): 580–593.

De Dreu, C. K. (2012). Oxytocin modulates cooperation within and competition between groups: an integrative review and research agenda. *Hormones and Behavior* 61(3): 419–428.

De Freitas, J., Sarkissian, H., Newman, G. E., Grossmann, I., De Brigard, F., Luco, A., & Knobe, J. (2018). Consistent belief in a good true self in misanthropes and three interdependent cultures. *Cognitive Science* 42: 134–160.

DeGrazia, D. (2000). Prozac, enhancement, and self-creation. *Hastings Center Report* 30(2): 34–40.

DeGrazia, D. (2014). Moral enhancement, freedom, and what we (should) value in moral behaviour. *Journal of Medical Ethics* 40: 361–368.

De Haan, S., Rietveld, E., Stokhof, M., & Denys, D. (2017). Becoming more oneself? Changes in personality following DBS treatment for psychiatric disorders: experiences of OCD patients and general considerations. *PLoS One* 12(4): e0175748.

Delgado, J. M. R. (1969). *Physical control of the mind: toward a psychocivilized society*. World Bank Publications.

Demaree-Cotton, J., & Kahane, G. (2018). The neuroscience of moral judgment. In A. Z. Zimmerman, K. Jones, & M. Timmons (Eds.), *The Routledge handbook of moral epistemology*. Routledge, pp. 84–104.

Dennett, D. (1978). Brain writing and mind reading. In *Brainstorms: philosophical essays on mind and psychology*. Penguin Books, pp. 43–56.

De Ridder, D., Laere, K., Dupont, P., Menovsky, T., & Heyning, P. (2007). Visualizing out-of-body experience in the brain. *New England Journal of Medicine* 357(18): 1829–1833.

Devinsky, J., Sacks, O., & Devinsky, O. (2010). Klüver–Bucy syndrome, hypersexuality, and the law. *Neurocase* 16(2): 140–145.

Dima, D., Roiser, J. P., Dietrich, D. E., Bonnemann, C., Lanfermann, H., Emrich, H. M., & Dillo, W. (2009). Understanding why patients with schizophrenia do not perceive the hollow-mask illusion using dynamic causal modelling. *Neuroimage* 46(4): 1180–1186.

Ditto, P. H., Liu, B. S., Clark, C. J., Wojcik, S. P., Chen, E. E., Grady, R. H., et al. (2019). At least bias is bipartisan. *Perspectives on Psychological Science* 14(2): 273–291.

Ditto, P. H., Pizarro, D. A., & Tannenbaum, D. (2009). Motivated moral reasoning. In D. M. Bartels, C. W. Bauman, L. J. Skitka, & D. L. Medin (Eds.), *The psychology of learning and motivation*. Vol. 50. Elsevier, pp. 307–338.

Dooley, R. (2020). Nielsen makes major neuromarketing cuts due to pandemic. *Forbes*. https://www.forbes.com/sites/rogerdooley/2020/09/07/nielsen-neuromarketing-cuts/.

Doris, J. (2015). *Talking to our selves: reflection, ignorance, and agency*. Oxford University Press.

Douglas, T. (2008). Moral enhancement. *Journal of Applied Philosophy* 25: 228–245.

Duarte, J. L., Crawford, J. T., Stern, C., Haidt, J., Jussim, L., & Tetlock, P. E. (2015). Political diversity will improve social psychological science. *Behavioral and Brain Sciences* 38(e130): 1–54.

Dubiel, H. (2009). *Deep in the brain: living with Parkinson's disease*. Europa Editions.

Dubljevic, V., & Racine, E. (2017). Moral enhancement meets normative and empirical reality: assessing the practical feasibility of moral enhancement neurotechnologies. *Bioethics* 31: 338–348.

Duffy, K., & Chartrand, T. (2017). From mimicry to morality. In W. Sinnott-Armstrong & C. B. Miller (Eds.), *Moral psychology*. Vol. 5. MIT Press, pp. 439–464.

Duhigg, C. (2012). How companies learn your secrets. *The New York Times*. https://www.nytimes.com/2012/02/19/magazine/shopping-habits.html.

Duncan, S., & Barrett, L. F. (2007). Affect is a form of cognition: a neurobiological analysis. *Cognition and Emotion* 21(6): 1184–1211.

Dworkin, R. (1993). *Life's dominion*. Alfred A. Knop.

Eagleman, D. (2015). *The brain: the story of you*. Pantheon.

Eagleman, D. (2020). *Livewired: the inside story of the ever-changing brain*. Vintage.

Earp, B. D., Douglas, T., & Savulescu, J. (2018). Moral neuroenhancement. In Johnson & Rommelfanger (Eds.), pp.166–184.

Earp, B. D., Sandberg, A., Kahane, G., & Savulescu, J. (2014). When is diminishment a form of enhancement? Rethinking the enhancement debate in biomedical ethics. *Frontiers in Systems Neuroscience* 8(12): 1–8.

Earp, B., & Savulescu, J. (2020). *Love drugs: the chemical future of relationships*. Redwood Press.

Eklund, A., Nichols, T. E., & Knutsson, H. (2016). Cluster failure: why fMRI inferences for spatial extent have inflated false-positive rates. *Proceedings of the National Academy of Sciences* 113(28): 7900–7905.

Elliott, C. (1996). *The Rules of insanity: moral responsibility and the mentally ill offender*. SUNY Press.

Elliott, C. (1998). The tyranny of happiness: ethics and cosmetic psychopharmacology. In E. Parens (Ed.), *Enhancing human traits. ethical and social implications*. Georgetown University Press, pp. 177–188.

Elliott, K. C. (2017). *A tapestry of values: an introduction to values in science*. Oxford University Press.

Engber, D. (2018). The Dartmouth sexual harassment allegations are so much worse than I thought. *Slate.* https://slate.com/technology/2018/11/dartmouth-sexual-assault-harassment-lawsuit-psychology.html.

Estes, S. (2012). The myth of self-correcting science. *The Atlantic.* http://www.theatlantic.com/health/archive/2012/12/the-myth-of-self-correcting-science/266228/.

Ewing, M. (2017). The court system shouldn't interrupt the treatment process. *The Atlantic.* https://www.theatlantic.com/politics/archive/2017/12/opioids-massachusetts-supreme-court/548480/.

Fanelli, D., Costas, R., & Ioannidis, J. P. A. (2017). Meta-assessment of bias in science. *Proceedings of the National Academy of Sciences* 114(14): 3714–3719.

Farahany, N. A. (2016). Neuroscience and behavioral genetics in US criminal law: an empirical analysis. *Journal of Law and the Biosciences* 2(3): 485–509.

Farwell, L. A., & Makeig, T. H. (2005). Farwell brain fingerprinting in the case of *Harrington v. State. Open Court* X (10): 3, 7–10, Indiana State Bar Assoc.

Feinberg, J. (1970). What is so special about mental illness? In J. Feinberg (Ed.), *Doing and deserving.* Princeton University Press, pp. 272–292.

Feltz, A., & May, J. (2017). The means/side-effect distinction in moral cognition: a meta-analysis. *Cognition* 166(September): 314–327.

Fine, C. (2010). *Delusions of gender: how our minds, society, and neurosexism create difference.* W. W. Norton.

Fine, C., & Kennett, J. (2004). Mental impairment, moral understanding and criminal responsibility: psychopathy and the purposes of punishment. *International Journal of Law and Psychiatry* 27(5): 425–443.

Firestone, C., & Scholl, B. J. (2016). Cognition does not affect perception: evaluating the evidence for "top-down" effects. *Behavioral and Brain Sciences* 39(e229): 1–77.

Fischer, J. M., & Ravizza, M. (1998). *Responsibility and control: a theory of moral responsibility.* Cambridge University Press.

Fiske, A. P., & Rai, T. S. (2014). *Virtuous violence: hurting and killing to create, sustain, end, and honor social relationships.* Cambridge University Press.

Fitz, N. S., Nadler, R., Manogaran, P., Chong, E. W., & Reiner, P. B. (2014). Public attitudes toward cognitive enhancement. *Neuroethics* 7(2): 173–188.

Flanagan, O. (2011). What is it like to be an addict? In J. Poland & G. Graham (Eds.), *Addiction and responsibility.* MIT Press, pp. 269–292.

Focquaert, F., Glenn, A., Raine, A. (2012). Free will, responsibility, and the punishment of criminals. In T. Nadelhoffer (Ed.), *The future of punishment.* Oxford University Press, pp. 247–274.

Foot, P. (1967). The problem of abortion and the doctrine of the double effect. *Oxford Review* 5: 5–15.

Forscher, P., Lai, C., Axt, J., Ebersole, C., Herman, M., Devine, P., & Nosek, B. (2019). A meta-analysis of procedures to change implicit measures. *Journal of Personality and Social Psychology* 117(3): 522–559.

Forstmann, M., Yudkin, D. A., Prosser, A. M., Heller, S. M., & Crockett, M. J. (2020). Transformative experience and social connectedness mediate the mood-enhancing effects of psychedelic use in naturalistic settings. *Proceedings of the National Academy of Sciences* 117(5): 2338–2346.

Foucault, M. (1988). *Madness and civilization: a history of insanity in the age of reason.* Vintage.

Fox, M. J. (2002). *Lucky man: a memoir.* Hyperion.

Franco, A., Malhotra, N., & Simonovits, G. (2014). Publication bias in the social sciences: unlocking the file drawer. *Science* 345(6203): 1502–1505.

Frankfurt, H. (1971). Freedom of the will and the concept of a person. *Journal of Philosophy* 68(1): 5–20.

Franzini, A., Marras, C., Ferroli, P., Bugiani, O., & Broggi, G. (2005). Stimulation of the posterior hypothalamus for medically intractable impulsive and violent behavior. *Stereotactic and Functional Neurosurgery* 83(2–3): 63–66.

Fraser, H., Parker, T., Nakagawa, S., Barnett, A., & Fidler, F. (2018). Questionable research practices in ecology and evolution. *PLoS One* 13(7): e0200303–16.

Frederick, S. (2005). Cognitive reflection and decision making. *The Journal of Economic Perspectives* 19(4): 25–42.

Fried, I., Mukamel, R., & Kreiman, G. (2011). Internally generated preactivation of single neurons in human medial frontal cortex predicts volition. *Neuron* 69(3): 548–562.

Garrett, B., & Hough, G. (2018). *Brain & behavior: an introduction to behavioral neuroscience* (5th ed.). SAGE.

Gaudet, L. M., Lushing, J. R., & Kiehl, K. A. (2014). Functional magnetic resonance imaging in court. *AJOB Neuroscience* 5(2): 43–45.

Gauthier, L., Taub, E., Perkins, C., Ortmann, M., Mark, V., Uswatte, G. (2008). Remodeling the brain: plastic structural brain changes produced by different motor therapies after stroke. *Stroke* 39(5): 1520–1525.

Gazzaniga, M. S. (1967). The split brain in man. *Scientific American* 217: 24–29.

Gazzaniga, M. S. (1983). Right hemisphere language following brain bisection. *American Psychologist* 38: 525–537.

Gazzaniga, M.S. (2005). *The ethical brain.* Dana Press.

Gazzaniga, M. S. (2012). Free will is an illusion, but you're still responsible for your actions. *The Chronicle of Higher Education.* https://www.chronicle.com/article/michael-s-gazzaniga-free/131167.

Gilbert, F., Goddard, E., Viaña, J. N. M., Carter, A., & Horne, M. (2017). I miss being me: phenomenological effects of deep brain stimulation. *AJOB Neuroscience* 8(2): 96–109.

Gilbert, F., Viaña, J. N. M., & Ineichen, C. (2021). Deflating the "DBS causes personality changes" bubble. *Neuroethics* 14: 1–17.

Gill, M. B. (2007). Moral rationalism vs. moral sentimentalism: is morality more like math or beauty? *Philosophy Compass* 2(1): 16–30.

Giubilini, A., & Sanyal, S. (2015). The ethics of human enhancement. *Philosophy Compass* 10: 233–243.

Glannon, W. (2007) Neurodiversity. *Journal of Ethics in Mental Health* 2: 1–5.

Glannon, W. (2009). Stimulating brains, altering minds *Journal of Medical Ethics* 35(5): 289–292.

Glannon, W. (2011). *Brain, body, and mind: neuroethics with a human face*. Oxford University Press.

Glannon, W. (2019). *Psychiatric neuroethics*. Oxford University Press.

Glenn, A. L., & Raine, A. (2014). Neurocriminology. *Nature Reviews Neuroscience* 15(1): 54–63.

Gliha, L. J. (2014). Forced sterilization nurse: "I can see now that it was so wrong." *Aljazeera America*. http://america.aljazeera.com/watch/shows/america-tonight/articles/2014/3/24/forced-sterilizationnurseicanseenowthatitwassowrong.html.

Gold, N., Colman, A. M., & Pulford, B. D. (2014). Cultural differences in responses to real-life and hypothetical trolley problems. *Judgment and Decision Making* 9(1): 65–76.

Goldin, C., & Rouse, C. (2000). Orchestrating impartiality: the impact of "blind" auditions on female musicians. *The American Economic Review* 90(4): 715–741.

Goldstein, J. L., & Godemont, M. M. (2003). The legend and lessons of Geel, Belgium: a 1500-year-old legend, a 21st-century model. *Community Mental Health Journal* 39(5): 441–458.

Goode, E. (1999). Mozart for baby? Some say, maybe not. *The New York Times*. https://www.nytimes.com/1999/08/03/science/mozart-for-baby-some-say-maybe-not.html.

Gopnik, A. (2015). How David Hume helped me solve my midlife crisis. *The Atlantic*. https://www.theatlantic.com/magazine/archive/2015/10/how-david-hume-helped-me-solve-my-midlife-crisis/403195/.

Graham, J., Haidt, J., Koleva, S., Motyl, M., Iyer, R., Wojcik, S. P., & Ditto, P. H. (2013). Moral foundations theory: the pragmatic validity of moral pluralism. *Advances in Experimental Social Psychology* 47: 55–130.

Grandin, T. (1995/2006). *Thinking in pictures: my life with autism* (Exp. ed.). Random House.

Grant, B. F., & Dawson, D. A. (1998). Age of onset of drug use and its association with DSM-IV drug abuse and dependence: results from the National Longitudinal Alcohol Epidemiologic Survey. *Journal of Substance Abuse* 10(2): 163–173.

Greely, H., Sahakian, B., Harris, J., Kessler, R. C., Gazzaniga, M., Campbell, P., & Farah, M. J. (2008). Towards responsible use of cognitive-enhancing drugs by the healthy. *Nature* 456(7223): 702–705.

Greene, J. D. (2009). The cognitive neuroscience of moral judgment. In M. S. Gazzaniga (Ed.), *The cognitive neurosciences*. MIT Press, pp. 987–999.

Greene, J. D. (2013). *Moral tribes: emotion, reason, and the gap between us and them*. Penguin.
Greene, J. D. (2014). Beyond point-and-shoot morality. *Ethics* 124(4): 695–726.
Greene, J. D. (2017). The rat-a-gorical imperative: moral intuition and the limits of affective learning. *Cognition* 167: 66–77.
Greene, J., & Cohen, J. (2004). For the law, neuroscience changes nothing and everything. *Philosophical Transactions of the Royal Society of London, Series B: Biological Sciences* 359(1451): 1775–1785.
Greene, J. D., Nystrom, L. E., Engell, A. D., Darley, J. M., & Cohen, J. D. (2004). The neural bases of cognitive conflict and control in moral judgment. *Neuron* 44(2): 389–400.
Greene, J. D., Sommerville, R. B., Nystrom, L. E., Darley, J. M., & Cohen, J. D. (2001). An fMRI investigation of emotional engagement in moral judgment. *Science* 293(5537): 2105–2108.
Greenwald, A. G., Poehlman, T. A., Uhlmann, E. L., & Banaji, M. R. 2009. Understanding and using the Implicit Association Test: III. *Journal of Personality and Social Psychology* 97(1): 17–41.
Grifell, M., & Hart, C. L. (2018). Is drug addiction a brain disease? *American Scientist* 106(3): 160–167.
Gurley, J. R., & Marcus, D. K. (2008). The effects of neuroimaging and brain injury on insanity defenses. *Behavioral Sciences & the Law* 26(1): 85–97.
Haas, J. (2020). Moral gridworlds: a theoretical proposal for modeling artificial moral cognition. *Minds and Machines* 30: 219–246.
Habermas, J. (2003). *The future of human nature*. Polity Press.
Hagerty, B. B. (2010). Inside a psychopath's brain: the sentencing debate. NPR Morning Edition. https://www.npr.org/templates/story/story.php?storyId=128116806.
Haidt, J. (2001). The emotional dog and its rational tail: a social intuitionist approach to moral judgment. *Psychological Review* 108(4): 814–834.
Haidt, J. (2012). *The righteous mind: why good people are divided by politics and religion*. Vintage.
Haidt, J., Koller, S. H., & Dias, M. G. (1993). Affect, culture, and morality, or is it wrong to eat your dog. *Journal of Personality and Social Psychology* 65: 613–628.
Han, H., Kim, J., Jeong, C., & Cohen, G. L. (2017). Attainable and relevant moral exemplars are more effective than extraordinary exemplars in promoting voluntary service engagement. *Frontiers in Psychology* 8: 1–14.
Hare, R. D. (1993). *Without conscience: the disturbing world of the psychopaths among us*. Guilford Press.
Hare, T. A., O'Doherty, J., Camerer, C. F., Schultz, W., & Rangel, A. (2008). Dissociating the role of the orbitofrontal cortex and the striatum in the computation of goal values and prediction errors. *Journal of Neuroscience* 28(22): 5623–5630.

Hari, J. (2015). The likely cause of addiction has been discovered, and it is not what you think. *The Huffington Post*. https://www.huffpost.com/entry/the-real-cause-of-addicti_b_6506936.

Harrington v. State of Iowa. (1997). No. 96–1232. https://caselaw.findlaw.com/us-8th-circuit/1385240.html.

Harris, J. (2011). Moral enhancement and freedom. *Bioethics* 25(2): 102–111.

Harris, S. (2012). *Free will*. Simon and Schuster.

Harris, R., & Gurel, L. (2012). A study of ayahuasca use in North America. *Journal of Psychoactive Drugs* 44(3): 209–215.

Hart, C. (2013). *High price: a neuroscientist's journey of self-discovery that challenges everything you know about drugs and society*. Harper.

Haslam, N., & Kvaale, E. P. (2015). Biogenetic explanations of mental disorder: the mixed-blessings model. *Current Directions in Psychological Science* 24(5): 399–404.

Hauser, M., Cushman, F., Young, L., Kang-Xing Jin, R., & Mikhail, J. (2007). A dissociation between moral judgments and justifications. *Mind & Language* 22(1): 1–21.

Haynes, J. D., & Rees, G. (2006). Decoding mental states from brain activity in humans. *Nature Reviews Neuroscience* 7(7): 523–534.

Head, M. L., Holman, L., Lanfear, R., Kahn, A. T., & Jennions, M. D. (2015). The extent and consequences of p-hacking in science. *PLoS Biology* 13(3): e1002106–15.

Hechtman, L., & Greenfield, B. (2003). Long-term use of stimulants in children with attention deficit hyperactivity disorder. *Pediatric Drugs* 5(12): 787–794.

Heinz, A. J., Wu, J., Witkiewitz, K., Epstein, D. H., & Preston, K. L. (2009). Marriage and relationship closeness as predictors of cocaine and heroin use. *Addictive Behaviors* 34(3): 258–263.

Henrich, J. (2015). *The secret of our success*. Princeton University Press.

Henrich, J. (2020). *The weirdest people in the world: how the West became psychologically peculiar and particularly prosperous*. Farrar, Straus and Giroux.

Heron, M. (2019). Deaths: leading causes for 2017. *National Vital Statistics Reports* 68(6): 1–76.

Heyman, G. M. (2009). *Addiction: a disorder of choice*. Harvard University Press.

Higgins, S. T., Budney, A. J., Bickel, W. K., Foerg, F. E., Donham, R., & Badger, G. J. (1994). Incentives improve outcome in outpatient behavioral treatment of cocaine dependence. *Archives of General Psychiatry* 51(7): 568–576.

Hirstein, W., Sifferd, K. L., & Fagan, T. K. (2018). *Responsible brains: neuroscience, law, and human culpability*. MIT Press.

Hochberg, L. R., Bacher, D., Jarosiewicz, B., Masse, N. Y., Simeral, J. D., Vogel, J., . . . & Donoghue, J. P. (2012). Reach and grasp by people with tetraplegia using a neurally controlled robotic arm. *Nature* 485(7398): 372.

Hoffman, G. A., & Bluhm, R. (2016). Neurosexism and neurofeminism. *Philosophy Compass* 11(11): 716–729.

Hohwy, J. (2013). *The predictive mind*. Oxford University Press.

Holton, R., & Berridge, K. C. (2013). Addiction between compulsion and choice. In N. Levy (Ed.), *Addiction and self-control*. Oxford University Press, pp. 239–268.

Horton, R. (2015). Offline: what is medicine's 5 sigma. *The Lancet* 385(9976): 1380.

Hsu, S. S. (2015). FBI admits flaws in hair analysis over decades. *The Washington Post*. https://www.washingtonpost.com/local/crime/fbi-ove rstated-forensic-hair-matches-in-nearly-all-criminal-trials-for-decades/ 2015/04/18/39c8d8c6-e515-11e4-b510-962fcfabc310_story.html.

Huebner, B. (2015). Do emotions play a constitutive role in moral cognition? *Topoi* 34(2): 427–440.

Hume, D. (1739/2000). *A treatise of human nature*. Edited by D. F. Norton & M. J. Norton. Oxford University Press.

Hutcherson, C. A., Montaser-Kouhsari, L., Woodward, J., & Rangel, A. (2015). Emotional and utilitarian appraisals of moral dilemmas are encoded in separate areas and integrated in ventromedial prefrontal cortex. *Journal of Neuroscience* 35(36): 12593–12605.

Hutzler, F. (2014). Reverse inference is not a fallacy per se: cognitive processes can be inferred from functional imaging data. *Neuroimage* 84: 1061–1069.

Hyman, S. E. (2005). Addiction: a disease of learning and memory. *American Journal of Psychiatry* 162(8): 1414–1422.

Hysek, C. M., Schmid, Y., Simmler, L. D., Domes, G., Heinrichs, M., Eisenegger, C., . . . & Liechti, M. E. (2014). MDMA enhances emotional empathy and prosocial behavior. *Social Cognitive and Affective Neuroscience* 9(11): 1645–1652.

Iacoboni, M., Freedman, J., & Kaplan, J. (2007). This is your brain on politics. *The New York Times*. https://www.nytimes.com/2007/11/11/opinion/11f reedman.html.

IIP John Jay (2021). Julie Eldred: a woman's experience with substance use disorder and the legal system [video]. Institute for Innovation in Prosecution. https://youtu.be/b9QoxXBAM0g.

Ioannidis, J. P. A. (2005). Why most published research findings are false. *PLoS Medicine* 2(8): e124-6.

James, W. (1890). *The principles of psychology*. Dover.

Jaworska, A. (1999). Respecting the margins of agency: Alzheimer's patients and the capacity to value. *Philosophy & Public Affairs* 28(2): 105–138.

Jefferson, A. (2022). Brain pathology and moral responsibility. In King & May (Eds.), pp. 63–85.

John, L. K., Loewenstein, G., & Prelec, D. (2012). Measuring the prevalence of questionable research practices with incentives for truth telling. *Psychological Science* 23(5): 524–532.

Johnson, L. S. M., & Rommelfanger, K. S. (Eds.) (2018). *The Routledge handbook of neuroethics*. Routledge.

Jones, K. (2003). Emotion, weakness of will and the normative conception of agency. *Royal Institute of Philosophy Supplement* 52: 181–200.

Jones, R., Tarter, R., & Ross, A. M. (2021). Greenspace Interventions, stress and cortisol: a scoping review. *International Journal of Environmental Research and Public Health* 18(6): 2802.

Joyce, R. (2006). *The evolution of morality*. MIT Press.

Just, M. A., Pan, L., Cherkassky, V. L., McMakin, D. L., Cha, C., Nock, M. K., & Brent, D. (2017). Machine learning of neural representations of suicide and emotion concepts identifies suicidal youth. *Nature Human Behaviour* 1(12): 911–919.

Kahan, D. M., Peters, E., Wittlin, M., Slovic, P., Ouellette, L. L., Braman, D., & Mandel, G. (2012). The polarizing impact of science literacy and numeracy on perceived climate change risks. *Nature Climate Change* 2(6): 732–735.

Kahane, G. (2011). Mastery without mystery: why there is no promethean sin in enhancement. *Journal of Applied Philosophy* 28(4): 355–368.

Kahane, G., Everett, J. A., Earp, B. D., Caviola, L., Faber, N. S., Crockett, M. J., & Savulescu, J. (2018). Beyond sacrificial harm: a two-dimensional model of utilitarian psychology. *Psychological Review* 125(2): 131–164.

Kahane, G., Wiech, K., Shackel, N., Farias, M., Savulescu, J., & Tracey, I. (2012). The neural basis of intuitive and counterintuitive moral judgment. *Social Cognitive and Affective Neuroscience* 7(4): 393–402.

Kahneman, D. (2011). *Thinking, fast and slow*. Farrar, Straus and Giroux.

Kamm, F. M. (2005). Is there a problem with enhancement? *The American Journal of Bioethics* 5(3): 5–14.

Kandel, E. (2018). *The disordered mind: what unusual brains tell us about ourselves*. Farrar, Straus and Giroux.

Kandel, E., Schwartz, J., Jessell, T., Siegelbaum, S. A., & Hudspeth, A. J. (2013). *Principles of neural science* (5th ed.). McGraw-Hill.

Kane, R. (1999). Responsibility, luck, and chance: reflections on free will and indeterminism. *Journal of Philosophy* 96(5): 217–240.

Kant, I. (1785/1997). *Groundwork for the metaphysics of morals*. Edited by M. Gregor & C. M. Korsgaard. Cambridge University Press.

Kaplan, R. M., & Irvin, V. L. (2015). Likelihood of null effects of large NHLBI clinical trials has increased over time. *PloS One* 10(8): e0132382.

Kapp, S. K., Gillespie-Lynch, K., Sherman, L. E., & Hutman, T. (2013). Deficit, difference, or both? Autism and neurodiversity. *Developmental Psychology* 49(1): 59–71.

Kass, L. R. (2003). Ageless bodies, happy souls: biotechnology and the pursuit of perfection. *The New Atlantis*. https://www.thenewatlantis.com/publications/ageless-bodies-happy-souls.

Katz, J. (2017). Drug deaths in America are rising faster than ever. *The New York Times*. https://www.nytimes.com/interactive/2017/06/05/upshot/opioid-epidemic-drug-overdose-deaths-are-rising-faster-than-ever.html.

Kean, S. (2014). *The tale of the dueling neurosurgeons*. Little, Brown.

Kelly, D. (2011). *Yuck! The nature and moral significance of disgust.* MIT Press.

Kelly, J. F., Greene, M. C., & Abry, A. (2021). A US national randomized study to guide how best to reduce stigma when describing drug-related impairment in practice and policy. *Addiction* 116(7): 1757–1767.

Kennett, J. (2006). Do psychopaths really threaten moral rationalism? *Philosophical Explorations* 9(1): 69–82.

Kennett, J. (2007). Mental disorder, moral agency, and the self. In Bonnie Steinbock (Ed.), *The Oxford handbook of bioethics.* Oxford University Press, pp. 90–113.

Kennett, J. (2013). Addiction, choice, and disease: how voluntary is voluntary action in addiction? In N. Vincent (Ed.), *Neuroscience and legal responsibility.* Oxford University Press, pp. 257–278.

Kennett, J., & Fine, C. (2008). Internalism and the evidence from psychopaths and "acquired sociopaths." In W. Sinnott-Armstrong (Ed.), *Moral psychology.* Vol. 3. MIT Press, pp. 173–190.

Kennett, J., & Fine, C. (2009). Will the real moral judgment please stand up? *Ethical Theory and Moral Practice* 12(1): 77–96.

Kiehl, K. A. (2006). A cognitive neuroscience perspective on psychopathy: evidence for paralimbic system dysfunction. *Psychiatry Research* 142(2–3): 107–128.

Kiehl, K., & Sinnott-Armstrong, W. (Eds.) (2013). *Handbook of psychopathy and law.* Oxford University Press.

King, M. (2014). Traction without tracing: a (partial) solution for control-based accounts of moral responsibility. *European Journal of Philosophy* 22 (3): 463–482.

King, M. (2020). Attending to blame. *Philosophical Studies* 177(5): 1423–1439.

King, M., & Carruthers, P. (2020). Responsibility and consciousness. In D. Nelkin & D. Pereboom (Eds.), *The Oxford handbook of moral responsibility.* Oxford University Press, pp. 448–467.

King, M., & May, J. (2018). Moral responsibility and mental illness: a call for nuance. *Neuroethics* 11(1): 11–22.

King, M., & May, J. (Eds.) (2022). *Agency in mental disorder: philosophical dimensions.* Oxford University Press.

Kitcher, P. (2001) *Science, truth, and democracy.* Oxford University Press.

Klaming, L., & Haselager, P. (2013). Did my brain implant make me do it? Questions raised by DBS regarding psychological continuity, responsibility for action and mental competence. *Neuroethics* 6(3): 527–539.

Koehler, J. (1993). The influence of prior beliefs on scientific judgments of evidence quality. *Organizational Behavior and Human Decision Processes* 56(1): 28–55.

Koenigs, M., Kruepke, M., Zeier, J., & Newman, J. P. (2012). Utilitarian moral judgment in psychopathy. *Social Cognitive and Affective Neuroscience* 7(6): 708–714.

Koenigs, M., Young, L. L., Adolphs, R., Tranel, D., Cushman, F. A., Hauser, M. D., & Damasio, A. R. (2007). Damage to the prefrontal cortex increases utilitarian moral judgements, *Nature* 446(7138): 908–911.

Koob, G. F., & Volkow, N. D. (2010). Neurocircuitry of addiction. *Neuropsychopharmacology* 35: 217–238.

Kosinski, M. (2021). Facial recognition technology can expose political orientation from naturalistic facial images. *Scientific Reports* 11(1): 1–7.

Koslowski, M., Johnson, M. W., Gründer, G., & Betzler, F. (2021). Novel treatment approaches for substance use disorders: therapeutic use of psychedelics and the role of psychotherapy. *Current Addiction Reports*, 1–11. DOI: 10.1007/s40429-021-00401-8.

Kotov, R., Krueger, R. F., Watson, D., Achenbach, T. M., Althoff, R. R., Bagby, R. M., ... & Zimmerman, M. (2017). The Hierarchical Taxonomy of Psychopathology (HiTOP): a dimensional alternative to traditional nosologies. *Journal of Abnormal Psychology* 126(4): 454.

Kreitmair, K. V. (2019). Dimensions of ethical direct-to-consumer neurotechnologies. *AJOB Neuroscience* 10(4): 152–166.

Krueger, R. F., Kotov, R., Watson, D., Forbes, M. K., Eaton, N. R., Ruggero, C. J., ... & Zimmermann, J. (2018). Progress in achieving quantitative classification of psychopathology. *World Psychiatry* 17(3): 282–293.

Kozuch, B., & McKenna, M. (2015). Free will, moral responsibility, and mental, illness. In D. D. Moseley & G. Gala (Eds.), *Philosophy and psychiatry problems, intersections, and new perspectives*. Routledge, pp. 89–113.

Kumar, V. (2016). Nudges and bumps. *Georgetown Journal of Law and Public Policy* 14: 861–876.

Kumar, V., & Campbell, R. (2022). *A better ape: the evolution of the moral mind and how it made us human*. Oxford University Press.

Kumar, V., Kodipady, A., & Young, L. (2022). A psychological explanation for the unique decline in anti-gay attitudes. Manuscript.

Kumar, V., & May, J. (2019). How to debunk moral beliefs. In J. Suikkanen & A. Kauppinen (Eds.), *Methodology & moral philosophy*. Routledge, pp. 25–48.

Kumar, V., & May, J. (2023). Moral Reasoning and moral progress. In D. Copp & C. Rosati (Eds.)., *The Oxford handbook of metaethics*. Oxford University Press.

Kunda, Z. (1990). The case for motivated reasoning. *Psychological Bulletin* 108(3): 480–498.

Kurth, C. (2018). *The anxious mind*. MIT Press.

Kurzban, R., Duckworth, A., Kable, J., & Myers, J. (2013). An opportunity cost model of subjective effort and task performance. *Behavioral and Brain Sciences* 36(6): 661–679.

Lam, B. (2018). Willful acts. Hi-Phi Nation [audio podcast], Season 2, Episode 8.

Latané, B., & Nida, S. (1981). Ten years of research on group size and helping. *Psychological Bulletin* 89(2): 308–324.

Leadbitter, K., Buckle, K. L., Ellis, C., & Dekker, M. (2021). Autistic self-advocacy and the neurodiversity movement: implications for autism early intervention research and practice. *Frontiers in Psychology* 12: 782.

Leentjens, A., Visser-Vandewalle, V., Temel, Y., Verhey, F. (2004). Manipulation of mental competence: an ethical problem in case of electrical stimulation of the subthalamic nucleus for severe Parkinson's disease. *Nederlands Tijdschrift voor Geneeskunde (The Dutch Journal of Medicine)* 148(28): 1394–1398.

Langleben, D. D. (2008). Detection of deception with fMRI: are we there yet? *Legal and Criminological Psychology* 13(1): 1–9.

Leshner, A. I. (1997). Addiction is a brain disease, and it matters. *Science* 278: 45–47.

Levy, D. A. (2003). Neural holism and free will. *Philosophical Psychology* 16(2): 205–228.

Levy, N. (2007). *Neuroethics: challenges for the 21st century*. Cambridge University Press.

Levy, N. (2013). Addiction is not a brain disease (and it matters). *Frontiers in Psychiatry* 4: 24.

Levy, N. (2014). *Consciousness and moral responsibility*. Oxford University Press.

Lewis, M. (2015). *The biology of desire: why addiction is not a disease*. PublicAffairs.

Lewis, M. (2017). A continuum is a continuum, and swans are not geese. Reply to Fenton & Wiers. *Neuroethics* 10(1): 167–168.

Libet, B. (1985). Unconscious cerebral initiative and the role of conscious will in voluntary action. *Behavioral and Brain Sciences* 8: 529–566.

Lidz, C. W., Mulvey, E. P., & Gardner, W. (1993). The accuracy of predictions of violence to others. *Journal of the American Medical Association* 269(8): 1007–1011.

Locke, J. (1689/1975). *An essay concerning human understanding*. Edited by P. H. Nidditch. Oxford University Press.

Loftus, E. F. (1997). Creating false memories. *Scientific American* 277(3): 70–75.

Longino, H. (1990). *Science as social knowledge*. Princeton University Press.

Lukianoff, G., & Haidt, J. (2015). The coddling of the American mind. *The Atlantic*. https://www.theatlantic.com/magazine/archive/2015/09/the-coddling-of-the-american-mind/399356/.

Lyons, T., & Carhart-Harris, R. L. (2018). Increased nature relatedness and decreased authoritarian political views after psilocybin for treatment-resistant depression. *Journal of Psychopharmacology* 32(7): 811–819.

Machery, E. (2014). In defense of reverse inference. *The British Journal for the Philosophy of Science* 65(2): 251–267.

Machery, E., & Doris, J. M. (2017). An open letter to our students. In B. G. Voyer & T. Tarantola (Eds.), *Moral psychology: a multidisciplinary guide*. Springer, pp. 127–147.

Macmillan, M. (2000). *An odd kind of fame: stories of Phineas Gage*. MIT Press.
Maguire, E. A., Woollett, K., & Spiers, H. J. (2006). London taxi drivers and bus drivers: a structural MRI and neuropsychological analysis. *Hippocampus* 16(12): 1091–1101.
Maibom, H. L. (2005). Moral unreason: the case of psychopathy. *Mind & Language* 20(2): 237–257.
Maibom, H. (2010). What experimental evidence shows us about the role of emotions in moral judgement. *Philosophy Compass* 5(11): 999–1012.
Mantione, M., Figee, M., & Denys, D. (2014). A case of musical preference for Johnny Cash following deep brain stimulation of the nucleus accumbens. *Frontiers in Behavioral Neuroscience* 8: 152.
Marcus, A., & Oransky, I. (2015). How the biggest fabricator in science got caught. *Nautilus*. http://nautil.us/issue/24/error/how-the-biggest-fabricator-in-science-got-caught.
Marsh, A. A., & Blair, R. J. R. (2008). Deficits in facial affect recognition among antisocial populations: a meta-analysis. *Neuroscience & Biobehavioral Reviews* 32(3): 454–465.
Maslen, H., Pugh, J., & Savulescu, J. (2015). The ethics of deep brain stimulation for the treatment of anorexia nervosa. *Neuroethics* 8(3): 215–230.
May, J. (2011). Egoism, empathy, and self-other merging. *Southern Journal of Philosophy* 49(s1): 25–39.
May, J. (2014a). On the very concept of free will. *Synthese* 191(12): 2849–2866.
May, J. (2014b). Does disgust influence moral judgment? *Australasian Journal of Philosophy* 92(1): 125–141.
May, J. (2016a). Emotional reactions to human reproductive cloning. *Journal of Medical Ethics* 42(1): 26–30.
May, J. (2016b). Repugnance as performance error: the role of disgust in bioethical intuitions. In S. Clarke et al. (Eds.), *The ethics of human enhancement: understanding the debate*. Oxford University Press, pp. 43–57.
May, J. (2018a). *Regard for reason in the moral mind*. Oxford University Press.
May, J. (2018b). The limits of appealing to disgust. In V. Kumar & N. Strohminger (Eds.), *The moral psychology of disgust*. Rowman & Littlefield, pp. 151–170.
May, J. (2021). Bias in science: natural and social. *Synthese* 199: 3345–3366.
May, J. (2023). Moral rationalism on the brain. *Mind & Language* 38(1): 237–255.
May, J., & Kumar, V. (2018). Moral reasoning and emotion. In K. Jones, M. Timmons, & A. Zimmerman (Eds.), *The Routledge handbook of moral epistemology*. Routledge, pp. 139–156.
May, J., & Kumar, V. (2023). Harnessing moral psychology to reduce meat consumption. *Journal of the American Philosophical Association*. DOI: 0.1017/apa.2022.2.

May, J., Workman, C., Haas, J., & Han, H. (2022). The neuroscience of moral judgment: empirical and philosophical developments. In. De Brigard & Sinnott-Armstrong (Eds.), pp. 17–47.

Mazar, N., Amir, O., & Ariely, D. (2008). The dishonesty of honest people: a theory of self-concept maintenance. *Journal of Marketing Research*, 45(6): 633–644.

Mazar, N., & Zhong, C. B. (2010). Do green products make us better people? *Psychological Science*, 21(4): 494–498.

McCabe, D. P., & Castel, A. D. (2008). Seeing is believing: the effect of brain images on judgments of scientific reasoning. *Cognition* 107(1): 343–352.

McCabe, D. P., Castel, A. D., & Rhodes, M. G. (2011). The influence of fMRI lie detection evidence on juror decision-making. *Behavioral Sciences & the Law*, 29(4): 566–577.

McConaughey, M. (2020). *Greenlights*. Crown.

McClure, S. M., Laibson, D. I., Loewenstein, G., & Cohen, J. D. (2004). Separate neural systems value immediate and delayed monetary rewards. *Science* 306(5695): 503–507.

McFarlane, J., & Illes, J. (2020). Neuroethics at the interface of machine learning and schizophrenia. *NPJ Schizophrenia* 6(1): 1–2.

McGrath, S. (2011). Normative ethics, conversion, and pictures as tools of moral persuasion. In M. Timmons (Ed.), *Oxford studies in normative ethics*. Vol. 1. Oxford University Press, pp. 268–294.

McGruder, J. (2002). Life experience is not a disease or why medicalizing madness is counterproductive to recovery. *Occupational Therapy in Mental Health* 17(3–4): 59–80.

McKibben, B. (2003). Designer genes. *Orion* (May–June). https://orionmagazine.org/article/designer-genes/.

McNamara, R. A., Willard, A. K., Norenzayan, A., & Henrich, J. (2019). Weighing outcome vs. intent across societies: how cultural models of mind shape moral reasoning. *Cognition* 182: 95–108.

Mele, A. (2014a). Free will and substance dualism: the real scientific threat to free Will? In W. Sinnott-Armstrong (Ed.), *Moral psychology*. Vol. 4. MIT Press, pp. 195–207.

Mele, A. (2014b). *Free: why science hasn't disproved free will*. Oxford University Press.

Mendez, M. F., Anderson, E., & Shapira, J. S. (2005). An investigation of moral judgement in frontotemporal dementia. *Cognitive and Behavioral Neurology* 18(4): 193–197.

Mercier, H., & Sperber, D. (2017). *The enigma of reason*. Harvard University Press.

Meynen, G. (2010). Free will and mental disorder: exploring the relationship. *Theoretical Medicine and Bioethics* 31(6):429–443.

Mikhail, J. (2011). *Elements of moral cognition*. Cambridge University Press.

Parmar, A., & Kaloiya, G. (2018). Comorbidity of personality disorder among substance use disorder patients: a narrative review. *Indian Journal of Psychological Medicine* 40(6): 517–527.
Pallesen, J. (2019). Orchestrating False beliefs about gender discrimination. Medium. https://medium.com/@jsmp/orchestrating-false-beliefs-about-gender-discrimination-a25a48e1d02.
Palop, J. J., Chin, J., & Mucke, L. (2006). A network dysfunction perspective on neurodegenerative diseases. *Nature* 443(7113): 768–773.
Parkinson, C., Sinnott-Armstrong, W., Koralus, P. E., Mendelovici, A., McGeer, V., & Wheatley, T. (2011). Is morality unified? Evidence that distinct neural systems underlie moral judgments of harm, dishonesty, and disgust. *Journal of Cognitive Neuroscience* 23(10): 3162–3180.
Paul, L. A. (2014). *Transformative experience*. Oxford University Press.
Payne, B. K. (2001). Prejudice and perception: the role of automatic and controlled processes in misperceiving a weapon. *Journal of Personality and Social Psychology* 81(2): 181–192.
Pellizzoni, S., Siegal, M., & Surian, L. (2010). The contact principle and utilitarian moral judgments in young children. *Developmental Science* 13(2): 265–270.
Persson, I., & Savulescu, J. (2008). The perils of cognitive enhancement and the urgent imperative to enhance the moral character of humanity. *Journal of Applied Philosophy* 25: 162–177.
Peterson, E. L. (2019). Can scientific knowledge sift the wheat from the tares? A brief history of bias (and fears about bias) in science. In K. McCain & K. Kampourakis (Eds.), *What is scientific knowledge? An introduction to contemporary epistemology of science*. Routledge, pp. 195–211.
Pew Research Center. (2009). Public praises science; scientists fault public, media. https://www.people-press.org/2009/07/09/public-praises-science-scientists-fault-public-media/.
Pickard, H. (2011). Responsibility without blame: empathy and the effective treatment of personality disorder. *Philosophy, Psychiatry, & Psychology* 18: 209–224.
Pickard, H. (2015). Psychopathology and the ability to do otherwise. *Philosophy and Phenomenological Research* 90(1): 135–163.
Pickard, H. (2017). Responsibility without blame for addiction. *Neuroethics* 10(1): 169–180.
Pickard, H. (2022). Is addiction a brain disease? A plea for agnosticism and heterogeneity. *Psychopharmacology* 239: 993–1007.
Pickard, H., & Pearce, S. (2013). Addiction in context. In N. Levy (Ed.), *Addiction and self-control*. Oxford University Press, pp. 165–189.
Petrie, B. F. (1996). Environment is not the most important variable in determining oral morphine consumption in Wistar rats. *Psychological Reports* 78(2): 391–400.

Poldrack, R. A. (2006). Can cognitive processes be inferred from neuroimaging data? *Trends in Cognitive Sciences* 10: 59–63.

Poldrack, R. (2018). *The new mind readers: what neuroimaging can and cannot reveal about our thoughts*. Princeton University Press.

Poldrack, R. A., Monahan, J., Imrey, P. B., Reyna, V., Raichle, M. E., Faigman, D., & Buckholtz, J. W. (2018). Predicting violent behavior: what can neuroscience add? *Trends in Cognitive Sciences* 22(2): 111–123.

Polich, J. (2007). Updating P300: an integrative theory of P3a and P3b. *Clinical Neurophysiology* 118(10): 2128–2148.

Pollan, M. (2018). *How to change your mind: what the new science of psychedelics teaches us about consciousness, dying, addiction, depression, and transcendence*. Penguin.

Pollan, M. (2021). *This is your mind on plants*. Penguin.

Presidential Commission for the Study of Bioethical Issues (2015). *Gray matters, Vol. 2: Topics At the intersection of neuroscience, ethics, and society*. Washington, DC. www.bioethics.gov.

President's Council on Bioethics (2003). *Beyond therapy: biotechnology and the pursuit of happiness*. Washington, DC.

Prinz, F., Schlange, T., & Asadullah, K. (2011). Believe it or not: how much can we rely on published data on potential drug targets? *Nature Reviews: Drug Discovery* 10(9): 712.

Prinz, J. J. (2006). The emotional basis of moral judgments. *Philosophical Explorations* 9(1): 29–43.

Prinz, J. J. (2016). Sentimentalism and the moral brain. In S. M. Liao (Ed.). *Moral brains*. Oxford University Press, pp. 45–73.

Pritschet, L., Powell, D., & Horne, Z. (2016). Marginally significant effects as evidence for hypotheses. *Psychological Science* 27(7): 1036–1042.

Pugh, J. (2019). No going back? Reversibility and why it matters for deep brain stimulation. *Journal of Medical Ethics* 45(4): 225–230.

Racine, E., Bar-Ilan, O., & Illes, J. (2005). fMRI in the public eye. *Nature Reviews Neuroscience* 6(2): 159–164.

Railton, P. (2014). The affective dog and its rational tale: intuition and attunement. *Ethics* 124(4): 813–859.

Railton, P. (2017). Moral learning: conceptual foundations and normative relevance. *Cognition* 167(Oct.): 172–190.

Ramachandran, V. S. (1996). The evolutionary biology of self-deception, laughter, dreaming and depression: some clues from anosognosia. *Medical Hypotheses* 47: 347–362.

Relkin, N., Plum, F., Mattis, S., Eidelberg, D., Tranel, D. (1996). Impulsive homicide associated with an arachnoid cyst and unilateral frontotemporal cerebral dysfunction. *Seminars in Clinical Neuropsychiatry* 3(1): 172–183.

Rini, R. (2017). Fake news and partisan epistemology. *Kennedy Institute of Ethics Journal* 27(2): E-43.

Robins, L., Helzer, J., Hesselbrock, M., & Wish, E. (2010). Vietnam veterans three years after Vietnam: how our study changed our view of heroin. *The American Journal on Addictions* 19(3): 203–211.

Rojas-Burke, J. (1993). PET scans advance as tool in insanity defense. *Journal of Nuclear Medicine* 34(1): 13N–26N.

Rosch, E. (1975). Cognitive representations of semantic categories. *Journal of Experimental Psychology: General* 104: 192–233.

Roskies, A. (2002). Neuroethics for the new millennium. *Neuron* 35(July): 21–23.

Roskies, A. (2006). Neuroscientific challenges to free will and responsibility. *Trends in Cognitive Sciences* 10(9): 419–423.

Roskies, A. L. (2007). Are neuroimages like photographs of the brain? *Philosophy of Science* 74(5): 860–872.

Rüsch, N., Angermeyer, M. C., & Corrigan, P. W. (2005). Mental illness stigma: concepts, consequences, and initiatives to reduce stigma. *European Psychiatry* 20(8): 529–539.

Rust, J., & Schwitzgebel, E. (2014). The moral behavior of ethicists and the power of reason. In H. Sarkissian & J. C. Wright (Eds.), *Advances in experimental moral psychology*. Bloomsbury, pp. 91–109.

Salzman, C. D., & Fusi, S. (2010). Emotion, cognition, and mental state representation in amygdala and prefrontal cortex. *Annual Review of Neuroscience* 33: 173–202.

Sandel, M. (2004). The case against perfection. *The Atlantic*. https://www.theatlantic.com/magazine/archive/2004/04/the-case-against-perfection/302927/.

Sanders, R. (2020). Neuroscientist John Ngai named director of NIH BRAIN Initiative. *Berkeley News*. https://news.berkeley.edu/story_jump/neuroscientist-john-ngai-named-director-of-nih-brain-initiative/

Sarkissian, H., Chatterjee, A., De Brigard, F., Knobe, J., Nichols, S., & Sirker, S. (2010). Is belief in free will a cultural universal? *Mind & Language* 25(3): 346–358.

Satel, S., & Lilienfeld, S. O. (2013). *Brainwashed: the seductive appeal of mindless neuroscience*. Basic Books.

Sauer, H. (2017). *Moral judgments as educated intuitions*. MIT Press.

Saver, J. L., & Damasio, A. R. (1991). Preserved access and processing of social knowledge in a patient with acquired sociopathy due to ventromedial frontal damage. *Neuropsychologia* 29(12): 1241–1249.

Scangos, K. W., Khambhati, A. N., Daly, P. M., Makhoul, G. S., Sugrue, L. P., Zamanian, H., . . . & Chang, E. F. (2021). Closed-loop neuromodulation in an individual with treatment-resistant depression. *Nature Medicine* 27(10): 1696–1700.

Schaefer, G. O. (2015). Direct vs. indirect moral enhancement. *Kennedy Institute of Ethics Journal* 25(3): 261–289.

Schermer, M. (2011). Ethical issues in deep brain stimulation. *Frontiers in Integrative Neuroscience* 5: 17.

Scheutz, M., & Malle, B. F. (2018). Moral robots. In Johnson & Rommelfanger (Eds.), pp. 363–377.

Schlag, A. K. (2020). Percentages of problem drug use and their implications for policy making: a review of the literature. *Drug Science, Policy and Law* 6: 1–9.

Schopp, R. F. (1991). *Automatism, insanity, and the psychology of criminal responsibility: a philosophical inquiry*. Cambridge University Press.

Schroeder, T. (2005). Moral responsibility and Tourette syndrome. *Philosophy and Phenomenological Research* 71 (1):106–123.

Schultz, W., Dayan, P., & Montague, P. R. (1997). A neural substrate of prediction and reward. *Science* 275: 1593–1599.

Schüpbach, M., Gargiulo, M., Welter, M., Mallet, L., Béhar, C., Houeto, J. L., ... & Agid, Y. (2006). Neurosurgery in Parkinson disease: a distressed mind in a repaired body? *Neurology* 66(12): 1811–1816.

Schurger, A., Sitt, J., Dehaene, S. (2012). An accumulator model for spontaneous neural activity prior to self-initiated movement. *Proceedings of the National Academy of Sciences* 109(42): E2904–E2913.

Schweitzer, N. J., & Saks, M. J. (2011a). Neuroimage evidence and the insanity defense. *Behavioral Sciences & the Law* 29(4): 592–607.

Schweitzer, N. J., Saks, M. J., Murphy, E. R., Roskies, A. L., Sinnott-Armstrong, W., & Gaudet, L. M. (2011b). Neuroimages as evidence in a mens rea defense: No impact. *Psychology, Public Policy, and Law* 17(3): 357–393.

Schwenkler, J., Byrd, N., Lambert, E., & Taylor, M. (2022). One: but not the same. *Philosophical Studies* 179: 1939–1951. DOI: 10.1007/s11098-021-01739-5.

Schwitzgebel, E., Cokelet, B., & Singer, P. (2020). Do ethics classes influence student behavior? Case study: teaching the ethics of eating meat. *Cognition* 203: 104397.

Selgelid, M. J. (2014). Moderate eugenics and human enhancement. *Medicine, Health Care and Philosophy* 17(1): 3–12.

Seligman, M. E. P., Railton, P., Baumeister, R. F., & Sripada, C. S. (2016). *Homo prospectus*. Oxford University Press.

Shenhav, A., & Greene, J. D. (2014). Integrative moral judgment: dissociating the roles of the amygdala and ventromedial prefrontal cortex. *Journal of Neuroscience*, 34(13): 4741–4749.

Shepard, J., & May, J. (2014). Does belief in dualism protect against maladaptive psychosocial responses to deep brain stimulation? An empirical exploration. *AJOB Neuroscience* 5(4): 40–42.

Shepherd, J. (2017). The folk psychological roots of free will. In D. Rose (Ed.), *Experimental metaphysics*. Bloomsbury, pp. 95–116.

Sher, G. (2009). *Who knew? Responsibility without awareness*. Oxford University Press.

Shoemaker, D. (2015). *Responsibility from the margins*. Oxford University Press.

Shoemaker, D. (2022). Disordered, disabled, disregarded, dismissed: the moral costs of exemptions from accountability. In King & May (Eds.), pp. 33–62.

Siddiqui, F., Osuna, E., & Chokroverty, S. (2009). Writing emails as part of sleepwalking after increase in Zolpidem. *Sleep Medicine* 10(2): 262–264.

Sifferd, K. (2022). Legal insanity and moral knowledge: why is a lack of moral knowledge related to a mental illness exculpatory? In King & May (Eds.), pp. 113–135.

Sikora, M., Nicolas, C., Istin, M., Jaafari, N., Thiriet, N., & Solinas, M. (2018). Generalization of effects of environmental enrichment on seeking for different classes of drugs of abuse. *Behavioural Brain Research* 341: 109–113.

Silberman, S. (2015). *NeuroTribes: the legacy of autism and the future of neurodiversity*. Avery.

Singer, J. (1999). "Why can't you be normal for once in your life?" From a problem with no name to the emergence of a new category of difference. In. M. Corker & S. French (Eds.), *Disability discourse*. Open University Press, pp. 59–67.

Singer, P. (2005). Ethics and intuitions. *The Journal of Ethics* 9: 331–352.

Sinnott-Armstrong, W. (2019). Consequentialism. In E. N. Zalta (Ed.), *The Stanford encyclopedia of philosophy*. https://plato.stanford.edu/archives/sum2019/entries/consequentialism/.

Sinnott-Armstrong, W., Roskies, A. L., Brown, T., & Murphy, E. (2008). Brain images as legal evidence. *Episteme* 5(3): 359–373.

Sitaram, R., Ros, T., Stoeckel, L., Haller, S., Scharnowski, F., Lewis-Peacock, J., . . . & Sulzer, J. (2017). Closed-loop brain training: the science of neurofeedback. *Nature Reviews Neuroscience* 18(2): 86–100.

Slingerland, E. (2021). *Drunk: how we sipped, danced, and stumbled our way to civilization*. Little, Brown Spark.

Smeding, H. M. M., Goudriaan, A. E., Foncke, E. M. J., Schuurman, P. R., Speelman, J. D., & Schmand, B. (2007). Pathological gambling after bilateral subthalamic nucleus stimulation in Parkinson disease. *Neurosurgery & Psychiatry* 78(5): 517–519.

Smith, H. (1983). Culpable ignorance. *Philosophical Review* 92: 543–571.

Solomon, M. (2001). *Social empiricism*. MIT Press.

Soon, C., Brass, M., Heinze, H., Haynes, J. (2008). Unconscious determinants of free decisions in the human brain. *Nature Neuroscience* 11(5): 543–545.

Sparrow, R. (2005). Defending deaf culture: the case of cochlear implants. *Journal of Political Philosophy* 13(2): 135–152.

Sparrow, R. (2014). Better living through chemistry? A reply to Savulescu and Persson on "moral enhancement." *Journal of Applied Philosophy* 31: 23–32.

Sripada, C. (2018). Addiction and fallibility. *The Journal of Philosophy* 115(11): 569–587.

Sripada, C. S. (2022a). Mental disorders involve limits on control, not extreme preferences. In King & May (Eds.), pp. 169–192.

Sripada, C. (2022b). Impaired control in addiction involves cognitive distortions and unreliable self-control, not compulsive desires and overwhelmed self-control. *Behavioural Brain Research* 418: 113639.

Sripada, C., & Taxali, A. (2020). Structure in the stream of consciousness: evidence from a verbalized thought protocol and automated text analytic methods. *Consciousness and Cognition* 85: 103007.

Stanley, M. L., Yin, S., & Sinnott-Armstrong, W. (2019). A reason-based explanation for moral dumbfounding. *Judgment and Decision Making* 14: 120–129.

Stanley, M. L., & De Brigard, F. (2019). Moral memories and the belief in the good self. *Current Directions in Psychological Science* 28(4): 387–391.

Starmans, C., & Bloom, P. (2018). Nothing personal: what psychologists get wrong about identity. *Trends in Cognitive Sciences* 22(7): 566–568.

Stegenga, J. (2018). *Medical nihilism*. Oxford University Press.

Stephens-Davidowitz, S. (2017). *Everybody lies: big data, new data, and what the internet can tell us about who we really are*. Dey Street Books.

Stitzer, M., & Petry, N. (2006). Contingency management for treatment of substance abuse. *Annual Review of Clinical Psychology* 2: 411–434.

Strawson, G. (1994). The impossibility of moral responsibility. *Philosophical Studies* 75(1–2): 5–24.

Strawson, P. F. (1962). Freedom and resentment. *Proceedings of the British Academy* 48:187–211.

Stroebe, W., Postmes, T., & Spears, R. (2012). Scientific misconduct and the myth of self-correction in science. *Perspectives on Psychological Science* 7(6): 670–688.

Strohminger, N., & Nichols, S. (2015). Neurodegeneration and identity. *Psychological Science* 26(9): 1469–1479.

Stroop, J. R. (1935). Studies of interference in serial verbal reactions. *Journal of Experimental Psychology* 18(6): 643.

Studerus, E., Kometer, M., Hasler, F., & Vollenweider, F. X. (2011). Acute, subacute and long-term subjective effects of psilocybin in healthy humans: a pooled analysis of experimental studies. *Journal of Psychopharmacology* 25(11): 1434–1452.

Summers, J. S. (2017). Post hoc ergo propter hoc: some benefits of rationalization. *Philosophical Explorations*, 20(sup1): 21–36.

Summers, J. S., & Sinnott-Armstrong, W. (2015). Scrupulous agents. *Philosophical Psychology* 28(7): 947–966.

Szasz, T. (1961/1974). *The myth of mental illness*. Harper and Row.

Szucs, D., & Ioannidis, J. P. (2020). Sample size evolution in neuroimaging research: an evaluation of highly-cited studies (1990–2012) and of latest practices (2017–2018) in high-impact journals. *NeuroImage* 221: 117164.

Tabb, K. (2015). Psychiatric progress and the assumption of diagnostic discrimination. *Philosophy of Science* 82(5): 1047–1058.

Tappolet, C. (2015). *Emotions, value, and agency*. Oxford University Press.
Terbeck, S., Kahane, G., McTavish, S., Savulescu, J., Cowen, P. J., & Hewstone, M. (2012). Propranolol reduces implicit negative racial bias. *Psychopharmacology* 222(3): 419–424.
Thomson, K. S., & Oppenheimer, D. M. (2016). Investigating an alternate form of the cognitive reflection test. *Judgment and Decision Making* 11(1): 99–113.
Trevena, J., & Miller, J. (2010). Brain preparation before a voluntary action: evidence against unconscious movement initiation. *Consciousness and Cognition* 19(1): 447–456.
Tse, W. S., & Bond, A. J. (2002). Serotonergic intervention affects both social dominance and affiliative behaviour. *Psychopharmacology* 161(3): 324–330.
Tullett, A. M. (2015). In search of true things worth knowing: Considerations for a new article prototype. *Social and Personality Psychology Compass* 9(4): 188–201.
Turner, A. J. (2010). Are disorders sufficient for reduced responsibility? *Neuroethics* 3 (2):151–160.
Twenge, J. M., Haidt, J., Joiner, T. E., & Campbell, W. K. (2020). Underestimating digital media harm. *Nature Human Behaviour* 4(4): 346–348.
Uddin, L. Q., Dajani, D. R., Voorhies, W., Bednarz, H., & Kana, R. K. (2017). Progress and roadblocks in the search for brain-based biomarkers of autism and attention-deficit/hyperactivity disorder. *Translational Psychiatry* 7(8): e1218–e1218.
Van IJzendoorn, M. H., & Bakermans-Kranenburg, M. J. (2012). A sniff of trust: meta-analysis of the effects of intranasal oxytocin administration on face recognition, trust to in-group, and trust to out-group. *Psychoneuroendocrinology* 37(3): 438–443.
Vargas, M. (2013). *Building better beings: A theory of moral responsibility*. Oxford University Press.
Vincent, N. (2013). Enhancing responsibility. In N. Vincent (Ed.), *Neuroscience and legal responsibility*. Oxford University Press, pp. 305–333.
Volkow, N. D., & Koob, G. (2015). Brain disease model of addiction: why is it so controversial? *Lancet Psychiatry* 2: 677–679.
Wakefield, J. C. (2020). Addiction from the harmful dysfunction perspective: how there can be a mental disorder in a normal brain. *Behavioural Brain Research* 389: 112665.
Waldman, A. (2017). *A really good day: how microdosing made a mega difference in my mood, my marriage, and my life*. Knopf.
Wallace, R. J. (1994). *Responsibility and the moral sentiments*. Harvard University Press.
Walters, G. D. (2000). Spontaneous remission from alcohol, tobacco, and other drug abuse: seeking quantitative answers to qualitative questions. *The American Journal of Drug and Alcohol Abuse* 26(3): 443–460.

Wang, J., Cherkassky, V. L., & Just, M. A. (2017). Predicting the brain activation pattern associated with the propositional content of a sentence: modeling neural representations of events and states. *Human Brain Mapping* 38(10): 4865–4881.

Washington, N. (2016). Culturally unbound: cross-cultural cognitive diversity and the science of psychopathology. *Philosophy, Psychiatry, & Psychology* 23(2): 165–179.

Washington, N., & Kelly, D. (2016). Who's responsible for this? Moral responsibility, externalism, and knowledge about implicit bias. In M. Brownstein & J. Saul (Eds.), *Implicit bias and philosophy*. Vol. 2. Oxford University Press, pp. 11–36.

Watson, Gary (1999). Disordered appetites: addiction, compulsion and dependence. In J. Elster (Ed.), *Addiction: entries and exits*. Russell Sage, pp. 3–28.

Wegner, D. M. (2003). *The illusion of conscious will*. MIT Press.

Weisberg, D. S., Keil, F. C., Goodstein, J., Rawson, E., & Gray, J. R. (2008). The seductive allure of neuroscience explanations. *Journal of Cognitive Neuroscience* 20(3): 470–477.

Wiesjahn, M., Jung, E., Kremser, J. D., Rief, W., & Lincoln, T. M. (2016). The potential of continuum versus biogenetic beliefs in reducing stigmatization against persons with schizophrenia: an experimental study. *Journal of Behavior Therapy and Experimental Psychiatry* 50: 231–237.

Wilholt, T. (2009). Bias and values in scientific research. *Studies in History and Philosophy of Science* 40(1): 92–101.

Winick, C. (1962). Maturing out of narcotic addiction. United Nations Office on Drugs and Crime, pp. 1–7.

Wolf, S. (1987). Sanity and the metaphysics of responsibility. In F. D. Schoeman (Ed.), *Responsibility, character, and the emotions*. Cambridge University Press, pp. 46–62.

Wolpe, P. R. (2002). Treatment, enhancement, and the ethics of neurotherapeutics. *Brain and Cognition* 50(3): 387–395.

Wolpe, P. R., Foster, K. R., & Langleben, D. D. (2005). Emerging neurotechnologies for lie-detection: promises and perils. *The American Journal of Bioethics* 5(2): 39–49.

Woodward, J. (2016). Emotion versus cognition in moral decision-making. In S. Matthew Liao (Ed.), *Moral brains: the neuroscience of ethics*. Oxford University Press, pp. 87–117.

Yoder, K. J., & Decety, J. (2014). Spatiotemporal neural dynamics of moral judgment: a high-density ERP study. *Neuropsychologia*, 60: 39–45.

Young, L. L., Camprodon, J. A., Hauser, M. D., Pascual-Leone, A., & Saxe, R. (2010). Disruption of the right temporoparietal junction with transcranial magnetic stimulation reduces the role of beliefs in moral judgments. *Proceedings of the National Academy of Sciences* 107(15): 6753–6758.

Young, L. L., Cushman, F. A., Hauser, M. D., & Saxe, R. (2007). The neural basis of the interaction between theory of mind and moral judgment. *Proceedings of the National Academy of Sciences* 104(20): 8235–8240.

Young, L., & Dungan, J. (2012). Where in the brain is morality? Everywhere and maybe nowhere. *Social Neuroscience* 7(1): 1–10.

Zollman, K. (2018). The credit economy and the economic rationality of science. *The Journal of Philosophy* 115(1): 5–33.

Index

For the benefit of digital users, indexed terms that span two pages (e.g., 52–53) may, on occasion, appear on only one of those pages.

Note: Tables and figures are indicated by *t* and *f* following the page number

abilism, 111
acquired sociopathy, 153–54, 161
addiction, 8, 11–12, 66, 73–74, 95–96, 119–45, 214–15, 245–46, 263, 268–69
    behavioral addictions, 69–70, 123, 142
    contingency management of, 129
    cooccurrence with other disorders, 137
    degrees of, 130–32
    deliberate abstinence, 129, 130
    disease vs. normality, 133–35
    dopamine hypothesis of, 123–28
    first characterized, 120–21
    hijacking the brain, 11–12, 129–30
    incentive salience, 127
    mature out of, 130
    moralization of, 120
    rates of, 135
    self-control in, 128–32
    spontaneous remission, 130
    withdrawal, 121*t*, 121–22, 126–27, 129, 133–34, 141
    See also brain disease model; tolerance
adjunctive role of drugs, 188
affect. *See* gut feelings
agency:
    bypassed, 41
    corporate model of, 56–59
    first described, 45–46
    ecological/scaffolded, 45–46
    enhanced in disorder, 99–102
    executive model of, 57

fluidity of, 109, 263–64, 267, 269–70
    See also cognitive continuity
Aharoni, Eyal, 150–51, 231, 232, 246–47, 248
alarmism xviii, 12, 200, 229, 253–56, 263–65. *See also* neurohype
Alexander, Bruce. *See* Rat Park study
Alloy, Lauren, 99–100
altruism, 176, 182, 190–91, 221. *See also* motivation
Alzheimer's disease, 5, 72–74, 79, 86, 88, 93, 99–100, 102, 105–6, 113, 129, 135, 142, 269–70
Amazon, 57
amygdala, 27–29, 152, 153, 156–57, 160–61, 167–68, 239, 261–62
amyotrophic lateral sclerosis (ALS), 73–74
Anderson, Elizabeth, 214–15, 222
animal welfare, 9–10, 180, 191, 200
anorexia nervosa, 66, 76–77
anosognosia, 207
anxiety, 8, 87, 98–100, 101, 103, 106–7, 108, 111–12, 113, 115, 121–22, 137, 142, 143, 144, 167, 184–85, 253, 263–64
applied ethics. *See* ethics
arachnoid cyst, 36–37, 62, 237
Ariely, Dan, 213, 252
Aristotle, 21, 194
Arpaly, Nomy, 58, 95, 98, 100–1, 108, 115–16
artificial intelligence (AI), 158–59

attention deficit hyperactivity disorder
   (ADHD), 95, 103–4, 105, 108, 135–
   36, 178–79
Aurelius, Marcus, 194
authenticity, 75, 76, 187–88
authoritarianism, 180, 183–84, 192
autism, 95, 99–100, 104, 105–6, 108, 109–
   10, 111–12, 117–18, 269–70, 271
automatism, 48, 60
autonomy:
   amid brain manipulation, 68–70
   in ethics, 21, 22, 199
   of patients, 68–70, 73, 109, 113, 117–
   18, 189–90
   See also free will
axon. See *neuron*
ayahuasca, 182–84, 188

Baars, Bernard, 54
Baggs, Mel, 109–10
Bargh, John, 49
Bartholow, Roberts, 69
basal ganglia, 28–29, 64, 86–87
base rates, 235–37, 247, 248
Batson, C Daniel, 182, 220, 221
Baylis, Françoise, 79
Berridge, Kent, 125–27, 132–33, 134–
   35, 138
beta-blockers, 184*t*, 191
bias:
   confirmation bias, 209–10, 224
   implicit bias, 56–57, 61, 184–85,
   189, 216–17
   partisan bias, 213
   racial bias, 181, 184*t*, 184–85, 189,
   191, 193
   in science, 214–19
bioethics, 4–5, 6, 9–10, 22, 71
   President's Council on, 71
   principles of, 22
bipolar disorder, 95–96, 100–1,
   104, 105–6
Blair, R J R, 152*f*, 155
blame. *See* responsibility
Bloom, Paul, 74–75
Bluhm, Robyn, 67, 70–71, 266
BOLD signal, 29–30
Bortolotti, Lisa, 99–100, 106, 226

brain (anatomy), 26–31
brain-computer interfaces, 16, 67, 182–
   83, 252–53, 254–55,
brain disease model (of addiction):
   characterization of, 122–23
   harms of, 138–41
   moral argument for, 139–40, 214–15
   vs. disorder model, 141–43
brain fingerprinting, 13–14, 230, 250
brain imaging:
   functional (fMRI), 29–30, 51–52, 231–
   32, 233, 234, 244–45, 248
   PET scan, 29–30, 36–37
   structural, 29–30, 36–37, 218
   See also reverse inference
BRAIN Initiative, 5–6
brain manipulation:
   autonomy, 65–67, 68–70
   direct vs. indirect, 66–67
   personality changes, 70–80
   safety/risk-benefit, 80–88
   See also DBS; ECT; tDCS; TMS
brain organoids, 9–10
brain overclaim syndrome, 242, 265–66
brain/mind reading:
   of consumers, 13–14, 251–56
   in courts, 229–32
   dangers/abuse of, 242–47
   lie detection, 235
   of political attitudes, 224–25
   privacy issues, 251–53, 255–56
   reliability of, 233–42
brainstem, 16, 64, 124, 125*f*
Brodmann areas, 26
Brownstein, Michael, 45–46, 49, 56, 58, 60
Buchanan, Allen, 178, 182, 191, 194, 195–
   96, 200, 256, 264–65
Buchanan's dictum, 264–65
Bucharest Early Intervention Study, 9–10
Buddhism, 194
bystander effect, 48–49

caffeine, 133–34, 187–88, 199, 264–65
Cajal, Santiago Ramón y, 24–25
Caramazza, Alfonso, 25, 161
cardiovascular disease, 83, 84*f*
Carol and Carl (split-brain patients), 206
Carruthers, Peter, 55

Caruso, Gregg, 46
Cash, Johnny, 75
cerebellum, 27f, 28–29
cerebral cortex, 26, 27f, 27, 28–29, 49, 198
Chartrand, Tanya, 48–49
Chatterjee, Anjan, 176, 194
choice. See free will
Christen, Markus, 66, 82–83
Churchland, Patricia, 61–62, 152, 157, 225
cingulate cortex, 28–29, 155–56, 167–68, 224–25, 246–47
Clapton, Eric, 131
Clark, Andy, 8, 19, 45–46
Clark v Arizona, 104–5
Clarke, Randolph, 38–39
Clarke-Doane Justin, 131–32, 270
Clinton, Hilary, 224–25
cochlear implants, 111, 264–65
Cochrane Collaboration, 82
cocktail party effect, 54
coercion, 81–82, 192
cognitive continuity, 109–10, 112, 113, 131–32, 142, 261, 268–72
Cognitive Continuum, 109, 113, 131, 233–34, 269–72
cognitive enhancers, 100–1, 176
cognitive liberty. See liberty
Cognitive Reflection Test, 165–66, 171–72
Cohen, Jonathan, 37–38, 167
coherence. See free will
comorbidity/co-occurrence, 105, 137
compass analogy, 162, 170
compassion, 11, 22–23, 74–75, 109, 112, 113, 116, 139, 143, 144, 158, 159–61, 175, 176, 182, 184t, 185–86, 189, 190–91, 193, 195–96, 267–68
compatibilism, 41
See also incompatibilism
concerns vs. arguments. See Buchanan's dictum
confabulation, 205–8, 226, 227, 251–52, 266–67
conflict of interest, 82, 83, 85, 211, 218–19, 226
Confucius, 21

consciousness:
 global workspace view of, 54–55, 56–57
 in free will, 54–59
consequentialism. See utilitarianism
consistency (reasoning), 13–14, 172–73, 210–11, 250
consumer neuroscience, 13–14, 185, 188, 200, 251–56
contingency management. See addiction
control. See free will
co-occurrence of disorders. See comorbidity
corporate model of agency. See agency
corpus collosum, 205–6
cosmetic neurology, 176
Coyne, Jerry, 35
CRISPR, 183
Crockett, Molly, 169–70, 180, 184t, 185
Cushman, Fiery, 169–70, 226
cyst. See arachnoid cyst

Damasio, Antonio, 49, 153, 154, 159
Daniels, Norman, 179, 233–34
Davidson, Donald, 210
Deaf culture, 110–11
De Brigard, Felipe, 23–24, 212–13
debunking arguments. See moral judgment
Decety, Jean, 155, 156–57
De Dreu, Carsten, 184t, 185–86
Deep Brain Stimulation (DBS), 64–65, 65f, 66, 67, 68, 69–70, 73, 75, 76–77, 79, 80, 81, 86–87, 88–89, 142–43, 184t, 185
deep self view. See coherence; true self
DeGrazia, David, 75, 178, 181, 189
Delgado, José. 65–66, 208
delusions, 97, 98–100, 104–6, 107, 108, 117, 159–60, 271
dementia, 66, 72, 73–74, 95, 99–100, 105–6, 129. See also Alzheimer's, FTD
dendrites. See neurons
Dennett, Daniel, 66
deontology, 21, 163
depression, 9, 11, 66, 77, 80, 83–85, 86, 87, 88, 93, 95, 104, 108, 111–12, 113, 115, 116, 117, 121–22, 137, 140, 143, 144, 176, 253, 269–70. See also Hamilton Rating Scale

Descartes, René, 15–17, 123–24, 272
desire. *See* motivation
determinism, 40–43, 44, 61–62, 273
diachronic agency. *See* agency
Dimitry (Parkinson's patient), 64–65, 67, 68, 69, 88–89
disability, models of, 110–12
disgust/repugnance, 162–63, 187
Ditto, Peter, 210, 212–13
domain-specific vs. general brain functions, 161
dopamine:
  in addiction, 123–28, 129, 130–33, 135–36, 137, 142
  in cognitive enhancement, 176
  down-regulation, 126–27
  in Parkinson's 64, 69–70
  pathways in the brain, 124–26, 125*f*
  in reinforcement learning, 124, 198
Doris, John, 45–46, 49, 58, 60–61, 180, 244
dorsolateral prefrontal cortex (dlPFC), 28*f*, 167–68, 171
dose-response curve, 185–86
Douglas, Thomas, 178, 181, 193, 196–97
drive to mastery, 193
drug courts, 144
dualism, 15–17, 44–45, 46, 68, 123–24
dual process theory of cognition, 165
Dubiel, Helmut, 80
Dugan, Brian, 149–51, 174, 231–32, 233–34

Eagleman, David, 25–26, 154
Earp, Brian, 99–100, 177–78, 182–83, 185, 188, 191
ecological agency. *See* agency
ego-dissolution, 176
Eldred, Julie, 119–20, 144
electroconvulsive therapy (ECT). *See* therapy
electroencephalography (EEG), 36–37, 49, 50*f*, 52, 156–57, 230, 233, 239–40, 250, 252
electromyography (EMG), 49–50
Elliott, Carl, 75, 98, 214
emotion. *See* moral judgment
empathy, 150, 174, 184*t*

enhancement:
  arms race, 197
  authenticity, 187–88
  character, 193–94
  fairness, 188–93
  permissive vs. restrictive views, 178
  safety, 196–99
  treatment/enhancement distinction, 178–80
environmental enrichment. *See* Rat Park study
epilepsy, 3, 13, 50–51, 88, 205
epiphenomenalism, 46–62, 273
essential-moral-self hypothesis, 74
ethicists, moral behavior of, 180
ethics
  applied vs. normative vs. meta, 20–23
  of neuroscience, 6–7
eugenics, 63, 81–82, 192
evidence:
  approaching with vigilance, 265–66
  corroborating role, 50–51, 157, 265, 272–73
  cumulative nature, 248
  FBI errors, 249
  Federal Rules of, 232
  probative value of neuroscience, 233–42
evolution of the mind, 23, 25, 162–63, 169–70, 187
executive model of agency, 57
exercise and the brain, 16–17, 66–67, 188, 192, 198, 265–66
extended mind hypothesis, 8
external validity, 52, 185–86, 235

Facebook, 252, 254–55
fairness, 21, 22, 182, 195–96, 232
  in enhancement, 195–96
  vs. other moral values, 22, 157
false conviction, 13–14, 250
false dichotomy, 143, 199
false memories. *See* memory
false positives and negatives, 82, 217–18, 235–37, 247
family resemblance concept, 39
Farahany, Nita, 231
Farwell, Larry. *See* brain fingerprinting

fatalism, 41
feminism and science, 214–15, 222, 266
Fine, Cordelia, 57, 60, 150–51, 154, 174, 222
Fischer, John Martin, 38–39, 68
Flanagan, Owen, 126, 129–30, 131
Fleabag (TV series), 59
fMRI. *See* brain imaging
Focquaert, Farah, 37–38
Foot, Philippa, 163
forward inference. *See* reverse inference
Foucault, Michel, 108
Fox, Michael J, 79
fragility. *See* resilience
Frankfurt, Harry, 39
fraud in science, 13, 215–16, 224, 226–27
freedom. *See* free will
Freeman, Walter. *See* lobotomy
free will:
    choice, 38, 40–43
    coherence, 39, 46–61
    consciousness/awareness, 35, 46–62, 68–69, 189–90, 266–67
    control/self-control, 4, 38–39, 45–46, 54, 56–57, 58, 59, 62, 68, 69, 95, 97, 114, 123, 128–32, 181, 231, 246–47, 261–62, 263, 267–69, 270
    initially defined, 38–40
    luck problem, 41–42
    See also responsibility
frontotemporal dementia (FTD), 73–74, 95, 99–100, 168

Gage, Phineas, 70, 153
gambling, 69–70, 86–87, 123, 142
gay rights. *See* homosexuality
Gazzaniga, Michael, 6, 43, 206, 226
genetic engineering, 182–83
genetic explanations, 142, 152–53, 170
gentle medicine, 85, 87, 205
Gilbert, Frederic, 67, 68, 70–71, 75
Glannon, Walter, 64, 68, 69, 100, 104, 110, 185–86, 232, 248
Glenn, Andrea, 152–53, 231, 232
global workspace view. *See* consciousness
Goals. *See* desires
Gopnik, Alison, 78

Grandin, Temple, 99–100, 104, 269–70, 271
Greene, Joshua, 37–38, 152, 156–57, 163, 165, 166–68, 169–70, 171–72, 173
group-to-individual problem, 233
growth hormone, 179
guilty. *See* insanity defense
gut feelings, 12, 60–61, 149, 151–73, 187
gyrus. *See* cerebral cortex

Haas, Julia Henke, 158–59
Habermas, Jürgen, 189
habit, 45–46, 48, 60, 120, 133–34, 140, 159–60, 166, 189–91, 194, 198–99, 267. *See also* ecological agency; neuroplasticity; reinforcement learning
Haggard, Ted, 76
Haidt, Jonathan, 22, 60–61, 159–60, 182–83, 194, 210
Hamilton Rating Scale for Depression, 83–84
Hare, Robert, 150–51, 154–55
Harrington, Terry, 229–31, 233, 241, 250
Harris, John, 181, 185–86, 189–90, 191
Harris, Sam, 35, 57
Hart, Carl, 129, 135–36, 140–41, 143, 222
Haynes, John-Dylan, 241–42
Heath, Robert, 179
Henrich, Joseph, 197, 201, 225, 233–34
Heyman, Gene, 129, 134–35, 141–42, 143
Hinckley Jr, John, 37
hippocampus, 28–29, 72,
Hirstein, William, 57, 98, 231
holism (of the mind), 66
Holton, Richard, 132–33
homeostasis, 133, 134, 139*t*, 197–98
homosexuality, 172–73, 179
Human Brain Project, 5–6
Hume, David, 78, 158, 162
humility, 85, 87–88, 193, 263, 265–66, 271
hypersexuality, 3, 87
hypomania, 87, 100–1

Iacoboni, Marco, 224–25
identity:
    and memory, 71–73
    moral traits, 73–77

identity: (*cont.*)
   numerical vs. qualitative, 74–75, 77, 88–89
   psychological continuity, 79
illusion:
   free will as, 35, 46,
   perceptual, 18–19, 18*f*,
   self as, 78
incentive salience. *See* addiction
incompatibilism, 41
inequality, 12, 180, 195–96, 200
innate (vs. learned), 25, 166, 169–70, 266–67. *See also* evolution of the mind
insanity defense, 11, 93–94, 117, 150–51, 231, 244
interactionism, 16–17. *See also* dualism
Ioannidis, John, 82, 217–18
irrationality, 158, 208, 210–11, 264, 266–67, 268–69
is-ought gap, 162

Jaworska, Agnieszka, 72–73
Jefferson, Anneli, 45–46
Jurassic Park (film), 5
Just, Marcel, 253–54

Kahane, Guy, 152, 167–68, 171, 193
Kahneman, Daniel, 165, 209–10, 237
Kamm, Frances, 191–92
Kandel, Eric, 17–18, 23–24, 71, 73–74, 86, 99–100
Kane, Robert, 38, 42
Kant, Immanuel, 21, 158
Kass, Leon, 71, 178, 187–89, 195
Kelly, Dan, 45–46, 58, 162–63
Kennett, Jeanette, 57, 60, 112, 130, 135, 150–51, 154, 158, 174
Kiehl, Kent, 152–53, 174, 238
King, Matt, 38, 55, 98–99, 114
kleptomania, 95–96, 103–4, 106
Klüver-Bucy Syndrome, 3–4, 7, 238, 261–62
Koenigs, Michael, 150–51, 155, 161, 168, 171
Kreitmair, Karola, 252–53, 255
Krueger, Robert F, 108
Kumar, Victor, 61, 160, 162–63, 172, 182, 192, 200, 201, 210–11, 225

Langleben, Daniel, 230, 235
Latané, Bibb, 48–49
learning:
   moral learning, 161, 171–73, 182–83, 185, 189–91
   from punishment, 159–60, 182
   trial-and-error, 170–71, 172, 187
   unconscious learning, 171–72, 264–65, 266–67
   See also amygdala; basal ganglia; dopamine; gut feelings; habit; reinforcement learning; neuroplasticity
Levy, Neil, 8, 48, 53, 54–55, 66–67, 130, 131–32, 135, 150–51, 179, 231–32, 235, 246, 250, 255
Lewis, Marc, 131, 134, 140
liberty:
   cognitive liberty, 13–14, 252–53, 255–56
   to enhance, 186
Libet, Benjamin, 49–50, 50*f*, 51*f*, 59–60
limbic system, 28–29, 153. *See also* mesolimbic pathway
lobotomy, 8–9, 63, 81
localization of function, 25–26, 239. *See also* reverse inference
Locke, John, 71, 73, 79
Loftus, Elizabeth, 248
LSD (lysergic acid diethylamide), 176, 177, 190–91, 199
luck problem. *See* free will

Machery, Edouard, 241, 244
Maibom, Heidi, 154–55, 158, 159–60
Malle, Bertram, 38, 45, 158–59
mania, 64–65, 68, 69, 86–87, 88–89, 98–99, 100–1. *See also* hypomania; kleptomania
marketplace of ideas, 205, 208, 226
Maslen, Hannah, 76–77
materialism. *See* physicalism
maturing out. *See* addiction
May, Joshua, 38, 39–40, 41–42, 61, 68, 82–83, 98–99, 131–32, 152, 157, 158, 159–60, 161, 162–63, 169–70, 171–72, 180, 181, 182, 187, 201, 210, 213, 220, 221, 244, 245
McConaughey, Matthew, 209

McGurk effect, 19
MDMA (ecstasy), 71–72, 176, 177–78, 184t
means vs. side-effect, 21, 165, 172
mechanism. *See* physicalism
medical nihilism, 85, 273. *See also* humility
melatonin, 188, 198–99, 200
Mele, Alfred, 44–45, 51–52
memory:
  false memories, 248–49
  and identity, 71–73
  recall, 241
  selective memory, 131,
  working memory, 54–55
  See also dementia
mental disorder:
  and blame, 11, 114–16
  and diminished agency, 102–5
  and enhanced agency, 99–102
  and stigma, 112–13
  variability within, 105–8
  See also addiction; anorexia nervosa; anxiety; attention deficit hyperactivity disorder (ADHD); autism; bipolar disorder; dementia; depression; mania; neurodiversity; obsessive-compulsive disorder (OCD); personality disorder; phobias; post-traumatic stress disorder (PTSD); psychopathy; schizophrenia; Scrupulosity; Tourette syndrome
Mercier, Hugo, 212, 226
mesolimbic pathway. *See* reinforcement learning
meta-ethics. *See* ethics
microdosing, 176–78, 190–91, 199, 264–65
Mikhail, John, 157, 164, 171–72
Mill, John Stuart, 20–21
mimicry, 48–49, 201, 267
mind-body problem, 15, 16
mind reading, 239, 240f, 246, 255, 265
  See also theory of mind
mind wandering, 55–56, 239, 240f
M'Naghten Rule. *See* insanity defense
Moll, Jorge, 152, 157

Montague, P Read, 43
moral brain. *See* moral judgment
moral dilemmas. *See* moral judgment
moral flabbiness, 194
moral incompetence. *See* psychopathy
moral judgment:
  brain areas involved in, 152–57
  debunking arguments, 162–63
  dual process theory of, 165
  emotion/reason dichotomy, 157–61
  moral dilemmas/trolley problem, 163–68
  reliability of, 169–73
  See also psychopathy
moral licensing. *See* motivated reasoning
moral progress, 180–81, 182, 200, 201
moral realism. *See* objectivity in ethics
moral values, 21–22, 73
Morse, Stephen, 98–99, 100–1, 104–5, 117, 232, 242, 246, 265–66
motivated reasoning:
  defined, 209–12
  moral licensing, 212–13
  motivated forgetting, 212–13
  post hoc vs. ante hoc, 210
  in science, 214–19
  wishful thinking, 211–12, 214–15, 220–21, 226
motivation:
  craving, 3, 45–46, 121–22, 121t, 123, 127–28, 130, 131–32, 133–34, 137, 139t, 140, 141, 169
  goals of scientists, 220–22, 221t, 223–26
  ultimate vs. instrumental goals, 220
  See also reinforcement learning
Mozart effect, 243
multiple comparisons. *See* statistical significance

Nahmias, Eddy, 40, 43, 44–45, 52, 61–62
naïve realism, 17
naïve view (about mental disorder), 95–97
narcolepsy, 102, 103, 105–6
National Institutes of Health (NIH), 83, 122–23
Nelkin, Dana, 60–61

Neuralink, 182–83, 252
neural prosthesis. *See* brain-computer interface
neurobabble, 242–46
neurocentrism, 8
neurodivergent. *See* neurodiversity
neurodiversity, 109–10, 111–12, 117–18, 191–92, 270–71
neuroethics (defined), 4–5
neurofeedback, 182, 184*t*, 185, 252
neurohype, 251, 255–56, 264. *See also* alarmism
neurological conditions. *See* acquired Alzheimer's; amyotrophic lateral sclerosis; anosognosia; arachnoid cyst; autism; epilepsy; frontotemporal dementia; Klüver-Bucy Syndrome; narcolepsy; Parkinson's; psychopathy; tetraplegia
neuromarketing, 251–56
neurons, 24–25
neuroplasticity, 25–26, 134, 251, 266–67
neuroprediction, 247
neuroredundancy, 123–24, 246–47, 256–57
neuroscience of ethics, 7
neurotransmitters, 24–25, 124, 126–27, 152–53, 182–83. *See also* dopamine; growth hormone; melatonin; serotonin; testosterone; opioids; oxytocin
neurotypical syndrome, 271. *See also* neurodiversity
Nichols, Shaun, 41–42, 44, 73–74, 78, 158, 159–60, 162, 172
Nielsen marketing firm, 252, 254–55
nootropics. *See* cognitive enhancers
normal vs. abnormal functioning, 37, 62, 109–10, 150, 152–53, 161, 173–74, 179, 233–35, 268–69. *See also* neurodiversity
normative ethics. *See* ethics
Nosek, Brian, 214, 216, 220–21, 226
nuanced neuroethics, 14, 98–99, 131, 261, 262–63, 266, 268
nucleus accumbens, 124, 125*f*, 198
null hypothesis. *See* statistical significance

objectivity, 22–23, 205, 209–10, 211
obsessive-compulsive disorder (OCD), 11, 66, 75, 81, 88, 93, 95–96, 101, 103, 108, 142, 269*f*, *See also* Scrupulosity
Odysseus, story of, 45–46
Olds & Milner study, 124
Open Science Collaboration, 49, 215, 244
opioids, 11–12, 81–82, 119–20, 124, 125–26, 127, 139, 141, 144
Oreskes, Naomi, 83, 225–26
oscilloscope, 49–50
out-of-body experiences, 15–16
oxytocin, 184*t*, 184–86, 191, 198

P300 brain wave. *See* brain fingerprinting
Parfit, Derek, 79
parity argument, 229, 250
Parity Principle, 67, 183
Parkinson's disease, 64–65, 69–70, 75, 79, 80, 86, 88–89, 132–33, 140–41
Parks, Kenneth. *See* somnambulism
Paul, Laurie, 77
personality disorder, 98, 111–12, 137
  anti-social personality disorder, 105–6, 116, 118, 150, 159–60, 174
  borderline personality disorder, 137, 143
p-hacking. *See* statistical significance
phlogiston, 44
phobias, 97, 105–6, 108, 113, 143
physicalism (or materialism), 16–17, 43–44, 62
Pickard, Hanna, 98–99, 113, 114, 129, 130, 135, 137, 139, 140, 143, 270
Pickard's Principle, 270
pituitary gland, 179, 184–85
Plato, 158, 181
Poldrack, Russell, 29–30, 218, 224–25, 232, 233, 238–39, 241, 247
Pollan, Michael, 133–34, 176, 188
positron emission tomography (PET), 29–30
posterior Superior Temporal Sulcus (pSTS), 27–28
post-traumatic stress disorder (PTSD), 71–72, 94, 95–96, 105–6, 108, 117

predictive processing, 19
prefrontal cortex, 26, 152, 156*t*, 167, 185
pre-registration (of studies), 83, 84*f*, 227
President's Council on Bioethics. *See* bioethics
principles of bioethics. *See* bioethics
principle of moral psychology, 22
principles of neuroethics, 262–63
Prinz, Jesse, 158, 159–60
psilocybin (magic mushrooms), 176, 177, 184*t*, 190–91, 198
psychedelics, 12, 71–72, 77–78, 142–43, 176, 177, 179–80, 183–84, 188, 190–91, 262, 264–65
psychopathology. *See* mental disorder
psychopathy, 12, 95–96, 98, 149–51, 152–53, 154–56, 159–60, 171, 174, 231–32, 237, 238, 246–47
psychotherapy. *See* therapy
puberty, 77–78, 262, 264
punishment, 35, 47, 96, 119–20, 140, 143, 150, 153, 159–60, 182, 231–32, 262
p-value. *See* statistical significance

questionable research practices, 13, 208, 212–13, 214, 216–19, 227

Racine, Eric, 185–86, 197–98, 242
Rafferty, Mary, 69
Railton, Peter, 56, 171–72
Raine, Adrian, 152–53, 231, 232
Ramachandran, V. S., 207
rationalism, 158–61
rationalization. *See* motivated reasoning
Rat Park study, 136
Ravizza, Mark, 38–39, 68
reactive attitudes, 96
 See also resentment
readiness potential (RP), 49, 50*f*, 52
reason vs. emotion. *See* moral judgment; rationalism
reasoning. *See* consistency reasoning; dual process theory of cognition; motivated reasoning; rationalism
reinforcement learning, 124, 159, 169, 190–91, 198
relapse, 120, 121*t*, 121–22, 127, 132, 133–34, 137–38, 143, 144, 246–47

relativism. *See* objectivity in ethics
reliability of moral intuition. *See* moral judgment
replication (crisis), 13, 216, 219, 226, 227, 272–73. *See also* Open Science Collaboration
repugnance. *See* disgust
Research Domain Criteria, 108
resentment, 96, 263–64
resilience, 194
responsibility;
 amid manipulation, 68–70
 hyper-responsibility, 100
 vs. legal responsibility, 94
 taking it, 113
 tracing it, 57–58, 60, 69
 without blame, 114, 143, 270
 See also free will
reverse inference, 157, 224–25, 238–42, 240*f*, 248, 250, 272–73
reward system. *See* reinforcement learning
risk-benefit ratio/analysis, 67, 70–71, 74–75, 79, 80–88, 197, 264
Robbins, Lee. *See* Vietnam Veterans study
Roskies, Adina, 6, 30, 43, 234
Routh, Eddy Ray, 94, 117

safety:
 of biomedical enhancement, 196–99, 256, 264–65
 of medical interventions, 81–85
Saks, Elyn, 107
Salmon fMRI study, 218
same-sex marriage. *See* homosexuality
sample size, 82, 217–18, 227, 244
Sandel, Michael, 178, 193, 195
Sarkissian, Hagop, 38, 41
Satel, Sally, 123–24, 129, 140–41, 143, 231–32, 234, 235, 246, 251
Savulescu, Julian, 177–78, 180, 182, 191–92
schizophrenia, 18–19, 81, 93, 94, 95–96, 102–3, 104–5, 106, 107, 110–11, 113, 271–72
Schroeder, Timothy, 96–97
Schwitzgebel, Eric, 180
Scrupulosity, 198

searchlight view. *See* agency, executive model of
selective serotonin reuptake inhibitors (SSRIs), 83–84
self-control, 4, 26, 62, 68, 69–70, 95, 97, 119, 120, 129, 130, 144, 181, 231–32, 238, 261–62, 268–69. *See also* free will
self-correction in science, 226
self-deception, 13, 205–8, 211
Selgelid, Michael, 81, 195, 197
sentimentalism. *See* rationalism
serotonin, 24–25, 75, 83–84, 85, 184–85
sexual misconduct, 3, 52–53, 71–72, 149–50, 215–16, 231–32, 238, 261–63
Shepard, Jason, 68
Shepherd, Joshua, 54
Sher, George, 57, 58
Shoemaker, David, 98, 113, 150–51
Sifferd, Katrina, 117
Singer, Peter, 163, 169
Sinnott-Armstrong, Walter, 20–21, 23–24, 101, 102–3, 152–53, 231, 232, 234, 244–45
situationism, 48–49
sleepingwalkng. *See* somnambulism
sociopathy. *See* acquired sociopathy; psychopathy
somatic markers, 159
somnambulism, 47
sourcehood principle, 97
Sparrow, Rob, 111, 178, 189, 192
spectrum. *See* autism; cognitive continuum
split-brain patients, 205–8, 227
spontaneous remission. *See* addiction
Sripada, Chandra, 55–56, 97, 114, 130, 131–32
standard deviation, 234, 234f, 254
Stanford Prison Experiment, 217
Star Trek, 20–21
statistical significance:
explained, 30
marginal significance, 216–17
multiple comparisons, 218
p-hacking, 216, 218–19, 225
p-value, 216–17

See also base rates; external validity; questionable research practices; replication (crisis)
Stegenga, Jacob, 81–82, 83–84, 85, 86, 214
steroids, 178–79, 197–98
stigma. *See* mental disorder
stoicism, 194–68, 271
Strawson, Galen, 95–96, 97
Strawson, P. F., 96
stroke, 5, 16, 25–26, 81–82, 83, 161, 252
Stroop task, 166, 171–72
substance use disorder. *See* addiction
substantia nigra, 64, 125f
subthalamic nucleus (STN), 64
suicide, 35–36, 87, 117, 131
sulcus. *See* cerebral cortex
Summers, Jesse, 101, 102–3, 226
superior temporal sulcus (STS). *See* temporoparietal junction
Superman, 16
synapse. *See* neurons
Szasz, Thomas, 108

Tabb, Kathryn, 108, 131–32, 270
taboo violations, 210
Target (retail company), 255
temporoparietal junction (TPJ), 16, 27–28, 155, 156t, 239
testosterone, 197–98, 222
tetraplegia, 16
The Good Place (TV series), 179–80
theory of mind, 155, 239
therapeutic communities, 143
Therapy
 adjunctive role with drugs, 188
 cognitive behavioral therapy, 45–46, 194
 electroconvulsive therapy (ECT), 86
 psychotherapy, 66–67, 71–72, 142–43, 179–80, 182, 188, 190–91, 196–97, 226
thought-action gap, 237–38
tolerance
 of drugs, 121, 121t, 126–27, 129, 133–34, 197–98
 of people, 182, 184t, 185–86

Tourette syndrome, 66, 95–96
tracing principle. *See* responsibility: tracing it
transcranial direct current stimulation (tDCS), 179–80, 184*t*, 185, 198
transcranial magnetic stimulation (TMS), 87, 155, 198
transformative experience, 63, 77–80, 88–89, 111, 262, 264, 267–68, 273
treatment/enhancement distinction. *See* enhancement
trolley problem, 163–68, 273
Tullett, Alexa, 220–21
tu quoque replies, 199, 200, 226–27

utilitarianism, 20–21, 163, 169, 171, 173

values in science, 214–15
Vargas, Manuel, 41–42, 44, 45–46
ventral tegmental area (VTA), 124, 125*f*
ventromedial prefrontal cortex (vmPFC), 27–28, 153, 156*t*, 159, 161, 167, 171, 239
Vietnam Veterans study, 136, 137–38
Vincent, Nicole, 100

violence, aversion to, 169–70
virtue ethics, 21, 22, 194
Volkow, Nora, 121, 122–23, 126–27, 130–31, 138

Waldman, Ayelet, 177–78, 199–200
Washington, Natalia, 45–46, 58, 233–34
Watson, Gary, 131–32
Wegner, Daniel, 46, 47
Weinstein, Herbert, 35–38, 40, 62, 237, 238
wishful thinking. *See* motivated reasoning
witch, concept of, 44
withdrawal. *See* addiction
Wolf, Susan, 39
Wolpe, Paul, 86, 179, 196–97, 231–32, 235, 238–39, 250, 252–53
Woodward, James, 159

Yates, Andrea, 93–94, 117
Young, Liane, 134, 155

Zanzibar, 271–72
Zimbardo, Phil, 217

The manufacturer's authorised representative in the EU for product safety is Oxford
University Press España S.A. of El Parque Empresarial San Fernando de Henares,
Avenida de Castilla, 2 – 28830 Madrid (www.oup.es/en or product.safety@oup.com).
OUP España S.A. also acts as importer into Spain of products made by the manufacturer.

Printed in the USA/Agawam, MA
August 8, 2025

891696.001